Infections in the Intensive Care Unit

Guest Editors

MARIN H. KOLLEF, MD
SCOTT T. MICEK, PharmD

INFECTIOUS DISEASE CLINICS OF NORTH AMERICA

www.id.theclinics.com

Consulting Editor
ROBERT C. MOELLERING, Jr, MD

September 2009 • Volume 23 • Number 3

SAUNDERS an imprint of ELSEVIER, Inc.

W.B. SAUNDERS COMPANY
A Division of Elsevier Inc.
1600 John F. Kennedy Blvd., Suite 1800, Philadelphia, PA 19103-2899.
http://www.theclinics.com

INFECTIOUS DISEASE CLINICS OF NORTH AMERICA Volume 23, Number 3
September 2009 ISSN 0891-5520, ISBN-10: 1-4377-1231-2, ISBN-13: 978-1-4377-1231-5

Editor: Barbara Cohen-Kligerman

Infectious Disease Clinics of North America (ISSN 0891-5520) is published in March, June, September, and December (For Post Office use only: volume 23 issue 3 of 4) by Elsevier Inc., 360 Park Avenue South, New York, NY 10010-1710. Business and Editorial Offices: 1600 John F. Kennedy Blvd., Suite 1800, Philadelphia, PA 19103-2899. Customer Service Office: 6277 Sea Harbor Drive, Orlando, FL 32887-4800. Periodicals postage paid at New York, NY and additional mailing offices. Subscription prices are $218.00 per year for US individuals, $366.00 per year for US institutions, $109.00 per year for US students, $257.00 per year for Canadian individuals, $453.00 per year for Canadian institutions, $307.00 per year for international individuals, $453.00 per year for international institutions, and $151.00 per year for Canadian and international students. To receive student rate, orders must be accompanied by name of affiliated institution, date of term, and the *signature* of program/ residency coordinator on institution letterhead. Orders will be billed at individual rate until proof of status is received. Foreign air speed delivery is included in all *Clinics* subscription prices. All prices are subject to change without notice. **POSTMASTER**: Send address changes to *Infectious Disease Clinics of North America,* Elsevier Periodicals Customer Service, 11830 Westline Industrial Drive, St. Louis, MO 63146. **Customer Service: 1-800-654-2452 (US). From outside of the US, call 1-314-453-7041. Fax: 1-314-453-5170. E-mail: JournalsCustomerService-usa@elsevier.com (print support) or JournalsOnlineSupport-usa@elsevier.com (online support).**

Infectious Disease Clinics of North America is also published in Spanish by Editorial Inter-Médica, Junin 917, 1er A 1113, Buenos Aires, Argentina.

Reprints. For copies of 100 or more, of articles in this publication, please contact the Commercial Reprints Department, Elsevier Inc., 360 Park Avenue South, New York, New York 10010-1710. Tel. (212) 633-3812, Fax: (212) 462-1935, E-mail: reprints@elsevier.com.

Infectious Disease Clinics of North America is covered in *MEDLINE/PubMed (Index Medicus), Current Contents/ Clinical Medicine, Science Citation Alert, SCISEARCH,* and *Research Alert.*

Printed and bound by CPI Group (UK) Ltd, Croydon, CR0 4YY

Transferred to Digital Print 2011

Contributors

GUEST EDITORS

MARIN H. KOLLEF, MD
Professor of Medicine, Virginia J. and Sam E. Golman Chair in Respiratory Intensive Care, Division of Pulmonary & Critical Care Medicine, Washington University School of Medicine; and Director, Medical Intensive Care Unit, Director, Respiratory Care Services, Barnes-Jewish Hospital, St. Louis, Missouri

SCOTT T. MICEK, PharmD
Department of Pharmacy, Barnes-Jewish Hospital; and Adjunct Clinical Associate Professor, St. Louis College of Pharmacy, St. Louis, Missouri

AUTHORS

BRYAN T. ALEXANDER, PharmD
Postgraduate Year Two Specialty Pharmacy Resident, Barnes-Jewish Hospital, St. Louis, Missouri

ANTONIO ANZUETO, MD
Division of Pulmonary/Critical Care Medicine, South Texas Veterans Health Care System; and Division of Pulmonary/Critical Care Medicine, University of Texas Health Science Center at San Antonio, San Antonio, Texas

MARY C. BARSANTI, MD
Clinical Fellow in Infectious Diseases, Department of Internal Medicine, Division of Infectious Diseases, Washington University School of Medicine, St. Louis, Missouri

EMILI DIAZ, MD, PhD
Critical Care Department, Joan XXIII University Hospital, University Rovira i Virgili, IISPV, CIBER Enfermedades Respiratorias (CIBERES), Tarragona, Spain

GEORGE DIMOPOULOS, MD, PhD, FCCP
Professor, Department of Critical Care, University Hospital Attikon, Medical School, University of Athens; and Alfa Institute of Biomedical Sciences (AIBS), Athens, Greece

ERIK R. DUBBERKE, MD, MSPH
Assistant Professor, Division of Infectious Diseases, Department of Medicine, Washington University School of Medicine, St. Louis, Missouri

MATTHEW E. FALAGAS, MD, MSc, DSc
Alfa Institute of Biomedical Sciences (AIBS), Athens, Greece; Director, Infectious Diseases Clinic, "Henry Dunant" Hospital; and Adjunct Associate Professor, Department of Medicine, Tufts University School of Medicine, Boston, Massachusetts

RICARD FERRER, MD
Critical Care Center, Hospital Sabadell, Institut Universitari Parc Taulí, UAB, CIBER Enfermedades Respiratorias, Parc Taulí s/n, Sabadell, Spain

PATRICK M. FINNEGAN, PharmD, BCPS
Assistant Professor of Pharmacy Practice, St. Louis College of Pharmacy, St. Louis, Missouri

HITOSHI HONDA, MD
Fellow, Division of Infectious Diseases, Washington University of School of Medicine, St. Louis, Missouri

MARIN H. KOLLEF, MD
Professor of Medicine, Virginia J. and Sam E. Golman Chair in Respiratory Intensive Care, Division of Pulmonary & Critical Care Medicine, Washington University School of Medicine; and Director, Medical Intensive Care Unit, Director, Respiratory Care Services, Barnes-Jewish Hospital, St. Louis, Missouri

PETER K. LINDEN, MD
Professor of Critical Care Medicine, Department of Critical Care Medicine, University of Pittsburgh Medical Center; and Director Abdominal Organ Transplant ICU, University of Pittsburgh Medical Center, Pittsburgh, Pennsylvania

THIAGO LISBOA, MD
Critical Care Department, Joan XXIII University Hospital, University Rovira i Virgili, IISPV, CIBER Enfermedades Respiratorias (CIBERES), Tarragona, Spain

JOHN MAZUSKI, MD, PhD
Department of Surgery, Washington University School of Medicine, St. Louis, Missouri

JAY R. McDONALD, MD
Staff Physician, Infectious Disease Section, Specialty Care Service Line, St. Louis VA Medical Center; and Assistant Professor, Department of Internal Medicine, Division of Infectious Diseases, Washington University School of Medicine, St. Louis, Missouri

SCOTT T. MICEK, PharmD
Department of Pharmacy, Barnes-Jewish Hospital; and Adjunct Clinical Associate Professor, St. Louis College of Pharmacy, St. Louis, Missouri

MATTHEW R. MORRELL, MD
Division of Pulmonary and Critical Care Medicine, Washington University School of Medicine, Barnes-Jewish Hospital, St. Louis, Missouri

LENA M. NAPOLITANO, MD, FACS, FCCP, FCCM
Chief, Division of Acute Care Surgery [Trauma, Burns, Critical Care, Emergency Surgery]; Director, Trauma and Surgical Critical Care; Associate Chair and Professor of Surgery, Department of Surgery, University of Michigan Health System, Ann Arbor, Michigan

ROBERT C. OWENS, Jr, PharmD
Department of Clinical Pharmacy Services and Division of Infectious Diseases, Maine Medical Center, Portland, Maine; and Department of Medicine, University of Vermont, College of Medicine, Burlington, Vermont

JORDI RELLO, MD, PhD
Critical Care Department, Joan XXIII University Hospital, University Rovira i Virgili, IISPV,
CIBER Enfermedades Respiratorias (CIBERES), Tarragona, Spain

MARCOS I. RESTREPO, MD, MSc
Division of Pulmonary/Critical Care Medicine, South Texas Veterans Health Care System;
Veterans Evidence Based Research Dissemination and Implementation Center
(VERDICT); and Division of Pulmonary/Critical Care Medicine, University of Texas
Health Science Center at San Antonio, San Antonio, Texas

DAVID J. RIDDLE, MD
Fellow, Division of Infectious Diseases, Department of Medicine, Washington University
School of Medicine, St. Louis, Missouri

DAVID J. RITCHIE, PharmD, BCPS, FCCP
Clinical Pharmacist, Infectious Diseases, Barnes-Jewish Hospital; and Professor
of Pharmacy Practice, St. Louis College of Pharmacy, St. Louis, Missouri

ANDREW F. SHORR, MD, MPH
Division of Pulmonary and Critical Care Medicine, Washington Hospital Center, NW;
and Associate Professor of Medicine, Georgetown University School of Medicine,
Washington, DC

JOSEPH S. SOLOMKIN, MD
Professor of Surgery, Department of Surgery, University of Cincinnati College of
Medicine, Cincinnati, Ohio

MARTA ULLDEMOLINS, DPharm
Critical Care Department, Joan XXIII University Hospital, University Rovira i Virgili, IISPV,
CIBER Enfermedades Respiratorias (CIBERES), Tarragona, Spain

JORDI VALLÉS, MD, PhD
Critical Care Center, Hospital Sabadell, Institut Universitari Parc Taulí, UAB, CIBER
Enfermedades Respiratorias, Parc Taulí s/n, Sabadell, Spain

DAVID K. WARREN, MD, MPH
Assistant Professor of Medicine, Division of Infectious Diseases, Washington University
of School of Medicine, St. Louis, Missouri

KEITH F. WOELTJE, MD, PhD
Associate Professor, Department of Internal Medicine, Division of Infectious Diseases,
Washington University School of Medicine, St. Louis, Missouri

MARYA D. ZILBERBERG, MD, MPH
Adjunct Assistant Professor, School of Public Health and Health Sciences, University
of Massachusetts, Amherst; and President and CEO, EviMed Research Group, LLC,
Goshen, Massachusetts

Contents

Fever is a normal adaptive brain response to infectious and noninfectious causes involving a cytokine-mediated response, the generation of acute phase reactants, and the activation of numerous physiologic, endocrinologic and immunologic systems. Ninety percent of patients with severe sepsis in the intensive care unit (ICU) will experience fever during their hospitalization, while the half of the new detected febrile episodes are of noninfectious origin. In the ICU, fever should be treated in cardiorespiratory and neurosurgical patients and in those in whom temperature exceeds 40°C (104°F). Antipyretic therapy must be justified regardless of the metabolic cost (if fever exceeds its physiologic benefit), the result (if the symptomatic relief adversely affects the course of the febrile illness) and the side effects.

The diagnosis and management of severe sepsis and septic shock is a complex and dynamic process. Newer evidence-based interventions are constantly being developed and implemented with the purpose of improving morbidity and mortality. Current investigations are being performed in hospital environments to determine the change in behaviors and clinical impact with the most recent recommendations. The use of standardized treatment protocols in addition to newer diagnostic and treatment modalities in patients who have severe sepsis and septic shock can continue to improve patient-related outcomes and the damaging effect of these diseases on society.

Community-acquired pneumonia (CAP) is the leading cause of death from infectious diseases in the United States. It accounts for 500,000 hospitalizations and 45,000 deaths each year, and it represents one of the most common causes of ICU admission. The mortality rate due to severe CAP has shown little improvement over the past few years, with rates as high as 58% when patients were admitted to the ICU. Significant interest has focused on the sickest patients who have pneumonia treated in the ICU, regarding identification of need for ICU admission and therapies directed to improve outcomes in patients who have severe CAP. This article reviews epidemiologic, microbiologic, therapeutic, preventive, and outcomes data in patients who have CAP in the ICU.

Emili Diaz, Marta Ulldemolins, Thiago Lisboa, and Jordi Rello

Ventilator-associated pneumonia (VAP) management depends on the interaction between the infective agent, the host response, and the antimicrobial drug used. After the pathogen reaches the lungs, two outcomes are possible: either the microorganisms are eliminated by the host immune system, or they overcome the immune system and cause pulmonary infection. When a patient is thought to have VAP, two steps are strongly recommended: etiologic diagnostic testing and the immediate initiation of antibiotics. The daily management of VAP remains a challenge for physicians in the ICU. In recent years, a more dynamic approach has evolved, updating local epidemiology, evaluating VAP and diagnostic tools every day, and assessing host response using clinical and biochemical parameters.

Peter K. Linden

Despite significant advances in the prevention, diagnosis, and treatment of infection in the immunocompromised host, it remains a major cause of morbidity, increased length of stay, total costs, and of course mortality. Intensive care mortality rates are significantly higher among immunocompromised hosts in part due to the higher incidence of infection severity. The superimposition of the compromised host defenses and critical illness makes the detection and management of infections in such patients more difficult, but crucial toward salvaging patient outcome. Moreover, although there is a rapidly increasing evidence base in intensive care medicine, many interventional trials for the management of severe sepsis (activated protein C, adjunctive corticosteroids, goal-based resuscitation), acute lung injury (low stretch ventilation), and other organ failures have excluded immunocompromised hosts.

Jordi Vallés amd Ricard Ferrer

Hospital-acquired infections (HAI) occur in 5%–10% of patients admitted to hospitals in the United States, and HAIs remain a leading cause of morbidity and mortality. Patients admitted to ICUs account for 45% of all hospital-acquired pneumonias and bloodstream infections (BSIs), although critical care units comprise only 5% to 10% of all hospital beds. The severity of underlying disease, invasive diagnostic and therapeutic procedures that breach normal host defenses, contaminated life-support equipment, and the prevalence of resistant microorganisms are critical factors in the

high rate of infection in the ICUs. This article discusses the clinical importance of BSI, including hospital- and community-acquired episodes in the
ICU.

Severe Soft Tissue Infections

Lena M. Napolitano

Severe skin and soft tissue infections (SSTIs) frequently require management in the ICU, in part related to associated septic shock or toxic shock
syndrome or associated organ failure. Four fundamental management
principles are key to a successful outcome in caring for patients who
have severe SSTIs, including (1) early diagnosis and differentiation of necrotizing versus nonnecrotizing SSTI, (2) early initiation of appropriate empiric broad-spectrum antimicrobial therapy with consideration of risk
factors for specific pathogens and mandatory coverage for methicillin-
resistant *Staphylococcus aureus* (MRSA), (3) source control (ie, early aggressive surgical intervention for drainage of abscesses and debridement
of necrotizing soft tissue infections), and (4) pathogen identification and
appropriate de-escalation of antimicrobial therapy. MRSA has emerged
as the most common identifiable cause of severe SSTIs; therefore, initiation of empiric anti-MRSA antimicrobials is warranted in all cases of severe
SSTIs. In addition, appropriate critical care management—including fluid
resuscitation, organ support and nutritional support—is a necessary component in treating severe SSTIs.

Intra-abdominal Sepsis: Newer Interventional and Antimicrobial Therapies

Joseph S. Solomkin and John Mazuski

Complicated intra-abdominal infections are the second most common
cause of septic death in the intensive care unit. Although there have
been improvements in the outcome of sepsis regardless of etiology, this
is even more striking for intra-abdominal infections. From observation, recent advances in interventional techniques, including more aggressive use
of percutaneous drainage of abscesses and use of "open abdomen" techniques for peritonitis, have significantly affected the morbidity and mortality of physiologically severe complicated intra-abdominal infection.

Central Nervous System Infections: Meningitis and Brain Abscess

Hitoshi Honda and David K. Warren

Despite advances in antimicrobial and antiviral therapy, meningitis and
brain abscess are infections that result in significant morbidity and mortality. A multidisciplinary approach, including intensive care, is often required
in the treatment of these infections. Meningitis is defined by the presence
of the inflammation of the meninges, with characteristic changes in cerebrospinal fluid. Brain abscess is a focal infection of the brain parenchyma,
commonly caused by bacterial, fungal, and parasitic pathogens. This article reviews the common infectious etiologies of central nervous system infections, especially bacterial meningitis and brain abscess, and their
subsequent management in the intensive care unit.

Pulmonologists and intensivists often care for patients at risk for infections caused by both *Aspergillus* and *Candida*. Infection with either can lead to severe life-threatening disease, particularly in immunosuppressed patients, with mortality rates for invasive fungal disease often exceeding 30%. For both organisms, multiple diagnostic challenges remain while newer diagnostic modalities are being developed and tested. Fortunately, therapeutic paradigms are shifting, and clinicians have many new agents in their armamentarium for combating fungal infection. Given the rapidly changing literature in this broad area, it is imperative that physicians caring for immunosuppressed patients and for the critically ill remain abreast of this evolving field.

Acute infective endocarditis is a complex disease with changing epidemiology and a rapidly evolving knowledge base. To consistently achieve optimal outcomes in the management of infective endocarditis, the clinical team must have an understanding of the epidemiology, microbiology, and natural history of infective endocarditis, as well as a grasp of guiding principles of diagnosis and medical and surgical management. The focus of this review is acute infective endocarditis, though many studies of diagnosis and treatment do not differentiate between acute and subacute disease, and indeed many principles of diagnosis and management of infective endocarditis for acute and subacute disease are identical.

Timely provision of adequate antimicrobial coverage in an initial anti-infective treatment regimen results in optimal outcomes for bacterial and fungal infections. However, selection of appropriate antimicrobial regimens for treatment of infections in the intensive care unit (ICU) can be challenging due to expansion of resistance, which typically requires use of multidrug anti-infective regimens to provide adequate coverage of important pathogens commonly seen in the ICU setting. Indeed, a recent additional call to action by the Infectious Diseases Society of America (IDSA) has enforced the impact that antimicrobial-resistant pathogens can have on patient care. The term *ESKAPE* has been coined by this IDSA group to refer to *Enterococcus faecium, Staphylococcus aureus, Klebsiella pneumoniae, Acinetobacter baumanii, Pseudomonas aeruginosa*, and *Enterobacter* species, the etiologic causes of the majority of hospital-acquired infections in the United States that are able to effectively "escape" our antibiotic arsenal and that also mandate discovery of new antimicrobial agents. This article reviews select antibacterial agents and an antifungal agent in late stages of clinical development that appear to have potential for treatment of infections in the ICU.

Critical-care units can be barometers for appropriate antimicrobial use. There, life and death hang on empirical antimicrobial therapy for treatment of infectious diseases. With increasing therapeutic empiricism, triple-drug, broad-spectrum regimens are often necessary, but cannot be continued without fear of the double-edged sword: a life-saving intervention or loss of life following *Clostridium difficile* infection, infection from a resistant organism, nephrotoxicity, cardiac toxicity, and so on. While broadened initial empirical therapy is considered a standard, it must be necessary, dosed according to pharmacokinetic-pharmacodynamic principles, and stopped when no longer needed. Antimicrobial stewardship interventions shepherd these considerations in antimicrobial therapy. With pharmacists and physicians trained in infectious disease and critical care, clear-cut interventions can be focused on beginning or growing a stewardship program, or proposing future studies.

Hospital-acquired infections have profound social, economic, and personal costs to patients in the intensive care unit (ICU). Numerous risk factors, such as poor nutrition and hyperglycemia, directly involve patients. Meanwhile, hand hygiene, environmental cleaning, and appropriate hospital staffing can impact ICU infection rates. A multidirectional approach—including continuing staff education, minimizing risk factors, and implementing guidelines established by national committees—is necessary to decrease infections such as catheter-related bloodstream infections, urinary tract infections, ventilator-associated pneumonia, and *Clostridium difficile*. Infection-control committees can assist in implementing policies. This is an active area of research and we anticipate continued advancements to improve patient care.

Clostridium difficile infection (CDI) is becoming more common worldwide. The morbidity and mortality associated with *C difficile* is also increasing at an alarming rate. Critically ill patients are at particularly high risk for CDI because of the prevalence of multiple risk factors in this patient population. Treatment of *C difficile* continues to be a difficult problem in patients with severe or recurrent disease. This article seeks to provide a broad understanding of CDI in the intensive care unit, with special emphasis on risk factor identification, treatment options, and disease prevention.

VISIT THE CLINICS ONLINE!
Access your subscription at:
www.theclinics.com

Preface

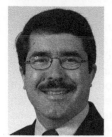 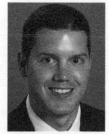

Marin H. Kollef, MD   Scott T. Micek, PharmD
Guest Editors

Despite advances in medical practice, serious infections, including severe sepsis and septic shock, remain responsible for significant morbidity and mortality. In the United States, approximately 450,000 cases of severe sepsis and septic shock occur each year, with an estimated mortality in excess of 30%. Many other serious infections also require intensive care, however, without the development of severe sepsis and septic shock. Additionally, newly acquired nosocomial infections are known to complicate the hospitalizations of critically ill patients, leading to greater morbidity and health care costs. Several decades of intense research aimed at identifying novel therapies for patients with pneumonia, septic shock, skin and skin structure infections, central nervous system infections, and intra-abdominal infections have failed to yield a "magic bullet." Nevertheless, advances in antimicrobial treatment and supportive care measures for these patients have improved patient outcomes by optimizing existing treatments.

Early, goal-directed cardiovascular resuscitation has been shown to decrease mortality in patients with severe sepsis and septic shock. In addition, the adequacy of initial empirical antibiotic treatment for patients with serious infections has been shown to affect mortality. Although getting the "right" antibiotic to patients seems to be a simple concept, implementation of this standard has been problematic. Some infections occurring in the intensive care unit do not present with specific signs or symptoms, promoting delayed administration of appropriate antimicrobial therapy. A common example is invasive fungal infection, which typically has delayed treatment associated with its occurrence. Antimicrobial resistance is another important issue limiting the timely administration of early appropriate antimicrobial treatment. Common gram-negative bacteria causing infections in critically ill patients (*Pseudomonas aeruginosa*, *Acinetobacter* sp, *Klebsiella* sp, and *Escherichia coli*) and gram-positive bacteria (methicillin-resistant *Staphylococcus aureus*, vancomycin-resistant enterococci) are often associated with inappropriate initial treatment resulting from clinicians' inability to identify the presence of health care–associated infection risk factors necessitating that these pathogens be empirically treated. Even if attempts are made initially to cover potentially antibiotic-resistant pathogens with an appropriate antimicrobial regimen, it may still be inadequate because of either low drug concentrations at the

Infect Dis Clin N Am 23 (2009) xiii–xiv
doi:10.1016/j.idc.2009.05.001
0891-5520/09/$ – see front matter © 2009 Elsevier Inc. All rights reserved.

infection site, higher minimum inhibitory concentrations of the pathogen for the antibiotics used, or both. Most clinicians treating patients in the intensive care unit are not provided with minimum inhibitory concentrations to assist them in selecting the most appropriate initial treatment regimen.

The prevention of serious infections in intensive care units is another key goal on which clinicians can focus. Intensive care units are important areas for the emergence and spread of nosocomial infections because of the frequent use of broad-spectrum antibiotics; the crowding of patients with high levels of disease acuity within relatively small, specialized areas; reductions in nursing staff and other support staff because of economic pressures, which increase the likelihood of person-to-person transmission of microorganisms; and the presence of more chronically and acutely ill patients who require prolonged hospitalizations and often harbor antibiotic-resistant bacteria. Increasingly, nosocomial infections, especially those acquired in the intensive care unit setting, are caused by antimicrobial-resistant pathogens that are associated with greater administration of inappropriate initial therapy and worse patient outcomes. Clinicians need to be aware of strategies that are not only aimed at prevention of nosocomial infections, but also aimed at the prevention of antimicrobial resistance. Many of the available prevention strategies are described in the Centers for Disease Control and Prevention 12-step program for the prevention of antimicrobial resistance (http://www.cdc.gov/drugresistance/healthcare). One of the key elements in this strategy is to consult experts in the field of nosocomial infections and antimicrobial resistance (eg, infectious disease experts, infection control practitioners, microbiologists) when designing interventions aimed at minimizing the emergence and spread of antibiotic-resistant pathogens. This issue of *Infectious Disease Clinics of North America* is aimed at providing an overview of the types of infections most often managed in the intensive care unit setting. The hope is to provide an up-to-date resource describing the optimal management of these infections, strategies for the prevention of commonly acquired infections among critically ill patients, and future areas in need of investigation.

Marin H. Kollef, MD
Division of Pulmonary and Critical Care Medicine
Washington University School of Medicine
Medical Intensive Care Unit
Respiratory Care Services
Barnes-Jewish Hospital
One Barnes-Jewish Hospital Plaza
St. Louis, MO 63110, USA

Scott T. Micek, PharmD
Department of Pharmacy
Barnes-Jewish Hospital
St. Louis College of Pharmacy
One Barnes-Jewish Hospital Plaza
St. Louis, MO 63110, USA

E-mail addresses:
mkollef@im.wustl.edu (M.H. Kollef)
stm8241@bjc.org (S.T. Micek)

Approach to the Febrile Patient in the ICU

George Dimopoulos, MD, PhD, FCCP[a,b,*],
Matthew E. Falagas, MD, MSc, DSc[b,c,d]

KEYWORDS

• Fever • Pathophysiology • Differential diagnosis
• Treatment • Critically ill

Thirty percent of medical patients will become febrile during their hospitalization, while up to 90% of critically ill patients with severe sepsis will experience fever during their stay in the intensive care unit (ICU).[1] This febrile response is a complex physiologic reaction to disease (inflammation and/or infection), which involves a cytokine-mediated rise in core body temperature, generation of acute phase reactants, and activation of numerous physiologic, endocrinologic and immunologic systems presenting from the other side beneficial and deleterious effects because of the increase of several parameters of immune function (cytokine production, T-cell activation, neutrophil, and macrophage function).[2]

Critically ill patients commonly present a newly elevated temperature at a certain time of their hospitalization, triggering a set of many diagnostic and laboratory tests. In these cases, a prudent and cost-effective manner of assessment is necessary, otherwise treatment is time-consuming, with elevated costs, and a disruptive result to the patient (eg, unneeded radiation, transport outside the controlled environment of the ICU, blood loss) and the caregiver staff are noted.[3] Fever in critically ill patients may be of infectious, noninfectious, or mixed origin and the confirmation of the source is often difficult, which leads to a diagnostic dilemma (ie, a difficult decision: "to treat or not to treat") and a variability of treating response from the medical and nursing staff institutionally.

In febrile, critically ill patients, traditionally a pharmacologic and/or mechanical antipyretic therapy is administered before the confirmation of the cause, indicating with this approach: (a) the misconceptions about the detrimental effects of fever especially

[a] Department of Critical Care, University Hospital Attikon, Medical School, University of Athens, 7 Kirpou Street, 14569, Athens, Greece
[b] Alfa Institute of Biomedical Sciences (AIBS), 9 Neapoleos Street, 151 23 Marousi, Athens, Greece
[c] Infectious Diseases Clinic, Henry Dunant Hospital, 7 Kirpou Street, Athens, Greece
[d] Department of Medicine, Tufts University School of Medicine, 136 Harrison Avenue, Boston, MA 02110, USA
* Corresponding author. Department of Critical Care, University Hospital Attikon, Medical School, University of Athens, 7 Kirpou Street, 14569, Athens, Greece.
E-mail address: dimop@vodafone.net.gr (G. Dimopoulos).

Infect Dis Clin N Am 23 (2009) 471–484
doi:10.1016/j.idc.2009.04.001
0891-5520/09/$ – see front matter © 2009 Elsevier Inc. All rights reserved.

in the children (eg, seizures, brain damage); and (b) the response on the part of the physicians to the psychological pressure, especially from the family.[3,4] This medical practice, despite the evidence that fever in the majority of the cases is a beneficial response to the disease, leads to an increased medical cost (eg, use of antipyretic drugs, icepacks, cooling blankets) and occasionally in organ dysfunction development (eg, volume-depleted patients, individuals with renal diseases).[4,5]

According to the American College of Critical Care Medicine of the Society of Critical Care Medicine and the Infectious Diseases Society of America, the goal for the treatment of a new temperature elevation in a previously afebrile, critically ill patient in whom the source of the fever is not obvious merits a detailed evaluation of the patient's medical history and a careful physical examination before the order of any laboratory or imaging procedure or before the administration of any drug; the goal is to promote the rational consumption of different resources and the efficient evaluation of the new event.[3]

DEFINITION, PHYSIOLOGY AND PATHOGENESIS OF THE FEVER

The mean body temperature in healthy individuals is 36.8°C (98.2 °F) with a range of 35.6°C (96 °F) to 38.0°C (100.8 °F) and a slight diurnal/circadian variation of between 0.5 and 1.0°C and during the heavy exercise a rise by 2° to 3°C is observed.[6] The presence of fever is defined when a core temperature >38.0°C (100.4 °F) is measured or when two consecutive measurements reveal elevations of temperature >38.3°C (101.0 °F). In neutropenic patients, a single measurement of oral temperature of > 38.3°C (101.0 °F) in the absence of an obvious environmental cause or an elevation of >38.0°C (100.4 °F) for a time period of more than 1 hour establishes the diagnosis of fever.[7] The body temperature is measured and monitored using a variety of methods and techniques (especially in ICU patients) at different body sites (Table 1).

After the action of exogenous stimuli (eg, infections, inflammatory or autoimmune diseases, vascular occlusive diseases, drugs), a release of large proteins (15.000–30.000 daltons) called "endogenous pyrogens" (interleukin-1 [IL-1], tumor necrosis factor [TNF]), IL-6, and interferons by monocytic cells is observed binding to specific receptors that are located in the preoptic region of the anterior hypothalamus.[8] At this

Table 1		
Measurement of fever using different techniques at different body sites		
Site	Method	Comments
Pulmonary artery	Mixed venous blood	Pulmonary artery catheter
Infrared ear	Thermometer	Values a few tenth below values in the pulmonary artery catheter and brain
Rectal temperature	Mercury thermometer or electrical probe	A few tenths higher than core temperature. Unpleasant and intrusive for patients
Oral measurement	Thermometer	Influenced by warmed gases delivered by respiratory devices, by eating and drinking
Axillary measurement	Thermometer	Underestimates core temperature, lacks reproducibility

site, a blood-brain barrier acts as a valve permitting the entrance of a limited quantity of those proteins into the brain. After the entrance, these pyrogens come into contact with neurons with the aid of small neuronal cells with fenestrated capillaries called "circumventricular organs" and a direct response of the neurons within the organum vasculosum of the lamina terminalis or of astrocytes or microglia to cytokines is noted, resulting in arachidonic acid metabolites production (prostaglandin E2 and thromboxane A2) and an up-regulation of the thermostatic set point.[9,10] The brain responds by sending signals able to activate effector mechanisms (through the spinal/supraspinal motor system or throughout the sympathetic nervous system), which in their turn generate heat, reduce heat loss, and increase core body temperature to match the up-regulation of the thermostatic set point. The activation of arachidonic acid metabolites act as substrate for the cyclo-oxygenase-2 (COX-2) pathway, which in turn leads to further elevation of prostaglandins levels, a decreased rate of firing of sensitive neurons, and an increased heat production. The role of COX-2 is important for the development of fever although its activity is inhibited by selective inhibitors, including nonsteroidal anti-inflammatory drugs (NSAIDS) and acetaminophen.[11]

Fever is characterized by beneficial and deleterious effects and by cardiovascular and metabolic demands (**Fig. 1**). The beneficial effects have been shown: (a) in mammalian models where the increased body temperature was associated to an enhanced resistance to infection; and (b) in clinical trials in adults where a positive correlation was recorded between maximum temperature on the bacteremia day and survival or between a temperature of >38°C and survival in spontaneous bacterial

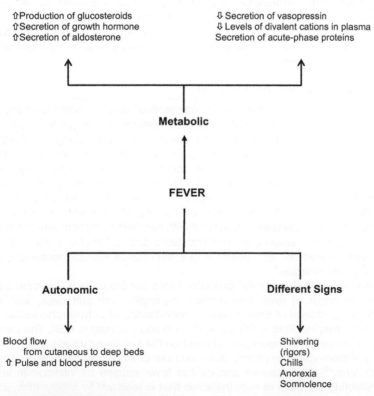

Fig. 1. Responses of different organs to fever.

peritonitis.[12,13] The deleterious effects of fever affect mainly: (a) patients with cardio-respiratory diseases because fever is poorly tolerated because of the increased cardiac output, the increased oxygen consumption, the elevated carbon dioxide production, and the increased energy expenditure; and (b) the neurosurgical patients who have head injuries and cerebrovascular accidents because moderate elevations of brain temperature exacerbate the injuries.[14,15] Upon the appearance of fever, elevated oxygen consumption (for each °C increase in body temperature a 13% increase in oxygen consumption is noted), increased heart rate, elevated cardiac output, and increased serum catecholamine production are noted, aiming to amelio-rate oxygen delivery to meet tissue demands.[16] According to the phase of fever, the patient manifests different signs and symptoms. During the initiation phase, chills in response to the elevation in temperature set point, increased insultation, decreased skin surface exposure, and shivering are associated with increased metabolic rate; during the plateau phase, the body temperature equilibrates the new thermostatic set point in the brain; and, during defervescence of the fever, effector mechanisms are activated, such as sweating, and the patient exhibits behaviors such as removing blankets with the aim to lose heat.[17]

CAUSES, DIAGNOSTIC APPROACH AND TREATMENT OF FEVER IN THE ICU

Generally, critically ill patients frequently show single spikes of elevated temperatures that return to normal without treatment. These events are considered without clinical significance and related to different interventions, enodtracheal suctioning, urinary catheter placement, and transfusion of blood products. The fever that is related to an invasive procedure or manipulation of an indwelling device with or without transient bacteremia frequently resolves spontaneously, while fever caused by underlying chronic diseases, current medical illness or its complications, or reactions following drug therapy may be persistent.

Noninfectious Causes of Fever in the ICU

Half of fever episodes in the ICU are of noninfectious origin, without the temperature usually exceeding 38.3°C, and additional necessary diagnostic procedures (**Table 2**).[18] The medical history, including recent interventions along with the physical examination, aids the clinician in narrowing down the differential diagnosis. However, the type of ICU population (eg, medical, surgical, trauma, neurosurgery and burn patients), the specific type of patients (eg, immunocompromised, elderly), the history of recent epidemics and the local epidemiology must be taken into account.[19]

In cardiac care units (CCUs), the main causes of noninfectious fever include: myocardial infraction, Dressler's syndrome with pericarditis, thromboemlolism, throm-bolytic therapy with hemorrhagic complications and antiarrythmic medication (eg, procainamide, quinidine), and deep venous thrombosis without necessarily routine venography performance.[1]

In neurosurgical ICU, patients' posterior fossa syndrome is a common cause of noninfectious origin of fever that mimics meningitis with stiff neck, low level of glucose/increased level of protein, and predominance of polymorphonuclear leuko-cytes in cerebrospinal fluid (CSF) as result of blood insertion in CSF. The differential diagnosis from bacterial meningitis is based on the negative cultures and the gradual lessening of meningeal symptoms as the number of red blood cells decreases in the CSF with time.[20] Other causes are: central fever caused by intracranial lesion or trauma affecting the brain or hypothalamus that is resistant to antipyretics, exceeds 39°C (106°F), and is characterized by absence of perspiration; the use of

Table 2
Main causes of fever in the ICU

System	Infectious Causes	Noninfectious Causes
CNS	Meningitis, encephalitis	Posterior fossa syndrome, central fever, seizures, cerebral infraction, hemorrhage, cerebrovascular accident
Cardiovascular	Central line, infected pacemaker, endocarditis, sterna osteomyelitis, viral pericarditis	Myocardial infarction, myocardial/perivalvular abscess, balloon pump syndrome, postpericardiectomy syndrome
Pulmonary	VAP, mediastinitis, tracheobronchitis, empyema	Pulmonary emboli, ARDS, atelectasis (without pneumonia), BOOP, bronchogenic carcinoma without postobstructive pneumonia, systemic lupus erythemaosus pneumonitis
Gastrointestinal	Intra-abdominal abscess, cholangiitis, cholecystitis, viral hepatitis, peritonitis, diarrhea (*Clostridium difficile*)	Pancreatitis, acalculus cholecystitis, ischemia of the bowel, bleeding, cirrhosis, ischemic colitis, irritable bowel syndrome
Urinary tract	Catheter-associated bacteremia, urosepsis, pyelonephritis, cystitis	Underestimates core temperature, lacks reproducibility
Skin/soft tissue	Decubitus ulcers, cellulitis, wound infection	—
Bone/joint	Chronic osteomyelitis, septic arthritis	Acute gout
Other	Transient bacteremia, sinusitis	Adrenal insufficiency, phlebitis/thrombophlebitis, neoplastic fever, alcohol/drug withdrawal, delirium tremens, drug fever, fat emboli, deep venous thrombosis, postoperative fever (48 h), fever after transfusion.

anticonvulsive medications; and deep venous thrombosis, including fat embolism in trauma patients. In the acute phase after head injury, the appearance of pyrexia is extremely frequent and deleterious for cerebral perfusion (CCP) and intracranial pressure (ICP); while lack of treatment by antipyretics has been correlated with a longer ICU stay.[21]

Acalculus cholecystitis, frequently unrecognized, is the result of gallbladder ischemia and bile stasis with an estimated incidence of 1.5%, especially in septic patients or in patients recovering from abdominal sepsis, because of the nonspecific clinical signs and laboratory workup (pain in the right upper quadrant, nausea, vomiting, fever).[22] The radiologic investigation using ultrasound (wall thickness >3 mm, intramural lucencies, gallbladder distension, pericholecystic fluid and intramural sludge) and CT scanning (high sensitivity and specificity) are helpful, while hepatobiliary scintigraphy is characterized by a high false-positive rate (>50%). Frequently, the diagnosis is delayed and the disease progresses to ischemia, gangrene and perforation, indicating in this manner that the necessary high index of suspicion from physicians' part, while the treatment choice is the percutaneous cholecystectomy.[23]

Fever caused by drug hypersensitivity or drug-related fever or "drug fever" is characterized by unknown incidence (3%–7% of febrile episodes are attributed to drug reactions, but many cases remain undiagnosed), a temperature ranged from 38.8°C(102 °F) to 40°C(104 °F), difficult diagnosis (usually established by exclusion because of the non-specific signs and laboratory tests), shaking chills and spiking temperatures.[1,23] A concomitant maculopapular rash makes the diagnosis simple but accompanies the fever in only 5%–10% of cases, while rarely an increased WBC count with a left shift, a moderate elevation of serum transaminases, peripheral eosinophilia, and a markedly elevated erythrocyte sedimentation rate (>100 mm/h) are recorded.[3] The signs that are associated with drug-fever are a lack of appropriate pulse rate response and a relative bradycardia in the absence of intrinsic conduction defects or beta-blockade. Any drug can cause fever due to hypersensitivity producing fever alone, with local inflammation at the site of administration (phlebitis, sterile abscess, soft tissue reaction) or because of the delivery systems (diluent intravenous fluid, intravascular delivery devices).[3] The high-risk agents for drug-fever are all antibiotics (especially β-lactams), anti-epileptic drugs (especially phenytoin), antiarrhythmics (mainly quinidine and procainamide), antihypertensives (a-methyldopa), diuretics, anti-seizures drugs, and stool softeners.[24] Antibiotics with lower risk for drug-fever development are: clindamycin, vancomycin, chloramphenicol, aztreonam, doxycycline, erythromycin, imipemen, quinolones, and aminoglycosides.[24] The time between initiating a drug and fever appearance is estimated to be 21 days (median 8 days) while the fever resolves usually within 72 hours after removing the offending drug. When a rash is present it persists for days or weeks.[2,3] The usual scenario of drug-fever in the ICU includes a patient in whom an already diagnosed infection is resolving and after an initial defervescence in temperature a recurrence of fever is noticed. In this patient, the antibiotics should be discontinued if the infection has been resolved or has not been detected another infectious site. If the patient is stable, but the infection has not been resolved, then the presumed offending agent should be removed and a modification to antibiotics, without potential sensitizing, according to the spectrum of pathogens should be performed.

Postoperative fever is common within the first 72 hours after surgery, usually caused by the release of endogenous pyrogens into the bloodstream. However, this type of fever warrants a careful evaluation to rule out infection, which is increasingly likely with time (after a patient is >96 hours febrile), while specific predisposing factors (type and site of surgery) and underlying comorbidities must be taken into account (pneumonia is common in upper abdominal surgery or thoracic surgery, wound infections in upper abdominal surgery, urinary infections in lower abdominal surgery).[25,26] In these patients, during the first 72 hours and if fever is the only indication, a chest radiograph or urine cultures are not mandatory, while surgical wounds should be examined daily for infection and a high level of suspicion should be maintained for obstructive vascular events (pulmonary embolism, deep venous thrombosis, superficial thrombophlebitis).[3]

Malignant hyperthermia (MH) and malignant neuroleptic syndrome (MNS) should be kept in mind in critically ill patients when fever is especially high. MH is more common in the operating room than in the ICU and occurs after general anesthesia with depolarizing agents including mutation in the calcium channel of sarcoplasmic reticulum.[3,9,27] MH can be caused by succinylcholine and inhaled anesthetics administration (especially halothane). MNS is a consequence of blockade of dopamine receptors from antipsychotic agents (phenothiazines, thioxanthenes, butyrophenones). Both, MH and MNS inhibit hypothalamic heat-conserving mechanisms generating high fever, muscular rigidity, and increased creatinine phosphokinase conentartions. The main difference among those two clinical entities is the initial muscle contraction (central in MNS) while frequently serotonin syndrome (excessive stimulation of the 5-HTIA-receptor by various psychiatric disorders), which may be exacerbated by the concomitant use of linezolid, is confused with MNS.[28] The treatment of MH and MNS include the removal of the offending drug and the administration of dantrolene or dopamine agonists (bromocryptine) to prevent tissue damage.

Other noninfectious causes of fever in critically ill patients are heatstroke (in patients under psychotropic medication or anticholinergic drugs needing discontinuation of the offending agent and external cooling of the body), withdrawal of certain drugs often with associated tachycardia, diaphoresis, and hyperreflexia (eg, alcohol, opiates, barbiturates, benzodiazepines), atelectasis or acute respiratory distress syndrome (ARDS) without pneumonia as a result of inflammatory process and blood transfusion (especially platelets), which is associated to an incidence of 0.5% and appears 30 min to 2 hours after the transfusion is begun and last 2–24 hours preceded by chills.[3,29]

Infectious Causes of Fever in the ICU

The ICU-acquired infections show a prevalence of between 10% (NNIS) and 20.6% (EPIC study) with ventilator-associated pneumonia (VAP) being the most common, followed by sinusitis, bloodstream and catheter-related infections, nosocomial diarrhea, and wound infections.[30,31]

Infections of the respiratory system
VAP occurs in 25% of mechanically-ventilated patients presenting with leukocytosis, purulent tracheal secretions ,and new or worsening infiltrates on the chest roentgenogram, while in immunocompomised patients, especially in solid organ transplant patients, VAP could be developed without the presence the above clinical manifestations.[32–34] The differential diagnosis includes ARDS, left ventricular failure (LVF), and tracheobronchitis because of the same pattern of the appeared pulmonary infiltrates. ARDS is characterized by the low lung volumes in chest radiographs and LVF from the immediate and permanent improvement of pulmonary infiltrates after the administration of aggressive, mainly diuretic, therapy.[2,3] The initial evaluation includes: (a) a chest imaging study with chest radiograph and CT scan; (b) cultures of secretions obtained from lower respiratory tract before antibiotics administration (expectorated sputum, tracheal secretions, Bronchoalveolar Lavage [BAL] obtained by fiberoptic bronchoscopy); and (c) in case of pleural effusion, stain culture and cytology of the pleural fluid.[35,36] Although the quantitative cultures have not been standardized sufficiently, they provide useful information, while blood cultures and other blood tests (PCR, CMV antigen, galactomannan and beta-D-glucan) could add in the diagnostic procedure.[3,35,36]

Catheter-related infections
Bloodstream infections originate mainly from gastrointestinal and genitourinary tracts in the absence of an IV-line or catheters, while catheter related are the infections caused by a pathogen that has colonized a vascular device.[2] The majority of ICU patients have

at least one central venous catheter (CVC), while most of them have some type of tunneled, cuffed CVCs, or subcutaneous central venous port. Catheter-related infections show an incidence of 10 infections/1.000 catheter days, while the relative risk for their appearance depends on the length of time with the catheter in situ, the number of ports, the number of manipulations, the type of the device, the patient population, and the techniques used in insertion.[37] The diagnosis is based on clinical signs including: the difficulty of drawing or infusing through the catheter, the presence of inflammation at the insertion site, and the recovery of microorganisms in multiple blood cultures.[38] For the evaluation of those signs, two peripheral blood cultures or one drawn percutaneously and one drawn through the catheter should be obtained, while blood cultures drawn through intravascular devices provide excellent sensitivity.[39] Different methods have been proposed aiming to reduce catheters' colonization, including topical administration of antibiotics and antimicrobial solutions, subcutaneous tunneling of catheters, and silver-impregnated subcutaneous cuffs.[40] The gold standard for the diagnosis and treatment is the removal and culture of the catheter with semiquantitative or quantitative catheter tip methods.[41]

Sinusitis

Sinusitis has an incidence of 5% of all nosocomial infections in the ICU affecting mainly trauma or neurosurgical patients, characterized by fever and leykocytosis, while purulent nasal discharge is often lacking (ie, it is present in only 25% of proved cases).[23,42] The predisposing factors for sinusitis development include: nasotracheal or nasogastric tube placement, nasal packing, facial fractures, and steroid administration, while the diagnosis is made by plain radiographs, CT scan or magnetic resonance imaging of the sinus.[43,44] Nasal endoscopy, in conjunction with plain radiography, increases the accuracy of diagnosis, depending on the skill of the practitioner.[45]

Nosocomial diarrhea

Critically ill patients frequently manifest diarrhea (ie, defined as more than two stools per day that conform to the container in which they are placed), which is caused by enteral feeding or by infectious causes. The commonest cause of febrile diarrhea in critically ill patients is *Clostridium difficile* (10%–25% of all cases of antibiotic-associated diarrhea), which ".....should be suspected in any patient with fever or leukocytosis and diarrhea who received an antibacterial agent or chemotherapy within 60 days before the onset of diarrhea.."[3,46,47] Nosocomial diarrhea caused by *C difficile* can be caused by any antibacterial agent, but the main causes are clindamycin, cepalosporins, and fluoroquinolones.[48] The gold standard for the diagnosis is the tissue culture assay, which presents, however, a 24–48 hour delay in results and high cost, while an enzyme immunoassay test (EIA) for toxin A and B is commercially available, easy to perform, and able to provide results within minutes to hours.[49] In case of severe illness and negative rapid tests for *C difficile* ,flexible sigmoidoscopy procedure remains a secure option for the diagnosis, while in HIV patients or patients exposed in different epidemiologic conditions, stool cultures for other pathogens is indicated.[50,51]

Intra-abdominal and surgical site infections

Intra-abdominal infections could be the main cause of ICU admission or a secondary cause after abdominal surgery (abscess formation, biliary sepsis). The diagnosis is facilitated by CT scan of the abdomen, ultrasound, and nuclear medicine techniques (gallium-67, indium-111 white blood cell scintigraphy).[2,23] CT scan and ultrasound are used for the detection of focal findings (CT scan is used mainly for mid-lower abdomen/peritoneal cavity, while ultrasound for infections in the pelvis and right upper quadrant abdomen).[52] Surgical site infections include mainly: the contamination of the surgical incision depending on the medical comorbitities of the patient; the duration of the operation; and whether antimicrobial prophylaxis was administered before incision.[26]

Fungal infections
Fungi (mainly *Candida* species) are a main cause of infections; development in critically ill patients is: associated with specific risk factors; characterized by difficult diagnosis because of the lack of a diagnostic tool able to discriminate colonization from infection; and showing an epidemiologic shift toward non-*albicans* species.[53–57] The definite diagnosis is made by the identification of the fungi from histologic or, sterile specimen obtained.

Other infections
Urinary tract infections In critically ill patients, urinary tract infections (UTIs) (mainly catheter-associated bacteriuria or candiduria) usually reflect colonization, are rarely symptomatic, and are not considered as a significant cause of morbidity or attributable mortality, while the traditional clinical signs and symptoms are rarely reported by the patient.[58,59]

Cytomegalovirus antigenemia, central nervous system infections During recent years, cytomegalovirus (CMV) antigenemia has been proposed as a cause of unexplained prolonged fever in severely ill, immunocompetent patients in the ICU, but the significance of CMV detection is unknown; however, patients with detectable CMV tend to have a higher morbidity and mortality compared with patients in whom the virus remains undetectable.[60] In neurocritical patients, fever occurs in 25% of the cases, but almost half of these fevers are of noninfectious origin. In these patients, the suspicion of infection development must be of high index because of the inherent limitations of the neurologic examination, the low yield of lumbar puncture in nonimmunocompromized patients, and the contraindications for lumbar puncture performance, which frequently are met in critically ill patients.[61,62] The diagnosis for a critically ill patient with a new episode of fever is made usually by imaging study (CT scan of the brain), culture of cerebrospinal fluid, and removal and culture of the placed catheter or other intracranial device.[63]

APPROACHING THE FEBRILE CRITICALLY ILL PATIENT AND TREATMENT OF THE FEVER

The initial approach to the febrile patient includes: (a) the overview of the medical record; (b) the physical examination; and (c) the evaluation of characteristics of the fever (magnitude, duration, relationship to patient's pulse rate, and temporal relationship to diagnostic and therapeutic interventions). In all febrile patients before the initiation of any treatment, at least two blood cultures by separate needles from different sites as well as other appropriate cultures must be obtained (**Fig. 2**). The clinician always has to consider that chills and fever appear 1–2 hours after the presence of microorganisms in the blood (initiating event), which explains the commonly observed negative blood cultures at the time of the temperature spike.[64]

   In the case of unexplained or unknown origin fever that is associated to unexplained leukocytosis, anion gap acidosis, hypotension or persistent tachycardia and tachypnea, the initial evaluation should be focused on ruling out septic syndrome development originated by urinary tract infection, VAP/nosocomial pneumonia, phlebitis, wound infections, or bacteremia.[2,23] In patients who have progressive signs of severe sepsis and in all neutropenic patients with fever, broad-spectrum antimicrobial therapy should be started immediately after cultures have been obtained, while all

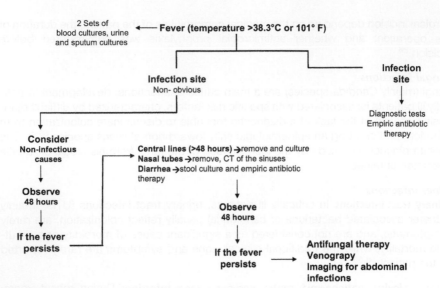

Fig. 2. Approach to the febrile patient in the ICU.

the central lines placed for > 48 hours and the nasal tubes should be removed and cultured using semiquantitative or quantitative cultures; however, in the case of diarrhea, stool cultures for WBC count and toxin against *C difficile* should be performed.[2,23] In patients who have abdominal sepsis or signs of abdominal infection, including tenderness and distension, CT scan of the abdomen is indicated. If the fever persists 48–96 hours after antibiotic treatment and without the cause or the source of the infection being identified, the patient must be reevaluated for risk factors associated with fungal infections (initiation of empiric antifungal treatment is indicated), while additional diagnostic tests, including venography, complete blood count (CBC) for eosinophils (drug fever), and abdominal imaging are indicated.[2,23]

During recent years, several biomarkers have been proposed as adjunctive markers for the evaluation of fever, aiming to discriminate true infection from noninfection or other inflammatory diseases. These biomarkers include: serum procalcitonin assays with variable cut-off points, endotoxin detection systems, trigering receptor expressed on myeloids cells-1 (TREM-1), C-reactive protein, tumor necrosis factor-α and Interleukin-6.[65–68] From all the above biomarkers, serum procalcitonin assay is approved for the early detection of bacterial infection/sepsis during the first day of ICU admission, while the rest of them have not yet been validated.[69]

The methods used for the suppression of the fever in the ICU include the administration of antipyretic agents (acetaminophen, cyclooxygenase 2 and nonsteroidal agents, metamizol and propacetamol) and external cooling techniques performance.[70,71] Antipyretic agents are agents able to block or reverse the cytokine-mediated rise in core temperature caused by fever without affecting body temperature and must be distinguished from hypothermic agents that are able to lower core temperature even in the absence of fever.[72] The external cooling methods include the placement of hypothermia blankets, which, however, are characterized by certain side effects including the large temperature fluctuations, the development of rebound hyperthermia, the appearance of hypermetabolism, and increased oxygen consumption, leading to elevated levels of epinephrine and norepinephrine.[73]

REFERENCES

1. Cunha BA, Shea KW. Fever in the intensive care unit. Infect Dis Clin North Am 1996;10:185–209.
2. Dimopoulos G. Approach to the febrile patient in the intensive care unit. In: Rello J, Kollef M, Diaz E, et al, editors. Infectious diseases in critical care. 2nd edition. Berlin: Heidelberg; 2007. p. 1–9.
3. O'Grady N, Barie PS, Bartlett JG, et al. Guidelines for evaluation of new fever in critically ill adult patients: 2008 update from the American College of Critical Care Medicine and the Infectious Diseases Society of America. Crit Care Med 2008;36(4):1330–49.
4. Ipp M, Jaffre D. Physicians' attitudes toward the diagnosis and management of fever in children 3 months to 2 years of age. Clin Pediatr (Phila) 1993;32:66–70.
5. Gozzoli V, Schottker P, Suter PM, et al. Is it worth treating fever in intensive care unit patients? Preliminary results from a randomized trial of the effect of external cooling. Arch Intern Med 2001;161:121–3.
6. Arbo MJ, Fine MJ, Hanusa BH, et al. Fever of nosocomial origin:etiology, risk factors and outcomes. Am J Med 1993;95:505–12.
7. Hudges WT, Armstrong D, Boddey GP, et al. 2002 guidelines for the use of anti-microbial agents in neutropenic patients with cancer. Clin Infect Dis 2002;34: 730–51.
8. Leon L. Cytokine regulation of fever: studies using gene knockout mice. J Appl Physiol 2002;92:2648–55.
9. Ryan M, Levy MM. Clinical review: fever in intensive care unit patients. Crit Care 2003;7:221–5.
10. Lubeshi GN. Cytokines and fever. Mechanisms and sites of action. Ann N Y Acad Sci 1998;856:83–9.
11. Simmons DL, Wagner D, Westover K. Nonsteroidal anti-inflammatory drugs, acet-aminophen, cyclooxygenase-2 and fever. Clin Infect Dis 2000;31(Suppl 5): S211–8.
12. Mackowiak PA. Brief history of antipyretic therapy. Clin Infect Dis 2000;31(Suppl 5):S154–6.
13. Weinstein MP, Iannini PB, Stratton CW, et al. Spontaneous bacterial peritonitis. A review of 28 cases with emphasis on improved survival and factors influencing prognosis. Am J Med 1978;64(4):592–8.
14. Manthaous CA, Hall JB, Olson D, et al. Effect of cooling on oxygen consumption in febrile critically ill patients. Am J Respir Crit Care Med 1995;151(1):10–4.
15. Ginsberg MD, Busto R. Combating hyperthermia in acute stroke: a significant clinical concern. Stroke 1998;29:529–34.
16. Ferguson A. Evaluation and treatment of fever in intensive care unit patients. Crit Care Nurs Q 2007;30(4):347–63.
17. Henker R, Kramer D, Rogers S. Fever. ACCN Clin Issues 1997;8:351–67.
18. Cunha BA. Intensive care, not intensive antibiotics. Heart Lung 1994;23:361–2.
19. O'Grady NP, Philip SB, Bartlett BC, et al. Practice guidelines for evaluating new fever in critically ill adult patients. Clin Infect Dis 1998;26:1042–59.
20. Cunha BA. Fever in the neurosurgical patient. Heart Lung 1996;17:608–15.
21. Stocchetti N, Rossi S, Roncati Zanier E, et al. Pyrexia in head-injured patients admitted to intensive care. Intensive Care Med 2002;28:1555–62.
22. Barie PS, Fischer E. Acute acalculus cholecystitis. J Am Coll Surg 1995;180: 232–4.
23. Marik PE. Fever in the ICU. Chest 2000;117(3):855–69.

24. Wood AJ. Adverse drug reactions. In: Fauci AS, Braunwald E, et al, editors. Harrison's principles of internal medicine. New York: McGraw-Hill; 1998. p. 422–30.
25. Garibaldi RA, Brodine S, Mathumiya S, et al. Evidence for the non-infectious etiology of early post-operative fever. Infect Control 1985;6:273–7.
26. Stevens DL, Bisno AL, Chambers HF, et al. Practice guidelines for the diagnosis and management of skin and soft-tissues infections. Clin Infect Dis 2005;41: 1373–406.
27. Heiman-Patterson TD. Neuroleptic malignant syndrome and malignant hyperthermia: important issues for the medical consultant. Med Clin North Am 1993; 77:477–92.
28. Lawrence KR, Adra M, Gillan PK, et al. Serotonin toxicity associated with the use of linezolid: a review of postmarketing data. Clin Infect Dis 2006;42:1578–83.
29. Saper CB, Breder CD. The neurologic basis of fever. N Engl J Med 1994;330: 1880–6.
30. Jarvis WR, Edwards JR, Culver DH, et al. Nosocomial infection rates in adult and pediatric intensive care units in the United States. National Nosocomial Infections Surveillance System. Am J Med 1991;91(3B):185S–91S.
31. Vincent JL, Bihari DJ, Suter PM, et al. The prevalence of nosocomial infection in Intensive Care Units in Europe. Results of the European Prevalence of Infection in Intensive Care (EPIC) study. EPIC International Advisory Committee. JAMA 1995; 274(8):639–44.
32. Chastre J, Fagon JY. Ventilator-associated pneumonia. Am J Respir Crit Care Med 2002;165:867–903.
33. Franquet T. High-resolution computed tomography (HRCT) of lung infections in non-AIDS immunocompromised patients. Eur Radiol 2006;16:707–18.
34. Pelletier SJ, Crabtree TD, Cleason TC, et al. Characteristics of infectious complications associated with mortality after solid organ transplantation. Clin Transplant 1999;13:260–5.
35. Rello J, Diaz E, Rodriguez A, et al. Advances in the management of pneumonia in the intensive care unit: review of the current thinking. Clin Microbiol Infect 2005; 11(Suppl 5):30–8.
36. Heyland D, Dodek P, Muscedere J, et al. A randomized trial of diagnostic techniques for ventilator associated pneumonia. N Engl J Med 2006;355:2619–30.
37. Maki DG, Kluger DM, Crinch CJ. The risk of bloodstream infection in adults with different intravascular devices: a systematic review of 200 published prospective studies. Mayo Clin Proc 2006;81:1159–71.
38. Safdar N, Maki DG. Inflammation at the insertion site is not predictive of catheter bloodstream infection with shorterm, noncuffed central venous catheters. Crit Care Med 2002;30:2632–5.
39. Safdar N, Fine JP, Maki DG. Meta-analusis: methods for diagnosing intravascular device-related bloodstream infection. Ann Intern Med 2005;142:451–66.
40. McConell SA, Gubbins PO, Anaissie EJ. Are antimicrobial-impregnated catheters effective? Replace the water and grab your washcloth, because we have a baby to wash. Clin Infect Dis 2004;39(12):1829–33.
41. Catton JA, Dobbins BM, Kite P, et al. In situ diagnosis of intravascular catheter-related bloodstream infection: a comparison of quantitative culture, differential time to positivity and endoluminal brushing. Crit Care Med 2005;33:787–91.
42. Caplan ES, Hoyt NJ. Nosocomial sinusitis. JAMA 1982;247:639–41.
43. Vargas F, Bui HN, Boyer A, et al. Trasnasal puncture based on echographic sinusitis evidence in mechanically ventilated patients with suspicion of nosocomial maxillary sinusitis. Intensive Care Med 2006;32:858–66.

44. Kountakis SE, Skoulas IG. Middle meatal vs antral lavage cultures in intensive care unit patients. Otolaryngol Head Neck Surg 2002;126:377–81.
45. Roberts DN, Hampal S, East CA, et al. The diagnosis of inflammatory sinonasal disease. J Laryngol Otol 1995;109:27–30.
46. Bartlett JC. Narrative review: the new epidemic of Clostridium difficile –associated enteric disease. Ann Intern Med 2006;145:758–64.
47. Pepin J, Valiquette L, Alary ME, et al. Clostridium difficle-associated diarrhea in a region of Quebec from 1991 to 2003: a changing pattern of disease severity. CMAJ 2004;171:466–72.
48. Pepin J, Saheb N, Coulombe MA, et al. Emergence of fluoroquinolones as the predominant risk factor for Clostridium difficile –associated diarrhea: a cohort study during an epidemic in Quebec. Clin Infect Dis 2005;41:1254–60.
49. Ticehurst JR, Aird DZ, Dam LM, et al. Effective detection of toxigenic Clostridium difficile by a two-step algotithm including tests for antigen and cytoxin. J Clin Microbiol 2006;44:1145–9.
50. Hogenauer C, Langner C, Beubler E, et al. Klebsiella oxytoca as a causative organism of antibiotic-associated hemorrhagic colitis. N Engl J Med 2006;355: 2418–26.
51. Warny M, Pepin J, Fang A, et al. Toxin production by an emerging strain of Clostridium difficile associated with outbreaks of severe diasease in North America and Europe. Lancet 2005;366:1079–84.
52. Meduri GU, Belechia JM, Massie JD, et al. The role of gallium-67 scintigraphy in diagnosing sources of fever in ventilated patients. Intensive Care Med 1996;22: 395–403.
53. Dimopoulos G, Vincent JL. Candida and Aspergillus infections in critically ill patients. Clin Intensive Care 2002;13(1):1–12.
54. Peres-Bota D, Rodriguez-Villalobos H, Dimopoulos G, et al. Infections with Candida spp. in critically ill patients are primarily related to the length of stay in the intensive care unit. Clin Microbiol Infect 2004;10(6):550–5.
55. Dimopoulos G, Karabinis A, Samonis G, et al. Candidemia in inimmunocompromised and immunocompetent critically ill patients: a prospective comparative study. Eur J Clin Microbiol Infect Dis 2007;26(6):377–84.
56. Dimopoulos G, Ntziora F, Rachiotis G, et al. Candida albicans versus non- albicans bloodstream infection in critically ill patients: differences in risk factors and outcomes. Anesth Analg 2008;106(2):523–9.
57. Holley A, Dulhunty JM, Blot SI, et al. Temporal trends, risk factors and outcome in albicans and non-albicans candidaemia: an epidemiological study in 4 internationally independent multi-disciplinary intensive care units. Intern J Antimicrob Agents 2009;33(6):554.
58. Laupland KB, Bagshaw SM, Gregson DB, et al. Intensive care unit-acquired urinary tract infections in a regional critical care system. Crit Care 2005;9(2):R60–5.
59. Gaynes R, Edwards JR. National Nosocomial Infections Surveillance System Overview of nosocomial infections caused by gram-negative bacilli. Clin Infect Dis 2005;41(6):848–54.
60. Jaber S, Chanques G, Borry J, et al. Cytomegalovirus infection in critically ill patients: associated factors and consequences. Chest 2005;127:233–41.
61. Commichau C, Scarmeas N, Mayer SA. Risk factors for fever in the neurologic intensive care unit. Neurology 2003;60:837–41.
62. Jackson WL, Shorr AF. The yield of lumbar puncture to exclude nosocomial meningitis as aetiology for mental status changes in the medical intensive care unit. Anaesth Intensive Care 2006;34:21–4.

63. Tunkel AR, Hartman BJ, Kaplan SL, et al. Practice guidelines for the management of bacterial memingitis. Clin Infect Dis 2004;39:1267–84.
64. Pronovost PJ, Holzmueller CG. Partnering for quality. J Crit Care 2004;19(3): 121–9.
65. Suprin E, Camus C, Gacouin A, et al. Procalcitonin: a valuable indicator of infection in a medical ICU? Intensive Care Med 2000;26:1232–8.
66. Selberg O, Hecker H, Martin M, et al. Discrimination of sepsis and systemic inflammatory response syndrome by determination of circulating plasma concentrations of procalcitonin, protein complement 3a and interleukin-6. Crit Care Med 2008;28:2793–8.
67. Marshall JC, Walker PM, Foster DM, et al. Measurement of endotoxin activity in critically ill patients using whole blood neutrophil dependent chemiluminescence. Crit Care 2002;6:342–8.
68. Cohen J. The detection and interpretation of endotoxaemia. Intensive Care Med 2000;26(Suppl 1):S51–6.
69. Marshall JC, Foster D, Vincent JL, et al. Diagnostic and prognostic implications of endotoxemia in critical illness: results of the MEDIC study. J Infect Dis 2004;190: 527–34.
70. Thompson HJ. Fever: a concept analysis. J Adv Nurs 2005;51(5):484–92.
71. Manthous CA. Toward a more thoughtful approach to fever in critically ill patients. Chest 2000;117(3):627–8.
72. Gozzoli V, Treggiari MM, Kleger GR, et al. Randomized trial of the effect of antipyretics by metamizol, propacetamol or external cooling on metabolism, hemodynamics and inflammatory response. Intensive Care Med 2004;30(3):401–7.
73. Mackowiak PA. Physiological rationale for suppression of fever. Clin Infect Dis 2000;31(Suppl 5):S185–9.

The Management of Severe Sepsis and Septic Shock

Matthew R. Morrell, MD[a],*, Scott T. Micek, PharmD[b], Marin H. Kollef, MD[a]

KEYWORDS

- Severe sepsis • Septic shock • Goal-directed therapy
- Empiric antibiotics • Vasoactive agents • Biomarkers

Severe sepsis and septic shock persist as major health care problems despite ongoing research to improve overall outcomes. Overall mortality from severe sepsis or septic shock ranges from 30% to 60% despite aggressive medical care and accounts for 9.3% of all deaths in the United States.[1–3] In fact, severe sepsis and septic shock is the 10th leading cause of death in the United States.[4] More than 750,000 cases of sepsis occur each year in the United States, resulting in more than 380,000 intensive care admissions and initiation of mechanical ventilation in 130,000 cases. The number of cases of severe sepsis and septic shock has been estimated to reach 934,000 and 1,110,000 cases by the years 2010 and 2020. Severe sepsis and septic shock also consume considerable health care resources with the average cost per case being $22,000. Annual total costs associated with the care of patients who have sepsis have been estimated to be near $17 billion.[1] These annual costs will most likely increase in the upcoming years because of the overall aging population, emergence of newer antimicrobial-resistant bacteria, and increasing use of invasive therapeutic measures.

Sepsis is defined by a systemic inflammatory response syndrome, such as fever, tachypnea, tachycardia, or leukocytosis, in response to a culture-proven or clinically suspected infection. The clinically suspected infections may include a wound with purulent discharge, community-acquired pneumonia in a previously healthy individual, or ruptured bowel with free air or bowel contents in the peritoneum. More recently the grading system of sepsis was modified to include severe sepsis, septic shock, and refractory septic shock.[3,5] Severe sepsis includes the previously mentioned clinical criteria for sepsis in addition to at least one sign of organ hypoperfusion or

This manuscript was supported in part by the Barnes-Jewish Hospital Foundation.

[a] Division of Pulmonary and Critical Care Medicine, Department of Medicine, Washington University School of Medicine, Barnes-Jewish Hospital, 660 South Euclid Avenue, Campus Box 8052, St. Louis, MO 63110, USA

[b] Department of Pharmacy, Washington University School of Medicine, Barnes-Jewish Hospital, 660 South Euclid Avenue, Campus Box 8052, St. Louis, MO 63110, USA

* Corresponding author.

E-mail address: mmorrell@dom.wustl.edu (M.R. Morrell).

Infect Dis Clin N Am 23 (2009) 485–501
doi:10.1016/j.idc.2009.04.002
0891-5520/09/$ – see front matter © 2009 Elsevier Inc. All rights reserved.

id.theclinics.com

dysfunction, such as cardiac dysfunction, acute lung injury, or altered mental status. Septic shock is defined by severe sepsis in addition to a systemic mean blood pressure less than 60 mm Hg (or <80 mm Hg if previous hypertension) after an attempt at adequate fluid resuscitation or a need for vasopressors to maintain a systemic mean blood pressure greater than 60 mm Hg (or >80 mm Hg if previous hypertension). Finally, refractory septic shock exists if dopamine greater than 15 μg/kg/min or norepinephrine or epinephrine greater than 0.25 μg/kg/min is required to maintain a mean blood pressure greater than 60 mm Hg (80 mm Hg if previous hypertension). These definitions were established to facilitate early diagnosis, follow physiologic responses, aide entry into clinical trials, and help staging and prognostication.

The occurrence of septic shock seems to peak in the sixth decade of life. Predisposing factors include male sex, non-white ethnic origin in North Americans, comorbid diseases, malignancy, immunodeficiency or immunocompromised state, chronic organ failure, alcohol dependence, and genetic factors.[1,6–8] The most common sites of infection include the respiratory tract, genitourinary system, and abdomen.[1,6] In 25% of individuals who have severe sepsis or septic shock, multiple sites of infection can account for the clinical presentation. Twenty percent of individuals have severe sepsis or septic shock with site unknown.[1,6]

The causative organism of severe sepsis and septic shock depends on multiple factors, including endemic microbial pathogens (eg, malaria in Southeast Asia), patient comorbid conditions (HIV, malignancy), and possible microbial colonization. Gram-positive bacteria account for most pathogens associated with severe sepsis and septic shock with a range of 30% to 50%.[6] Severe sepsis and septic shock due to gram-negative bacteria have been diminishing, but still account for 25% to 30% of cases, with a higher prevalence in genitourinary infections.[8] Over the past decade, the percentage of multidrug-resistant (MDR) bacteria has significantly increased. In addition, the number of cases of severe sepsis or septic shock due to fungi has also significantly increased. In fact, MDR bacteria and fungi account for 25% of cases of severe sepsis and septic shock.[6,8] Viruses and parasites are identified in 2% to 4% of cases; however, this may be an underestimate. In 20% to 30% of cases, a causative organism is not identified, which may be affected by the relatively low sensitivity of blood cultures and preadministration of antibiotics.

INITIAL ASSESSMENT

Sepsis is the result of complex interactions between the infecting microorganism and host immune, inflammatory, and coagulation responses. Sepsis has been divided into phases, early and late, by fluctuations in these specific host responses and to facilitate further targeted therapies.[9] The early stage of sepsis, defined as the first 6 hours, is highlighted by an early diagnosis of severe sepsis or septic shock and institution of early, goal-directed therapy.[10,11] Early goal-directed therapy allows for ongoing patient assessment and results in a decrease in both in-hospital and overall mortality.[10,12] Many critical first-line therapies should be administered during this crucial period in severe sepsis and septic shock (**Fig. 1**).

The first priority in a patient who has severe sepsis or septic shock involves stabilization of the airway and breathing. Supplemental oxygen should be provided to the patient and institution of mechanical ventilation should be performed if necessary. Second, an assessment of perfusion should be performed. Blood pressure should be assessed by a sphygmomanometer or arterial catheter if blood pressure is labile. However, attempts at placing an arterial line to obtain an accurate assessment of blood pressure should not delay further management of severe sepsis or septic shock.

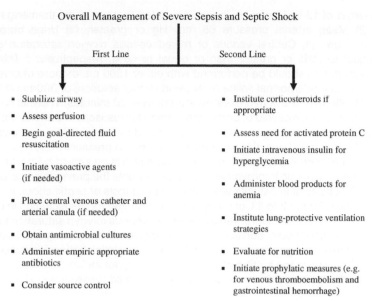

Overall Management of Severe Sepsis and Septic Shock

First Line — Second Line

First Line

- Stabilize airway
- Assess perfusion
- Begin goal-directed fluid resuscitation
- Initiate vasoactive agents (if needed)
- Place central venous catheter and arterial canula (if needed)
- Obtain antimicrobial cultures
- Administer empiric appropriate antibiotics
- Consider source control

Second Line

- Institute corticosteroids if appropriate
- Assess need for activated protein C
- Initiate intravenous insulin for hyperglycemia
- Administer blood products for anemia
- Institute lung-protective ventilation strategies
- Evaluate for nutrition
- Initiate prophylatic measures (e.g. for venous thromboembolism and gastrointestinal hemorrhage)

Fig. 1. Therapies used in the treatment of severe sepsis and septic shock.

Once hypoperfusion is documented, early restoration of perfusion is necessary to limit secondary organ dysfunction and reduce mortality (**Fig. 2**). Goals of initial resuscitation of sepsis-induced hypoperfusion should include: (1) Central venous pressure of 8 to 12 mm Hg. If a patient is mechanically ventilated, a higher central venous

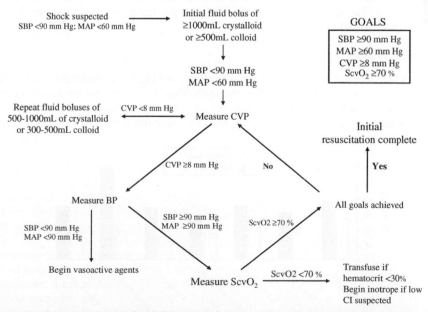

Shock suspected
SBP <90 mm Hg; MAP <60 mm Hg

Initial fluid bolus of ≥1000mL crystalloid or ≥500mL colloid

GOALS

SBP ≥90 mm Hg
MAP ≥60 mm Hg
CVP ≥8 mm Hg
$ScvO_2$ ≥70 %

SBP <90 mm Hg
MAP <60 mm Hg

Repeat fluid boluses of 500-1000mL of crystalloid or 300-500mL colloid

CVP <8 mm Hg

Measure CVP

Initial resuscitation complete

CVP ≥8 mm Hg   No   Yes

Measure BP

SBP ≥90 mm Hg
MAP ≥90 mm Hg

$ScvO2$ ≥70 %

All goals achieved

SBP <90 mm Hg
MAP <90 mm Hg

Begin vasoactive agents

Measure $ScvO_2$ $ScvO2$ <70 %

Transfuse if hematocrit <30%
Begin inotrope if low CI suspected

Fig. 2. Initial resuscitation with goal-directed therapy in the initial stage of severe sepsis and septic shock. CVP, central venous pressure; MAP, mean arterial pressure; SBP, systolic blood pressure; $ScvO_2$, central venous oxygen saturation.

pressure target of 12 to 15 mm Hg is recommended to account for the filling imped-iment;[13] (2) Mean arterial pressure 65 mm Hg or greater; (3) Urine output 0.5 mL/kg/h or more; (4) Central venous or mixed venous oxygen saturation greater than or equal to 70% or greater than or equal to 65%, respectively.[11] This initial volume resuscitation should be performed with either 1000 mL or more of crystalloid (0.9% sodium chloride/normal saline or lactated Ringer solution) or 300 to 500 mL of colloids (5% albumin or 6% hydroxyethyl starch) over 30 minutes. There is no differ-ence in outcomes when colloid or crystalloid is used for resuscitative efforts; however, hydroxyethyl starch has been associated with reports of renal failure and increased bleeding.[14–16] Volume status, tissue perfusion, and blood pressure must be assessed after the initial fluid challenge and further fluid administration should be continued as long as the hemodynamic improvement continues or until the previous goals are met. Large fluid deficits exist in patients who have severe sepsis or septic shock and up to 6 to 10 L of crystalloid or 2 to 4 L of colloid may be required for resuscitation in the first 24 hours.[10] If the goals for central venous or mixed venous oxygen saturations are not met during the initial 6 hours, consideration can be given to transfusing red blood cells to achieve a hematocrit greater than or equal to 30% or administration of a dobutamine infusion.[10,11] Finally, in the setting of life-threatening hypotension, vasoactive agents may be required for supportive care during the initial fluid resuscitation stage.

DIAGNOSIS

Appropriate antimicrobial cultures should be obtained on initial presentation of severe sepsis or septic shock. At least two blood cultures should be obtained with at least one drawn percutaneously and one drawn through each vascular access device, unless the device was recently placed within the last 48 hours.[11] Cultures from other sites that may be the source of infection, such as urine and sputum, should be also obtained. Although obtaining these cultures is essential to confirm infection and allow tapering of antibiotic regimens, they should not delay the administration of early and appropriate antibiotics.

ANTIBIOTIC THERAPY

Multiple studies have documented the critical nature of early administration of broad-spectrum antibiotics and the effect on mortality (**Fig. 3**).[17–19] In a recent retrospective cohort study in patients who had septic shock, increasing delays in the initiation of effective antimicrobial therapy after the onset of hypotension were associated with

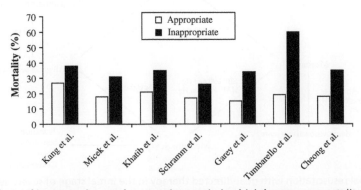

Fig. 3. Effects of inappropriate and appropriate antimicrobial therapy on mortality in severe sepsis and septic shock. (*Data from* references.[24,77–82])

a significantly increased risk for death. The median time to initiation of effective therapy was also shown to be a significant predictor of mortality.[20] The most recent guidelines from the Surviving Sepsis Campaign recommend starting intravenous antibiotic therapy as early as possible because each hour delay in administration of effective antibiotics is associated with a measurable increase in mortality.[11,17,20]

The increasing prevalence of fungi, methicillin-resistant *Staphylococcus aureus*, vancomycin-resistant enterococcus, highly resistant gram-negative bacilli, and local patterns of antibiotic susceptibility should be considered in the choice of initial antibiotic regimens for severe sepsis and septic shock.[21,22] The initial selection of antimicrobial therapy should be broad enough to cover all likely pathogens and be able to penetrate in adequate concentrations into the presumed source of sepsis (**Fig. 4**). In areas with a relatively high prevalence of *Candida* species, an echinocandin to cover fluconazole-resistant *Candida glabrata* and *krusei* should be included in the antimicrobial milieu for presumed fungal sepsis.[17,23] Patient factors, such as recent antibiotic administration, underlying comorbid conditions, risk factors for colonization with MDR pathogens, and documented drug intolerances also play a crucial role in initial selection of antibiotic therapy. Initial treatment of presumed MDR pathogens as a source of severe sepsis and septic shock should include combination therapy with two antimicrobial agents to increase the likelihood of providing appropriate treatment and resultant improved mortality.[24] In locations with MDR pathogens, such as *Klebsiella pneumoniae* carbapenemase (KPC) gram-negative bacteria, and pan-resistant *Pseudomonas aeruginosa*, antimicrobial treatment with alternative regimens, such as colistin, should be considered. Knowledge of local susceptibilities and pathogen minimum inhibitory concentration (MIC) is also critical when selecting the initial antimicrobial regimen. One recent study found that empiric therapy with piperacillin-tazobactam for treatment of *pseudomonas* bacteremia with reduced susceptibility was associated with increased mortality, despite being appropriate.[25] If high MICs to cefepime and piperacillin-tazobactam are prevalent, broader coverage with

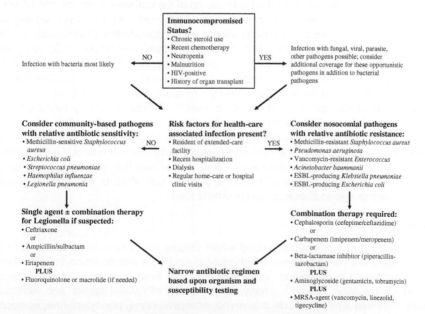

Fig. 4. Initial antibiotic selection for severe sepsis and septic shock.

a carbapenem may be more appropriate rather than use of inferior therapies. Consideration can also be given to different antimicrobial dosing strategies, such as continuous infusion, to maximize the time above the MIC for treatment of causative pathogens.[26]

Patients who have severe sepsis or septic shock warrant broad-spectrum therapy until the causative organism is identified. Once culture results and antimicrobial susceptibility data return, further therapy should be pathogen directed and all unnecessary antibiotics should be discontinued in accordance with good antimicrobial stewardship to avoid drug toxicities and the development of nosocomial superinfections with *Candida* species, *Clostridium difficile*, or vancomycin-resistant *enterococcus.*[27] Such de-escalation approaches in patients who have severe sepsis and septic shock have been shown to have improved outcomes.[28] The duration of antibiotic therapy is somewhat controversial; however, current recommendations are to continue therapy for 7 to 10 days. Longer courses of therapy may be appropriate in patients who have a slow clinical response, undrainable focus of infection, or immunologic deficiencies, such as neutropenia.[11] In most cases of severe sepsis or septic shock, antimicrobial cultures are negative and thus the decision to continue, taper, or stop antibiotic therapy must be made on the basis of clinical information.[6,8]

CATHETERS

Frequently in severe sepsis and septic shock, blood pressure readings from a noninvasive arm cuff are inaccurate. Systolic pressure with an arm cuff often overreads at low pressures (<60 mm Hg) and the use of an arterial cannula provides a more accurate and reproducible measurement of true arterial pressure. In addition, an indwelling arterial cannula provides continuous analysis so that decisions regarding therapy can be based on immediate and accurate information. Vasoactive agents are required once fluid resuscitation does not restore adequate hemodynamic function. These agents should be administered through a central venous catheter as soon as one is available. Once appropriately placed with the tip of the catheter at the cavoatrial junction, frequent assessments of the central venous pressure and mixed venous oxygen saturation can be obtained to assist in volume resuscitation efforts in the early stages of septic shock. Often in severe sepsis and septic shock, empiric antibiotics are given during the early phases of volume resuscitation/vasopressor initiation and multiple venous accesses are required. Placement of a multilumen catheter can alleviate this potential problem. Use of pulmonary artery catheters has declined over the past 2 decades due to the lack of a definitive benefit.[29] Pulmonary artery catheters can provide potentially useful information, such as an assessment of cardiac function in patients who have severe sepsis and septic shock; however these advantages are plagued by results that are subject to interpretation and may not reflect the true hemodynamic status.[30] Although pulmonary artery catheter insertion may be appropriate in select cases, the routine use of pulmonary artery catheters in patients who have severe sepsis or septic shock is not recommended.

VASOACTIVE THERAPY

Vasopressors and inotropes are used when volume expansion alone is not able to restore adequate hemodynamic function or during fluid resuscitation in the setting of life-threatening hypotension. Vasopressors differ from inotropes, which increase cardiac contractility; however, many drugs have both vasopressor and inotropic effects. Potential agents include dopamine, norepinephrine, phenylephrine, epinephrine, and vasopressin. Using these therapies, the mean arterial pressure (MAP) should be maintained at 65 mm Hg or greater, because this has been shown to preserve tissue perfusion in severe sepsis and septic shock.[31] Currently, there is no definitive evidence of the superiority of one vasopressor over another toward patient-oriented outcomes.[32] The choice of vasopressor should depend on the desired physiologic effect, subsequent response, and possible adverse effects.

Norepinephrine is a strong α-adrenergic agonist with less pronounced β-adrenergic effects; as a result, a significant increase in MAP and systemic vascular resistance, with little change in cardiac rate or output, is observed.[33] Because of its potent vaso-constrictive activity, it is commonly used as an initial vasoactive agent in severe sepsis and septic shock. Dopamine is a natural precursor of norepinephrine and epinephrine and possesses distinct dose-dependent pharmacologic effects. At lower doses, it acts on dopaminergic receptors resulting in selective vasodilatation in renal mesen-teric and coronary beds. Further increases in the dose result in stimulation of β1-adrenergic receptors resulting in an increase in heart rate and cardiac contractility. At higher doses, α1-adrenergic effects predominate, leading to arterial vasoconstric-tion.[33] Low-dose dopamine should not be used to preserve renal function because there is no difference in urine output, need for renal replacement, or survival compared with placebo.[34] Dopamine is also more arrhythmogenic and should be used with caution in patients who have underlying heart disease.[35] Epinephrine has potent β1-adrenergic and moderate β2- and α1-adrenergic effects. Increases in cardiac output result at lower doses with vasoconstriction predominating at higher doses. The degree of splanchnic vasoconstriction and risk for dysrhythmias seems to be greater with epinephrine compared with other vasoactive agents.[36] Phenylephrine has purely α-adrenergic agonist activity and results in vasoconstriction with minimal cardiac inotropy or chronotropy. As a result, phenylephrine may be a good choice when tachy-arrhythmias limit therapy with other vasopressors.[33]

Recent studies have shown that vasopressin levels in septic shock are lower than anticipated for a shock state, which may contribute to persistent hypotension.[37] Current evidence documents the efficacy of adding low-dose vasopressin in severe sepsis and septic shock that is refractory to other vasopressors.[38,39] A recent study, however, failed to show any benefit on mortality when used in combination with norepinephrine.[40] Potential complications from vasopressin infusion include coronary and mesenteric ischemia.

Dobutamine is not a vasopressor but is an inotrope that has variable effects on blood pressure. Primarily it has both β1- and β2-adrenergic effects resulting in an increase in heart rate and cardiac contractility. Dobutamine should be considered for patients who have low cardiac output in the presence of adequate left ventricular filling pressure and adequate mean arterial pressure.[11] Other vasopressors, such as dopamine, norepi-nephrine, and epinephrine, also have inotropic effects in addition to their vasoconstric-tive effects. An inotrope should be considered to maintain an adequate cardiac index, mean arterial pressure, mixed venous oxygen content, and urine output.[33]

SOURCE CONTROL

Eradication of the inciting infection is essential to the successful treatment of severe sepsis and septic shock. Source control represents a key component of success and involves the drainage of infected fluids, removal of infected devices, debridement of infected soft tissues, and definitive measures to correct anatomic derangement resulting in ongoing antimicrobial contamination.[41] Every patient presenting with severe sepsis or septic shock should be evaluated as soon as possible for the pres-ence of a focus of infection amenable to source control measures.[11,42] These infectious foci should be controlled with the least physiologic upset possible (eg, percutaneous rather than surgical drainage of an abscess) because certain source control interventions may cause further complications. If intravascular access devices are believed to be a possible source of severe sepsis or septic shock, they should be removed as soon as possible. The risks and benefits of the specific intervention plus the risks of transfer should be evaluated on an individualized basis.[43]

CORTICOSTEROIDS

The role of corticosteroids in the treatment of severe sepsis and septic shock has been controversial. The therapeutic role of corticosteroids arose from the theory that severe sepsis or septic shock results from an exaggerated and uncontrolled host inflammatory response. Another theory suggested that critically ill patients can suffer from a relative adrenal insufficiency. Early randomized controlled studies documented a decrease in the time to shock resolution; however, a reduction in overall mortality was not observed with high-dose corticosteroids.[44,45] Further studies using lower, more physiologic doses of steroids further documented a reduction in the time of shock reversal and cessation of vasopressor use.[46] A subsequent larger multicenter randomized controlled trial of patients who had vasopressor-unresponsive septic shock showed a reduction in mortality rate in all patients with a further reduction in time to shock resolution in patients who had relative adrenal insufficiency as defined by a suboptimal adrenocorticotropic hormone (ACTH) cortisol response.[47] The Corticosteroid Therapy of Septic Shock (CORTICUS) trial, a large multicenter trial in which patients who had septic shock were randomized to either hydrocortisone or placebo, showed a faster reversal of shock among all patients.[48] The trial failed to show a mortality benefit with steroid therapy, and in fact showed an increased incidence of superinfections, including new episodes of sepsis or septic shock.

Current recommendations from the Surviving Sepsis Campaign advocate that steroids should only be used in the setting of septic shock if a patient's blood pressure is poorly responsive to both adequate fluid resuscitation and vasopressor support.[11] An ACTH stimulation test has been used early in the course of sepsis to identify those patients who have a relative adrenal insufficiency who should then receive supplemental steroids. In the CORTICUS trial, however, the overall population of patients seemed to benefit regardless of ACTH stimulation test outcome.[48] As a result, the ACTH stimulation test is no longer recommended to identify those patients who should receive steroids.[11,49] Hydrocortisone should be used preferentially over dexamethasone because of a possible prolonged suppression of the hypothalamic-pituitary-adrenal axis after administration of dexamethasone.[50] Doses of corticosteroids comparable to 200 to 300 mg/d of hydrocortisone should be used for the purpose of treating septic shock; however, there is no consensus regarding the duration and method of cessation (abrupt versus tapering) of steroids. Cessation of steroid administration should be considered when vasopressors are no longer required for the treatment of severe sepsis and septic shock.

RECOMBINANT ACTIVATED PROTEIN C

Activated protein C is an endogenous protein that is associated with fibrinolysis and the inhibition of coagulation and inflammation. Activated protein C inactivates factors Va and VIIIa, preventing the generation of thrombin, which inhibits platelet activation, neutrophil recruitment, and mast cell degranulation.[9] During severe sepsis, the activation of protein C is inhibited by inflammatory cytokines and decreased levels of activated protein C have been associated with an increased risk for death.[51] In a recent study evaluating the efficacy of recombinant human-activated protein C (RHAPC) in severe sepsis, patients were randomized to receive either RHAPC or placebo. Premature cessation of the study occurred before completion because of the significant mortality benefit from RHAPC, although treated patients did have a higher bleeding diathesis.[52] A subsequent open-label trial documented similar improvements in mortality, especially when RHAPC is administered within the first 24 hours of severe sepsis.[53] Finally, a randomized placebo-controlled trail evaluating the efficacy of RHAPC in patients who had severe sepsis with a low risk for death as defined by an Acute Physiology and Chronic Health Evaluation (APACHE II) score less than 25 was terminated early because of the lack of any mortality benefit. This study also documented an increase in serious bleeding episodes in those patients treated with RHAPC.[54] After compiling the results of the previously mentioned trials, RHAPC should be considered in patients who have severe sepsis with a high risk for death as defined by an APACHE II score of 25 or greater or multiorgan failure, if there are no contraindications, such as recent surgery, intracranial hemorrhage, or previous risk for bleeding.[11] RHAPC is not recommended for patients who have severe sepsis and low risk for death.

INTRAVENOUS INSULIN

Hyperglycemia associated with severe sepsis and septic shock results from the counterregulatory hormone and cytokine responses associated with severe illness, coupled with the administration of excess dextrose in intravenous fluids and total parenteral nutrition. Hyperglycemia impairs the phagocytic function of neutrophils and macrophages and results in endothelial dysfunction. The exact protective mechanism of insulin in sepsis is unknown; however, it is believed to be a modulator of numerous inflammatory pathways and an inhibitor of apoptosis.[55] Supplemental insulin has been shown to improve the morbidity and mortality of critically ill patients. In 2001, a randomized controlled trial showed that mechanically ventilated patients treated with an intensive intravenous regimen had a reduction in all-cause mortality from 8.0% to 4.6%. The greatest reduction in mortality was seen in patients who had multiorgan failure and a septic focus.[56] The intensive intravenous insulin regimen also reduced the number of episodes of bacteremia, incidence of acute renal failure requiring hemodialysis, number of transfusions, and incidence of polyneuropathy. A subsequent study showed that an intensive intravenous insulin regimen improved mortality in patients who stayed in the ICU for more than 3 days. In a subgroup of patients who stayed in the ICU less than 3 days, an intensive intravenous insulin regimen increased mortality. In addition, the intensive regimen also had a threefold higher rate of hypoglycemia than the conservative treatment arm.[57] More recently, the Volume Substitution and Insulin Therapy in Severe Sepsis (VISEP) trial, which randomized patients to intensive intravenous insulin or conventional therapy as well as two methods of volume resuscitation, showed similar results after an interim analysis showed higher rates of hypoglycemia (17.0% versus 4.1%), higher rates of serious adverse events, and no difference in mortality.[58] All of these previously mentioned trials with intensive intravenous insulin had a targeted glucose level of 80 to 110 mg/dL. Currently there is a lack of consensus about optimal dosing of intravenous insulin and target glucose levels and current trials are underway to evaluate any differences in clinical outcomes between regimens. Current recommendations for patients who have severe sepsis and hyperglycemia admitted to the ICU are to administer intravenous glucose after initial hemodynamic stabilization with a target glucose level less than 150 mg/dL. Patients on intravenous insulin should have frequent blood glucose assessments to avoid the adverse consequences of hypoglycemia and consideration should be given to administering a glucose calorie source concurrently with the intravenous insulin.

BLOOD PRODUCTS ADMINISTRATION

Anemia is a common problem in severe sepsis and septic shock. Frequent blood sampling for laboratory testing, blood loss from surgical procedures to obtain source control, decreased red blood cell synthesis, and possibly increased red blood cell destruction can contribute to the development of anemia. Decreased red blood cell synthesis may result from the increased septic levels of tumor necrosis factor-α and interleukin-1β that decrease the expression of erythropoietin. Although administration of recombinant human erythropoietin may reduce transfusion requirements, its use does not affect clinical outcomes, such as mortality.[59] If patients have coexisting conditions that warrant its use, consideration can be given to continuing the use of erythropoietin. No target hemoglobin level exists in the setting of severe sepsis and septic shock. During the first 6 hours of septic shock, a target hematocrit of 30% is recommended in patients who have low central venous oxygen saturations.[10] Once tissue hypoperfusion has resolved and there are no extenuating circumstances, such as hemorrhage, myocardial ischemia, or severe hypoxemia, the goal hemoglobin level is subject to debate. In the Transfusion Requirements in Critical Care trial, euvolemic critically ill patients were randomized to a restricted target hemoglobin of greater than 7 g/dL or greater than 10 g/dL and were transfused to maintain these targets. Overall mortality was similar between the two groups; however, younger patients who had lower APACHE II scores had overall lower mortality rates with the restricted target when compared with the liberal hemoglobin target.[60] Current recommendations are to maintain a target hemoglobin of 7.0 to 9.0 g/dL and to institute red blood cell transfusions when the hemoglobin decreases to less than 7.0 g/dL.[11] Although no randomized trials exist in severe sepsis and septic shock, recommendations for platelet transfusions are to administer platelets when counts are less than 5000/μL. Higher platelet counts (>50,000/μL) are frequently required for invasive procedures or surgery. Similarly, fresh frozen plasma should be administered in the presence of active bleeding or before surgical or invasive procedures if there is a documented deficiency of coagulation factors as demonstrated by an elevated prothrombin time, partial thromboplastin time, or international normalized ratio.[11]

MECHANICAL VENTILATION

Another complication of severe sepsis and septic shock is acute lung injury (ALI) as defined by a partial pressure of oxygen in arterial blood to inspired fraction of oxygen ratio (Pa_{O_2}/F_{IO_2}) of less than 300 mm Hg. Often this lung injury progresses to worsening respiratory failure requiring the initiation of mechanical ventilation. Lung-protective ventilation using relatively low tidal volumes (6 mL/kg predicted body weight) decreases mortality and is beneficial in septic acute lung injury, resulting in lower organ dysfunction and decreased levels of inflammatory cytokines.[61,62] High tidal volumes and high plateau pressures should be avoided in ALI. The upper limit goal for plateau pressures in a passively inflated patient should be 30 cm H_2O or less, with consideration given to chest wall compliance.[11] When appropriate, permissive hypercapnia (elevated partial pressure of carbon dioxide above the baseline) may be allowed to minimize plateau pressures and tidal volumes. Attention should also be given toward maintaining a positive end expiratory pressure (PEEP) level to avoid alveolar collapse and resultant ventilator-induced lung injury. A PEEP level greater than 5 cm H_2O is usually required to avoid alveolar collapse.[63] Caution should be exercised to avoid overdistension and higher plateau pressures while titrating PEEP. To date, no randomized trials have shown any benefit to one single mode of ventilation when compared to any other mode of ventilation in severe sepsis and septic shock.

NUTRITION

Severe sepsis and septic shock are characterized by high energy expenditure, catabolism, and negative nitrogen balance. The use of enteral or parenteral nutrition in severe sepsis and septic shock to correct this problem has been somewhat controversial. Critical illness is associated with gastric dysmotility and bowel ileus, which complicates enteral feeding.[64] In addition, parenteral nutrition has been associated with significant morbidity, such as an increased risk for infection and hepatic dysfunction. Initiation of nutrition is thus often delayed in the critical care setting. More recent studies have suggested that early enteral feeding may reduce morbidity from severe sepsis and septic shock. Early nutrition has been demonstrated to improve wound healing, host immune function, nitrogen balance, and preserve intestinal mucosal integrity. In addition, early enteral nutrition is associated with a lower incidence of infection and shorter hospital length of stay.[65] No improvement in mortality has been documented with initiation of early nutrition, however. In general, the enteral route is preferred over the parenteral route because the parenteral route is more likely to cause hyperglycemia, biliary stasis, and infectious complications. If bowel obstruction, severe acute pancreatitis, major gastrointestinal hemorrhage, or significant hemodynamic instability complicates severe sepsis or septic shock, the enteral route should be avoided. Parenteral nutrition is indicated for patients who have a contraindication to enteral nutrition or when a patient consistently fails enteral feeding trials.[66]

PROPHYLACTIC MEASURES

Patients who have severe sepsis or septic shock are at risk for additional complications, such as the development of deep venous thrombosis (DVT), gastrointestinal bleeding, and aspiration of gastric and oral contents. Multiple studies have documented the benefit of DVT prophylaxis in reducing the incidence of venous thromboembolism.[67,68] All patients who have severe sepsis or septic shock should receive DVT prophylaxis with either low-dose unfractionated heparin or low molecular weight heparin. If a contraindication for anticoagulation exists, patients should receive mechanical prophylaxis with compression stockings or intermittent compression devices. Patients who have severe sepsis or septic shock often require mechanical ventilation, or have a coagulopathy or significant hypotension, all of which are risk factors for gastrointestinal bleeding.[69] Stress ulcer prophylaxis using a proton pump inhibitor or histamine type-2 antagonists should be given to patients who have severe sepsis or septic shock to prevent upper gastrointestinal bleeding. The benefits of acid suppression and prevention of gastrointestinal bleeding should be weighed against the increased stomach pH that results from acid suppression and the incidence of ventilator-associated pneumonia.[70] In addition, the head of the hospital bed should be elevated 30 to 45 degrees in patients who have severe sepsis and septic shock requiring mechanical ventilation to reduce the risk for aspiration and development of ventilator-associated pneumonia.[71] The head of the bed should also be elevated in patients receiving enteral feedings.

Occasionally patients who have severe sepsis or septic shock develop secondary infections throughout the course of the disease. Prior antibiotic use has been associated with the development of fungal infections, which can have significant morbidity and mortality, especially if appropriate antibiotic therapy is delayed.[17] In addition, the development of cytomegalovirus viremia and *C difficile* colitis has been reported in patients who have severe sepsis and septic shock. Particular attention should be paid to patients who have prior risk factors (eg, organ transplant recipients and neutropenic patients) for developing secondary infections and opportunistic infections. Consideration can be given to prophylactic use of antibiotics in these high-risk patients, although no recommendations currently exist.

BIOMARKERS

As sepsis progresses to more severe forms of septic shock, global tissue hypoxia emerges with subsequent inflammation, organ dysfunction, and increased mortality. This progression is accompanied by a progression of proinflammatory, anti-inflammatory and apoptotic biomarkers. One failure in the management of sepsis is the difficulty in recognizing the early stages of disease and determining which patients will progress and develop a more severe form of illness. The use of biomarkers has significantly improved the diagnosis and management of other acute diseases, such as coronary artery disease and pulmonary embolism; at present, however, there is no single accepted biomarker or combination of biomarkers for use in patients who have suspected sepsis. Current biomarkers under investigation include pro–brain natriuretic peptide, transcription growth factor β, C-reactive protein, procalcitonin, interleukin-1 receptor antagonist, and intercellular adhesion molecule-1, among others.[72,73] Procalcitonin and C-reactive protein have been shown to reflect the severity of sepsis and septic shock and can be used to tailor antimicrobial therapies; however, their usefulness in the early phase of sepsis remains questionable.[74,75] At present the role of biomarkers for diagnosis and prognosis in severe sepsis and septic shock remains undefined.[11]

SUMMARY

The diagnosis and management of severe sepsis and septic shock is a complex and dynamic process. Newer evidence-based interventions are constantly being developed and implemented with the purpose of improving morbidity and mortality. Current investigations are being performed in hospital environments to determine the change in behaviors and clinical impact from the most recent Surviving Sepsis recommendations. With the recent updated guidelines, medical institutions frequently follow sepsis protocols incorporating early empiric antibiotics, restoration of tissue perfusion, initiation of vasopressor support, and other supportive measures that have been shown to improve patient outcomes, including overall mortality.[28] A recent study assessing the value of a standardized protocol for patients who have severe sepsis and septic shock demonstrated that those patients who received care adherent to standardized protocols were more likely to receive antimicrobials within 3 hours of presentation, receive appropriate initial antimicrobial treatment, and have a shorten mean length of stay.[28] In another study, patients who had sepsis treated with standardized order sets also have reduced morbidity, such as lower incidence of renal failure and cardiovascular failure and overall improved in-hospital mortality.[76] The use of standardized treatment protocols in addition to newer diagnostic and treatment modalities in patients who have severe sepsis and septic shock can continue to improve patient-related outcomes and the damaging effect of these diseases on society.

REFERENCES

1. Angus DC, Linde-Zwirble WT, Lidicker J, et al. Epidemiology of severe sepsis in the United States: analysis of incidence, outcome, and associated costs of care. Crit Care Med 2001;29(7):1303–10.

2. Sasse KC, Nauenberg E, Long A, et al. Long-term survival after intensive care unit admission with sepsis. Crit Care Med 1995;23(6):1040–7.

3. Annane D, Aegerter P, Jars-Guincestre MC, et al. Current epidemiology of septic shock: the CUB-Réa network. Am J Respir Crit Care Med 2003;168(2):165–72.

4. Kung HC, Hoyert DL, Xu J, et al. Deaths: final data for 2005. Natl Vital Stat Rep 2008;56(10):1–120.

5. Levy MM, Fink MP, Marshall JC, et al. 2001 SCCM/ESICM/ACCP/ATS/SIS international sepsis definitions conference. Crit Care Med 2003;31(4):1250–6.

6. Annane D, Bellissant E, Cavaillon JM. Septic shock. Lancet 2005;365(9453): 63–78.

7. Lin MT, Albertson TE. Genomic polymorphisms in sepsis. Crit Care Med 2004; 32(2):569–79.

8. Alberti C, Brun-Buisson C, Burchardi H, et al. Epidemiology of sepsis and infection in ICU patients from an international multicentre cohort study. Intensive Care Med 2002;28(2):108–21.

9. Hotchkiss RS, Karl IE. The pathophysiology and treatment of sepsis. N Engl J Med 2003;348(2):138–50.

10. Rivers E, Nguyen B, Havstad S, et al. Early goal-directed therapy in the treatment of severe sepsis and septic shock. N Engl J Med 2001;345(19):1368–77.

11. Dellinger RP, Levy MM, Carlet JM, et al. Surviving sepsis campaign: international guidelines for management of severe sepsis and septic shock: 2008. Crit Care Med 2008;36(1):296–327.

12. Nguyen HB, Corbett SW, Steele R, et al. Implementation of a bundle of quality indicators for the early management of severe sepsis and septic shock is associated with decreased mortality. Crit Care Med 2007;35(4):1105–12.

13. Bendjelid K, Romand JA. Fluid responsiveness in mechanically ventilated patients: a review of indices used in intensive care. Intensive Care Med 2003; 29(3):352–60.

14. Finfer S, Bellomo R, Boyce N, et al. A comparison of albumin and saline for fluid resuscitation in the intensive care unit. N Engl J Med 2004;350(22):2247–56.

15. Schortgen F, Lacherade JC, Bruneel F, et al. Effects of hydroxyethyl starch and gelatin on renal function in severe sepsis: a multicentre randomized study. Lancet 2001;357(9260):911–6.

16. De Jonge E, Levi M. Effects of different plasma substitues on blood coagulation: a comparative review. Crit Care Med 2001;29(6):1261–7.

17. Morrell M, Fraser VJ, Kollef MH. Delaying the empiric treatment of candida bloodstream infection until positive blood culture results are obtained: a potential risk factor for hospital mortality. Antimicrob Agents Chemother 2005;49(9):3640–5.

18. Ibrahim EH, Sherman G, Ward S, et al. The influence of inadequate antimicrobial treatment of bloodstream infections on patient outcomes in the ICU setting. Chest 2000;118(1):146–55.

19. Kollef MH, Sherman G, Ward S, et al. Inadequate antimicrobial treatment of infections: a risk factor for hospital mortality among critically ill patients. Chest 1999; 115(2):263–74.

20. Kumar A, Roberts D, Wood KE, et al. Duration of hypotension before initiation of effective antimicrobial therapy is the critical determinant of survival in human septic shock. Crit Care Med 2006;34(6):1589–96.

21. National Nosocomial Infections Surveillance System. National Nosocomial Infections Surveillance (NNIS) System Report, data summary from January 1992 through June 2004, issued October 2000. Am J Infect Control 2004;32(8): 470–85.

22. Rosenthal VD, Maki DG, Mehta A, et al. International Nosocomial Infection Control Consortium report, data summary for 2002–2007, issued January 2008. Am J Infect Control 2008;36(9):627–37.
23. Labelle AJ, Micek ST, Roubinian N, et al. Treatment-related risk factors for hospital mortality in Candida bloodstream infections. Crit Care Med 2008; 36(11):2967–72.
24. Micek ST, Lloyd AE, Ritchie DJ, et al. Pseudomonas aeruginosa bloodstream infection: importance of appropriate initial antimicrobial treatment. Antimicrob Agents Chemother 2005;49(4):1306–11.
25. Tam VH, Gamez EA, Weston JS, et al. Outcomes of bacteremia due to Pseudomonas aeruginosa with reduced susceptibility to piperacillin-tazobactam: implications on the appropriateness of resistance breakpoint. Clin Infect Dis 2008; 46(6):862–7.
26. Boselli E, Breilh D, Rimmelé T, et al. Alveolar concentrations of piperacillin/tazobactam administered in continuous infusion to patients with ventilator-associated pneumonia. Crit Care Med 2008;36(5):1500–6.
27. Dellit TH, Owens RC, McGowan JE Jr, et al. Infectious Diseases Society of America and the Society for Healthcare Epidemiology of America guidelines for developing an institutional program to enhance antimicrobial stewardship. Clin Infect Dis 2007;44(2):159–77.
28. Micek ST, Roubinian N, Heuring T, et al. Before-after study of a standardized hospital order set for the management of septic shock. Crit Care Med 2006; 34(11):2707–13.
29. Wiener RS, Welch HG. Trends in the use of pulmonary artery catheter in the United States, 1993–2004. JAMA 2007;298(4):423–9.
30. Osman D, Ridel C, Ray P, et al. Cardiac filling pressure are not appropriate to predict hemodynamic response to volume challenge. Crit Care Med 2007; 35(1):64–8.
31. LeDoux D, Astiz ME, Carpati CM, et al. Effects of perfusion pressure on tissue perfusion in septic shock. Crit Care Med 2000;28(8):2729–32.
32. Müllner M, Urbanek B, Havel C, et al. Vasopressors for shock. Cochrane Database Syst Rev 2004;(3):CD003709.
33. Hollenberg SM, Ahrens TS, Annane D, et al. Practice parameters for hemodynamic support of sepsis in adult patients. Crit Care Med 2004;32(9):1928–48.
34. Bellomo R, Chapman M, Finfer S, et al. Low dose dopamine in patients with early renal dysfunction: a placebo-controlled randomized trial. Australian and New Zealand Intensive Care Society (ANZICS) Clinical Trials Group. Lancet 2000; 356(9248):2139–43.
35. Regnier B, Rapin M, Gory G, et al. Haemodynamic effects of dopamine in septic shock. Intensive Care Med 1977;3(2):47–53.
36. De Backer D, Creteur J, Silva E, et al. Effects of dopamine, norepinephrine, and epinephrine on the splanchnic circulation in septic shock: which is best? Crit Care Med 2003;31(6):1659–67.
37. Landry DW, Levin HR, Gallant EM, et al. Vasopressin deficiency contributes to the vasodilation of septic shock. Circulation 1997;95(5):1122–5.
38. Patel BM, Chittock DR, Russell JA, et al. Beneficial effects of short-term vasopressin infusion during severe septic shock. Anesthesiology 2002;96(3): 576–82.
39. Holmes CL, Walley KR, Chittock DR, et al. The effects of vasopressin on hemodynamics and renal function in severe septic shock: a case series. Intensive Care Med 2001;27(8):1416–21.

40. Russell JA, Walley KR, Singer J, et al. Vasopressin versus norepinephrine infusion in patients with septic shock. N Engl J Med 2008;358(9):877–87.
41. Marshall JC, Maier RV, Jimenez M, et al. Source control in the management of severe sepsis and septic shock: an evidence-based review. Crit Care Med 2004;32(11 Suppl):S513–26.
42. Jimenez MF, Marshall JC. Source control in the management of sepsis. Intensive Care Med 2001;27(Suppl 1):S49–62.
43. Evans A, Winslow BH. Oxygen saturation and hemodynamic response in critically ill mechanically ventilated adults during intra-hospital transport. Am J Crit Care 1995;4(2):106–11.
44. Sprung CL, Caralis PV, Marcial EH, et al. The effect of high-dose corticosteroids in patients with septic shock. A prospective, controlled study. N Engl J Med 1984; 311(18):1137–43.
45. Effect of high-dose glucocorticoid therapy on mortality in patients with clinical signs of systemic sepsis. The Veterans Administration Systemic Sepsis Cooperative Study Group. N Engl J Med 1987;317(11):659–65.
46. Briegel J, Forst H, Haller M, et al. Stress doses of hydrocortisone reverse hyperdynamic septic shock: a prospective, randomized, double-blind, single-center study. Crit Care Med 1999;27(4):723–32.
47. Annane D, Sebille V, Charpentier C, et al. Effect of treatment with low doses of hydrocortisone and fludrocortisone on mortality in patients with septic shock. JAMA 2002;288(7):862–71.
48. Sprung CL, Annane D, Keh D, et al. Hydrocortisone therapy for patients with septic shock. N Engl J Med 2008;358(2):111–24.
49. Marik PE, Pastores SM, Annane D, et al. Recommendations for the diagnosis and management of corticosteroid insufficiency in critically ill adult patients: consensus statements from an international task force by the American College of Critical Care Medicine. Crit Care Med 2008;36(6):1937–49.
50. Reincke M, Allolio B, Würth G, et al. The hypothalamic-pituitary-adrenal axis in critical illness: response to dexamethasone and corticotrophin-releasing hormone. J Clin Endocrinol Metab 1993;77(1):151–6.
51. Lorente JA, García-Frade LJ, Landín L, et al. Time course of hemostatic abnormalities in sepsis and its relation to outcome. Chest 1993;103(5):1536–42.
52. Bernard GR, Vincent JL, Laterre PF, et al. Efficacy and safety of recombinant human activated protein C for severe sepsis. N Engl J Med 2001;344(10): 699–709.
53. Vincent JL, Bernard GR, Beale R, et al. Drotrecogin alfa (activated) treatment in severe sepsis from the global open-label trial ENHANCE: further evidence for survival and safety and implications for early treatment. Crit Care Med 2005; 33(10):2266–77.
54. Abraham E, Laterre PF, Garg R, et al. Drotrecogin alfa (activated) for adults with severe sepsis and a low risk of death. N Engl J Med 2005;353(13):1332–41.
55. Gao F, Gao E, Yue TL, et al. Nitric oxide mediates the antiapoptotic effect of insulin in myocardial ischemia-reperfusion: the roles of PI3-kinase, Akt, and endothelial nitric oxide synthase phosphorylation. Circulation 2002;105(12):1497–502.
56. Van den Berghe G, Wouters P, Weekers F, et al. Intensive insulin therapy in critically ill patients. N Engl J Med 2001;345(19):1359–67.
57. Van den Berghe G, Wilmer A, Hermans G, et al. Intensive insulin therapy in the medical ICU. N Engl J Med 2006;354(5):449–61.
58. Brunkhorst FM, Engel C, Bloos F, et al. Intensive insulin therapy and pentastarch resuscitation in severe sepsis. N Engl J Med 2008;358(2):125–39.

59. Corwin HL, Gettinger A, Rodriguez RM, et al. Efficacy of recombinant human erythropoietin in the critically ill patient: a randomized, double-blind, placebo-controlled trial. Crit Care Med 1999;27:2346–50.

60. Hébert PC, Wells G, Blajchman MA, et al. A multicenter, randomized controlled trial of transfusion requirements in critical care. N Engl J Med 1999;340(6): 409–17.

61. Ventilation with lower tidal volumes as compared with traditional tidal volumes for acute lung injury and the acute respiratory distress syndrome. The Acute Respiratory Distress Syndrome Network. N Engl J Med 2000;342(18):1301–8.

62. Ranieri VM, Suter PM, Tortorella C, et al. Effect of mechanical ventilation on inflammatory mediators in patients with acute respiratory distress syndrome: a randomized controlled trial. JAMA 1999;282:54–61.

63. Gattinoni L, Caironi P, Cressoni M, et al. Lung recruitment in patients with the acute respiratory distress syndrome. N Engl J Med 2006;354(17):1775–86.

64. Nguyen NQ, Fraser RJ, Bryant LK, et al. Diminished functional association between proximal and distal gastric motility in critically ill patients. Intensive Care Med 2008;34:1246–55.

65. Marik PE, Zaloga GP. Early enteral nutrition in acutely ill patients: a systematic review. Crit Care Med 2001;29(12):2264–70.

66. Roberts SR, Kennerly DA, Keane D, et al. Nutrition support in the intensive care unit. Adequacy, timeliness and outcomes. Crit Care Nurse 2003;23(6):49–57.

67. Halkin H, Goldberg J, Modan M, et al. Reduction of mortality in general medical in-patients by low-dose heparin prophylaxis. Ann Intern Med 1982; 96(5):561–5.

68. Pingleton SK, Bone RC, Pingleton WW, et al. Prevention of pulmonary emboli in a respiratory intensive care unit: efficacy of low-dose heparin. Chest 1981; 79(6):647–50.

69. Cook DJ, Fuller HD, Guyatt GH, et al. Risk factors for gastrointestinal bleeding in critically ill patients. Canadian Critical Care. N Engl J Med 1994;330(6):377–81.

70. Kahn JM, Doctor JN, Rubenfeld GD. Stress ulcer prophylaxis in mechanically ventilated patients: integrating evidence and judgment using a decision analysis. Intensive Care Med 2006;32:1151–8.

71. Metheny NA, Clouse RE, Chang YH, et al. Tracheobronchial aspiration of gastric contents in critically ill tube-fed patients: frequency, outcomes, and risk factors. Crit Care Med 2006;34(4):1007–15.

72. Rivers EP, Kruse JA, Jacobsen G, et al. The influence of early hemodynamic optimization on biomarker patterns of severe sepsis and septic shock. Crit Care Med 2007;35(9):2016–24.

73. Shapiro NI, Trzeciak S, Hollander JE, et al. A prospective, multicenter derivation of a biomarker panel to assess risk of organ dysfunction, shock, and death in emergency department patients with suspected sepsis. Crit Care Med 2009; 37(1):1–9.

74. Nobre V, Harbarth S, Graf JD, et al. Use of procalcitonin to shorten antibiotic treatment duration in septic patients: a randomized trial. Am J Respir Crit Care Med 2008;177(5):498–505.

75. Castelli GP, Pognani C, Meisner M, et al. Procalcitonin and C-reactive protein during systemic inflammatory response syndrome, sepsis and organ dysfunction. Crit Care 2004;8(4):R234–42.

76. Thiel SW, Asghar MF, Micek ST, et al. Hospital-wide impact of a standardized order set for the management of bacteremic severe sepsis. Crit Care Med 2009;37(3):819–24.

77. Kang CI, Kim SH, Park WB, et al. Bloodstream infections caused by antibiotic-resistant gram-negative bacilli: risk factors for mortality and impact of inappropriate initial antimicrobial therapy on outcome. Antimicrob Agents Chemother 2005;49(2):760–6.
78. Khatib R, Saeed S, Sharma M, et al. Impact of initial antibiotic choice and delayed appropriate treatment on the outcome of Staphylococcus aureus bacteremia. Eur J Clin Microbiol Infect Dis 2006;25(3):181–5.
79. Schramm GE, Johnson JA, Doherty JA, et al. Methicillin-resistant Staphylococcus aureus sterile-site infection: the importance of appropriate initial antimicrobial treatment. Crit Care Med 2006;34(8):2239–41.
80. Garey KW, Rege M, Pai MP, et al. Time to initiation of fluconazole therapy impacts mortality in patients with candidemia: a multi-institutional study. Clin Infect Dis 2006;43(1):25–31.
81. Tumbarello M, Sanguinetti M, Montuori E, et al. Predictors of mortality in patients with bloodstream infections caused by extended-spectrum-beta-lactamase-producing Enterobacteriaceae: importance of inadequate initial antimicrobial treatment. Antimicrob Agents Chemother 2007;51(6):1987–94.
82. Cheong HS, Kang CI, Wi YM, et al. Inappropriate initial antimicrobial therapy as a risk factor for mortality in patients with community-onset Pseudomonas aeruginosa bacteraemia. Eur J Clin Microbiol Infect Dis 2008;27(12):1219–25.

Severe Community-Acquired Pneumonia

Marcos I. Restrepo, MD, MSc[a,b,c,*], Antonio Anzueto, MD[a,c]

KEYWORDS

- Community-acquired infections • Pneumonia
- Therapeutics • Intensive care unit

Community-acquired pneumonia (CAP) is a serious condition that could lead to poor outcomes, including death, longer hospital stay, and high health care cost. The sickest patients who have CAP are those who require hospitalization and are usually admitted to the ICU. CAP and influenza are the first leading causes of death from infectious diseases in the United States.[1,2] CAP represents one of the most common causes of ICU admission.[3] The term "severe CAP" identifies a group of patients who have severe disease, who are prone to have complications and poor outcomes, and who require a higher level of care. It is clear that the patients who require ICU admission differentiate from the less severe patients who have CAP in various ways. There is some controversy related to the term "severe," however, because it does not differentiate well if this is severe enough to be admitted to the hospital, severe enough to

Dr. Restrepo is supported by a Department of Veteran Affairs Veterans Integrated Service Network 17 new faculty grant and a KL2 program sponsored by the National Institute of Health. The views expressed in this article are those of the authors and do not necessarily represent the views of the Department of Veterans Affairs. This material is the result of work supported with resources and the use of facilities at the South Texas Veterans Health Care System. The funding agencies had no role in conducting the study, or role in the preparation, review, or approval of the manuscript.

Conflicts of interest: Dr. Antonio Anzueto has served in the speaker's bureaus of Pfizer, Boehringer Ingelheim, GlaxoSmithKline, Astra-Zeneca; and in the advisory board of Glaxo-SmithKline, Boehringer Ingelheim, Bayer-Schering Plough, and Pfizer. Dr. Marcos I. Restrepo has served on the speaker's bureau and advisory board for Ortho-McNeil-Janssen, Johnson & Johnson, Pfizer, and BARD, Inc.

[a] Division of Pulmonary/Critical Care Medicine, South Texas Veterans Health Care System, 7400 Merton Minter Boulevard, San Antonio, TX 78229, USA

[b] Veterans Evidence Based Research Dissemination and Implementation Center (VERDICT), and the South Texas Veterans Health Care System, 7400 Merton Minter Boulevard, San Antonio, TX 78229, USA

[c] Division of Pulmonary/Critical Care Medicine, University of Texas Health Science Center at San Antonio, TX, USA

* Corresponding author. Veterans Evidence Based Research Dissemination and Implementation Center (11C6) at the South Texas Veterans Health Care System Audie L. Murphy division at San Antonio, 7400 Merton Minter Boulevard (11C6), San Antonio, TX 78229.

E-mail address: restrepom@uthscsa.edu (M.I. Restrepo).

Infect Dis Clin N Am 23 (2009) 503–520
doi:10.1016/j.idc.2009.04.003
0891-5520/09/$ – see front matter. Published by Elsevier Inc.

require ICU admission, or severe enough because of the signs and symptoms that trigger a higher level of care despite the location in the hospital setting. The definition used in this article includes studies and information of patients severely ill with CAP who require ICU admission, have a higher risk for dying because of the condition, and require interventions that could only be provided in a higher-acuity level of care. The article reviews the most recent and relevant data regarding the epidemiology, microbiology, severity of the disease, therapeutic strategies, and preventive measures of severe CAP.

EPIDEMIOLOGY

CAP occurs in approximately 4 million adults in the United States[4] and it accounts for 10,000,000 physician visits, 500,000 hospitalizations, and 45,000 deaths each year.[5] CAP mortality is variable depending on the site of care; it is less than 1% in the outpatient setting, around 5% in inpatients not requiring ICU care, up to 25% in intubated patients, and near 50% in ICU patients requiring vasopressors.[6,7] Up to 36% of patients who have CAP require admission to the ICU[8,9] and despite advances in antimicrobial therapy and supportive measures the mortality in this group of patients ranges from 21% to 58%.[10] The main causes of death in patients who have severe CAP include refractory hypoxemia, refractory shock, and other pneumonia-related complications, predominantly multiorgan failure.[11–16] In addition, patients who have severe CAP tend to stay longer in the hospital, which is associated with higher hospital cost. It is estimated that patients in the ICU compared with ward patients carry higher cost driven by the longer length of stay: 23 days and $21,144 for ICU patients versus 6 days at a cost of approximately $7500 for ward patients.[6,17,18]

The recognition of patients at risk for severe CAP who may require ICU admission is critical. The most important risk factors associated with the need for hospitalization and particularly for admission to the ICU are patients who have CAP with prior comorbid conditions or received prior antibiotic therapy. Recent prior intravenous antibiotic therapy has been associated with multidrug-resistant pathogens, and in the Infectious Diseases Society of America (IDSA)/American Thoracic Society (ATS) clinical practice guidelines the recommendation is to call these patients health care–associated pneumonia (HCAP) patients, because of the similarity to pneumonia acquired in the hospital setting (hospital-acquired pneumonia or ventilator-associated pneumonia).[19] We limit our review to CAP only, and do not include HCAP studies; however, we consider prior antibiotic therapy as a risk factor for resistant pneumococcal disease. Advanced age has been associated with risk for acquiring severe CAP, particularly for those in whom comorbid conditions are also present. It is important to highlight the recent evidence associated with certain comorbid conditions, such as chronic obstructive pulmonary disease (COPD), alcohol abuse, renal failure, chronic heart failure, diabetes mellitus, coronary artery disease, malignancy, chronic neurologic disease, and chronic liver disease.[20,21] In the past few years, there has been interest in identifying certain risk factors associated with mortality even in patients who do not have comorbid conditions. These risk factors include signs of disease progression, multilobar lung disease, need for mechanical ventilation, and need for vasopressors. In addition, these patients have the greatest severity of the disease, which leads to higher mortality.[22]

MICROBIOLOGY

Multiple studies have evaluated the microbiology of patients who have severe CAP. Despite extensive laboratory testing, however, the causative pathogen remains unknown in 40% to 70% of cases.[23] It is estimated that the recognition of causative pathogens is higher in patients who have severe CAP, possibly because the laboratory testing is more available and there is a tendency toward higher testing in higher acuity levels. The most commonly recognized pathogen identified by far in ICU patients who have CAP is *Streptococcus pneumoniae*.[20,21,24] Other respiratory tract pathogens associated with CAP in the ICU include *Haemophilus influenza, Klebsiella pneumoniae, Legionella* spp, *Staphylococcus aureus*, and viral pneumonias. Mixed infections with typical and atypical pathogens occur in approximately 5% to 40% of cases and should always be considered to ensure patients are treated with appropriate empiric antimicrobial therapy.[25–32] The most common pathogens implicated with lethality are *S pneumoniae, S aureus* (particularly the community-associated methicillin-resistant strain CA-MRSA), *Legionella pneumophila*, and *Pseudomonas aeruginosa*. Extensive interest has focused on patients who have CAP due to drug-resistant *S pneumonia* (DRSP). Multiple studies were not able to confirm the association of DRSP and poor clinical outcomes. Rates of pneumonia due to *S aureus* have been increasing in the past 2 decades. Community-acquired MRSA pneumonia has been linked as a secondary bacterial infection in patients who have influenza infection.[33] Consequently, the Centers for Disease Control and Prevention has recommended empirically covering for MRSA in community-dwelling hosts who present with this viral infection.[34] *P aeruginosa* has been reported in patients who have severe CAP with specific risk factors, such as chronic or prolonged use of broad-spectrum antibiotic therapy, bronchiectasis, malnutrition, HIV, and immunosuppression.[29,35,36–38] **Table 1** shows the most common pathogens associated with severe CAP and their associated comorbid conditions.

SEVERITY ASSESSMENT AND CRITERIA FOR ICU ADMISSION

The site-of-care decision is critical for patients who have CAP because it affects the diagnostic work-up, the therapeutic interventions, and the clinical outcomes. Significant interest has been generated in this area of research over the past decade. In addition to the clinical prediction tools, there has been significant interest in the role of biomarkers as prognostic indicators in severe CAP. Several biomarkers have been suggested, but only few have enough clinical data to come up with substantial conclusions; the details go beyond the aims of this article and are therefore only briefly mentioned.[39] The two better biomarkers currently available are the C-reactive protein (CRP) and procalcitonin (PCT). Procalcitonin was superior to CRP to predict CAP from other conditions, and in one study was significantly related to the severity of disease.[39]

Several tools have been developed to predict mortality and accurately determine which patients could be sent home and treated safely with good clinical outcomes. Two extensively studied and validated tools have been recognized and are recommended by the multiple clinical practice guidelines related to CAP (**Table 2**).[8,24,40] The pneumonia severity of illness (PSI) score and the CURB-65 are the most frequently cited scores.[8,40] The PSI is based on 20 parameters that are evaluated at the time of clinical presentation and consist of three demographic, five comorbid conditions, five physical examination findings, and seven laboratory/imaging variables.[8] The goal of this tool is to identify patients who can be discharged safely and receive home treatment with antibiotic therapy. The PSI score is heavily influenced by age, and it does not include certain comorbid conditions that are frequently found in patients who have CAP, such as diabetes and COPD. In contrast, the second score is less complex; it is derived from the original CURB, but the addition of age converted it to a six-variable tool that includes Confusion, Urea, Respiratory rate, Blood pressure, and older than 65 years of age (CURB-65).[40,41] A simplified tool was suggested withdrawing

Table 1
Risk factors associated with selected pathogens in patients who have severe community-acquired pneumonia

Pathogen	Risk Factors
Streptococcus pneumoniae	Smoking, COPD, low socioeconomic status, sulfur dioxide air pollution, alcoholism, dementia, seizures, congestive heart failure, CVD, HIV infection
DRSP	Alcoholism, β-lactams within 3 months, presence of more than one coexisting disease, immunosuppressive illness
GNB and Pseudomonas aeruginosa	Diabetes mellitus, decreased functional status, comorbidities (cardiopulmonary, renal, central nervous system, hepatic, neoplasia), chronic aspiration, bronchiectasis
Staphylococcus aureus	Decreased functional status, CVD, intravenous drug use, diabetes mellitus, renal failure, influenza
Haemophilus influenzae	Bronchiectasis
CA-MRSA	Skin infections and prior influenza infection
Legionella spp	Chronic steroid use, hematologic malignancy, humid weather, male sex, smoking, diabetes mellitus, cancer, ESRD, HIV infection
Influenza	Air pollutants (nitrogen oxide, ozone, and particulate matter), winter season
Anaerobes	High dental plaque index or periodontal disease, aspiration

Abbreviations: CA-MRSA, community-associated methicillin-resistant S aureus; COPD, chronic obstructive pulmonary disease; CVD, cerebrovascular disease; DRSP, drug-resistant S pneumoniae; ESRD, end-stage renal disease; GNB, gram negative bacilli.

the only laboratory value needed to calculate the score (blood urea nitrogen) and named CRB-65, and it was validated with similar results.[41] The CURB-65 score does not recognize any comorbid conditions previously associated as risk factors for CAP, however, and it does not include low oxygen levels as one of the criteria. We therefore conclude that these tools are good to determine low-risk patients, but should not be extrapolated to the other end of the spectrum, the high-risk group of patients. Several studies try to determine which patients should be admitted to the ICU. To evaluate this, the ATS developed initial criteria to define the need for ICU admission based on the original studies by Ewig and colleagues.[42,43] Several changes were made to the initial criteria over the years, particularly in the minor criteria section. The most recent definition for severe CAP was suggested by the IDSA/ATS CAP guidelines in 2007.[24] These guidelines recommend the need for ICU admission for those patients who have one of the major criteria (mechanical ventilation with endotracheal intubation or septic shock requiring vasopressors) or for patients who have three of the nine minor criteria (**Table 3**). Several studies have validated these criteria to admit patients to the ICU and applied them also in other groups of patients, including elderly and HIV-infected patients.[6,37,42–46] The use of clinician experience and clinical judgment is always recommended in addition to the objective criteria.[47]

Several other tools have been evaluated to better predict the need for ICU admission and the risk for death in the highest severity group. Tools such as the

Table 2
Pneumonia severity index score and CURB-65 hospital admission risk class stratification scores.

Pneumonia Severity Index Score[a]				CURB-65[b]		
Risk Class	Points	Mortality (%)	Recommended Site of Care	Risk Class	Mortality (%)	Recommended Site of Care
I	—[c]	0.1	Outpatient	0	0.7	Outpatient
II	<70	0.6	Outpatient	1	2.1	Outpatient
III	71–90	2.8	Outpatient or brief inpatient	2	9.2	Inpatient
IV	91–130	8.2	Inpatient	3	14.5	Inpatient
V	>130	29.2	Inpatient	4–5	40–57	Inpatient (possible need for ICU care)

[a] Metlay and Fine[47] suggested a three-step process to decide the initial site of CAP treatment based on: (1) assessment of preexisting conditions that compromise safety of home care, (2) calculation of the pneumonia severity index score, and (3) clinical judgment[48]. *Data from* Fine MJ, Auble TE, Yealy DM, et al. A prediction rule to identify low-risk patients with community-acquired pneumonia. N Engl J Med 1997;336:243–50.
[b] CURB-65[40,41] related to Confusion (altered mental status); serum blood Urea nitrogen > 19.6 mg/dL; Respiratory rate > 30 breaths per minute; Blood pressure (BP) (systolic BP < 90 mm Hg or diastolic BP < 60 mm Hg); and age $\geq$ 65 years. Each criterion has a score of one, and the total score is added by the presence of each of the five criteria. Two or more criteria suggest severe CAP and admission to the hospital is recommended; a patient who has three or more criteria needs an assessment for ICU (more likely to be in scores 4 or 5).
[c] Risk class I: age < 50 years, no comorbidities, and absence of vital sign abnormalities.

PS-CURXO80, SMART-COP, and the PIRO-CAP scores have been created for this purpose. España and colleagues[48] developed and validated a clinical prediction rule to assess the diagnosis of severe CAP. This new prediction score was derived from the variables associated with severe CAP that include: arterial pH less than 7.30, Systolic blood pressure less than 90 mmHg, Confusion (or altered mental status), blood Urea nitrogen greater than 30 mg/dL, Respiratory rate greater than 30 breaths/min, multilobar/bilateral lung infiltrates (by X-ray), Oxygen arterial pressure less than 54 mm Hg or ratio of arterial oxygen tension to fraction of inspired oxygen less than 250 mm Hg, and age 80 years or older. The evaluation of severe CAP is based on the presence of one major criterion (PS) or two or more minor criteria (CURXO80). The model showed an area under the curve of 0.92 to accurately predict severe CAP.[48]

Charles and colleagues[49] developed the SMART-COP to predict the need for intensive respiratory and vasopressor support. The features statistically significantly associated with receipt of intensive respiratory care or vasopressor support were low Systolic blood pressure (1 point), Multilobar chest radiography involvement (1 point), low Albumin level (1 point), high Respiratory rate (age-adjusted) (1 point), Tachycardia (1 point), Confusion (1 point), poor Oxygenation (age-adjusted) (2 points), and low arterial pH (< 7.35) (2 points): SMART-COP. A SMART-COP score of 3 points or more identified 92% of patients who received intensive respiratory care or vasopressor support, including 84% of patients who did not need immediate admission to the ICU. This tool was validated externally in five different cohorts with consistent results and can assist the clinician in assessing the need for intensive respiratory care or vasopressor support and CAP severity.

Table 3
AmericanThoracic Society modified criteria and 2007 Infectious Diseases Society of America/ AmericanThoracic Society criteria

ATS 2001[29]	IDSA/ATS 2007[24]
Major criteria	
Need for mechanical ventilation	Need for mechanical ventilation
Requiring vasopressors (septic shock)	Septic shock with the need for vasopressors
Minor criteria	
Respiratory rate $\geq$ 30 breaths/min	Respiratory rate $\geq$ 30 breaths/min
PaO_2/FiO_2 ratio $\leq$ 250	New-onset confusion/disorientation
Bilateral or multilobar infiltrates	Thrombocytopenia (platelets < 100,000 cells/mL)
	Pao_2/Fio_2 ratio $\leq$ 250
	Uremia (BUN level > 20 mg/dL)
	Hypothermia (core temperature < 36°C)
	Bilateral or multilobar infiltrates
	Leukopenia (WBC count <4000 cells/mL)
	Hypotension requiring aggressive fluid resuscitation

The presence of at least one major criterion or at least two minor criteria defines pneumonia case severe enough to require ICU admission.
Abbreviations: BUN, blood urea nitrogen; Fio_2, fraction of inspired oxygen; WBC, white blood cell.
Data from References.[24,29,42,43,45]

Rello and colleagues[50] developed the CAP-PIRO score based on the score suggested for the risk for sepsis. This score evaluates variables related to the PIRO score that include: Predisposition, Infection, Response, and Organ dysfunction. The CAP-PIRO score intends to adjust for the complexity of the patients critically ill with CAP. CAP-PIRO score evaluates the following variables: Predisposition: comorbidities (COPD or immunocompromised) (1 point), age greater than 70 years (1 point); Infection: bacteremia (1 point), multilobar opacities (1 point); Response: shock (1 point), severe hypoxemia (1 point); and Organ dysfunction: acute respiratory distress syndrome (ARDS, 1 point), acute renal failure (1 point). Considering the observed mortality from each PIRO score, the patients were stratified in four levels of risk: (a) low, 0 to 2 points; (b) mild, 3 points; (c) high, 4 points; and (d) very high, 5 to 8 points. This score was able to consistently predict the ICU mortality and health care use in a cohort of 529 patients admitted to the ICU with CAP.[50]

In conclusion, the last four severity criteria scores have in common the overlap in the variables selected, and it is clear that the new concept of severe CAP goes beyond the lungs and looks for systemic organ dysfunction (**Table 4**). Future prospective validation studies are needed for these scores.

THERAPEUTIC STRATEGIES TO MANAGE SCAP PATIENTS

Traditionally the antimicrobial agents have been considered the cornerstone of therapy against severe CAP; however, with the purpose of understanding severe CAP as a systemic disease, there are other non-antimicrobial therapies that should be considered in this group of patients. Therapeutic strategies for managing patients who have severe CAP are summarized in **Box 1**.

Antimicrobial Therapies

Several professional organizations developed clinical practice guidelines with the objective of standardized therapy for CAP following an evidence-based medicine approach. The guidelines include specific recommendations for patients who have severe CAP usually managed in the ICU.[24–29,51] The guidelines emphasized the importance of appropriate, aggressive, and early management of patients who have CAP who are cared for in the ICU. Patients should be stratified according to the risk for *P aeruginosa* infection.[24] If a patient has no risk factors for pseudomonas infection, the treatment should always include two antibiotics, one (β-lactam) that covers pneumococcus (including drug-resistant isolates) and other likely respiratory pathogens, and therapy against atypical pathogens, especially *Legionella* spp, such as a macrolide (azithromycin or clarithromycin) or a respiratory fluoroquinolone (levofloxacin the highest dose of 750 mg/d or moxifloxacin).[24,25,27,29,52] If there are risk factors for *P aeruginosa*, the treatment should include at least three antibacterial medications: an initial empiric combination of appropriate antipseudomonal coverage (with a β-lactam antipseudomonal therapy) plus an antipseudomonas fluoroquinolone (levofloxacin 750 mg/d or ciprofloxacin 400 mg three times a day) or an antipseudomonal aminoglycoside.[24] The downside of a combination with an aminoglycoside is that atypicals, particularly *Legionella*, are not covered by this approach. In addition, the guidelines recommend including an antimicrobial agent with activity against atypical pathogens (eg, *L pneumophila*), using a regimen that includes a fluoroquinolone or, if fluoroquinolone is not present, the association of a macrolide. The failure to identify a pathogen has not been associated with a worse outcome particularly in the severely ill, but the empiric regimen should cover *S pneumoniae* and atypical pathogens.[53,54] In conclusion, the recommendation is to use empiric combination therapy with two or more antimicrobial agents according to the risk for pseudomonas infection and the constant atypical coverage mainly for legionella infection.

The data regarding the use of combination therapy are limited to a few randomized controlled trials, and most of the data come from observational studies that have evaluated the benefit of using combination therapy versus monotherapy in patients who have severe CAP admitted to the ICU.[55,56] From the limited data and significant heterogeneity between studies, we conclude that limited information is available to support the use of antimicrobial monotherapy in patients who have CAP in the ICU and further randomized controlled trials should be performed to clarify these questions.

Of all the combinations recommended by the guidelines, the one that has acquired a critical role is the use of macrolides in association with other antimicrobials. Initially, Waterer and colleagues[57] found that single effective drug therapy for severe bacteremic pneumococcal pneumonia was associated with a greater risk for death than dual effective therapy. Several other studies suggested a benefit to having a macrolide added to the β-lactam therapy in patients who have bacteremic pneumococcal pneumonia.[58–62] Not adding a macrolide to a β-lactam–based initial antibiotic regimen was an independent predictor of in-hospital mortality.[59] Recent studies suggest that macrolides may have beneficial effects for patients at risk for certain infections because of their immunomodulatory effects rather than antimicrobial properties.[60,61] In addition to these observations about noninfectious diseases, macrolides have been associated with better clinical outcomes in bacteremic pneumococcal pneumonia,[58,59,62] CAP,[7,58,59,63–66] and ventilator associated pneumonia.[67] Rodriguez and colleagues[7] found that in the subset of ICU patients who had CAP and shock, combination antibiotic therapy improved survival rates (odds ratio [OR] = 1.69; 95% CI, 1.09–2.60; P = .01), suggesting that combination therapy may be beneficial in more severe cases. This effect is presumed to be secondary to the immunomodulatory effect rather than the antimicrobial effects,[68] particularly associated with the host inflammatory response.[61,69]

On the other hand, there is enough clinical evidence that supports the clinical practice guideline recommendations[25,27,29] by demonstrating statistically significant

Table 4
Summary of variables evaluated by the different scoring systems to identify patients who have severe community-acquired pneumonia

	IDSA/ATSA 2007 (Minor Criteria)[24]	PS CURXO80[43]	SMART-COP[49]	CAP PIRO[50]
Age	—	≥ 80 y	—	Age > 70 y
Neurologic dysfunction	New-onset confusion/ disorientation	Confusion	Confusion	—
Respiratory dysfunction	Respiratory rate ≥ 30 bpm	Respiratory rate > 30 breaths/min	High respiratory rate (age-adjusted)	—
—	Pao_2/Fio_2 ratio ≤ 250	Pao_2/Fio_2 ratio ≤ 250[a]	Poor oxygenation (age-adjusted)	—
Circulatory dysfunction	Hypotension requiring aggressive fluid resuscitation	Systolic blood pressure < 90 mm Hg	Systolic blood pressure < 90 mm Hg	Shock
—	—	—	Tachycardia (heart rate ≥ 125 bpm)	—
Renal dysfunction	Uremia (BUN level > 20 mg/dL)	BUN > 30 mg/dL	—	Acute renal failure
Hematologic dysfunction	Leukopenia (WBC count < 4000 cells/mL)	—	—	—

Thrombocytopenia (platelets < 100,000 cells/mL)	—		—
Metabolic dysfunction	Arterial pH < 7.30	Arterial pH < 7.35	—
Nutritional dysfunction	—	Low albumin level < 3.5 g/dL	—
Temperature	Hypothermia (core temperature < 36°C)	—	—
Chest radiograph findings	Bilateral or multilobar infiltrates	Multilobar/bilateral lung affectation	Multilobar chest radiography involvement	Multilobar opacities
Laboratory	—	—	Bacteremia
Comorbidities	—	—	Comorbidities (COPD or immunocompromised)

Severe criteria (need for mechanical ventilation or septic shock with the need for vasopressors) by the 2007 IDSA/ATS were excluded from this table because there are no other places to care for these patients who have severe CAP.

[a] Hypoxemia: oxygen arterial pressure < 54 mm Hg or PaO_2/FiO_2 < 250 mm Hg.

> **Box 1**
> **Summary of therapeutic strategies to manage patients who have severe community-acquired pneumonia**
>
> Therapeutic and preventive strategies
>
> Pneumonia assessment for need for admission to the ICU
>
> Appropriate guideline-concordant antibiotic therapy
>
> Use of combination antibiotic therapy (coverage for typical and atypical pathogen)
>
> Early initiation of antibiotics (within 6 hours of presentation)
>
> Systemic corticosteroid therapy (still needs to be defined)
>
> Lung protective-ventilation strategy with low tidal volumes
>
> Recombinant human activated protein C
>
> CAP bundle (process measures, and so forth)
>
> Immunization (influenza or pneumococcal infection)

benefit for those patients receiving guideline-concordant therapies in patients who have CAP.[44,70–75] In addition, there are data to support the benefit of using a combination therapy of β-lactam agent plus a macrolide for initial empiric therapy to reduce mortality in patients who have CAP.[7,62,66,72] National practice guidelines strongly recommend that locally adapted guidelines should be implemented to improve process of care variables and relevant clinical outcomes.[24] Adherence to clinical practice guidelines for the treatment of CAP improves quality and efficiency of care.[76] Several studies report the use of a critical pathway to improve the treatment of CAP patients, including those who have severe disease.[77–82] Other publications[71,83–85] have consistently found a decrease in mortality with the introduction of guideline-concordant antimicrobial therapy or guideline-based protocols. Several of the quality indicators—early administration of antibiotics, appropriate antibiotic use following the clinical practice guidelines, use of a critical pathway, switch to oral therapy and early discharge—have all shown improved clinical outcomes in CAP.[25,26,29,86]

Non-Antimicrobial Therapies

Other non-antimicrobial therapies have focused on supporting patients who have evidence of severe CAP or sepsis due to CAP in a more comprehensive approach. These interventions are directed to early supportive therapy for patients who have severe sepsis correlating with improved survival, such as systemic corticosteroid therapy, lung protective-ventilation strategy, and recombinant human-activated protein C for severe sepsis.

Systemic steroids as adjunct therapy

Previous studies have shown increased pulmonary and systemic inflammatory cytokine levels in patients who have severe CAP.[87–89] Among ICU patients higher circulating inflammatory cytokine levels correlate with the presence of bilateral pneumonia,[90] bacteremia,[89] need for mechanical ventilation,[89] and higher Acute Physiology and Chronic Health Evaluation (APACHE) II and Multiple Organ Dysfunction Syndrome scores.[87,90] A balance between pro- and anti-inflammatory cytokines is critical in the host response. A randomized controlled trial[91] evaluated the efficacy and safety of 7 days of low-dose hydrocortisone infusion in 46 patients who had severe CAP admitted to the ICU. They found significant reduction in mortality (hydrocortisone group 0% versus placebo group 30%, $P = .009$) and length of ICU stay (hydrocortisone group 10 days versus placebo group 18 days, P = .01).[91] A retrospective study[92] that included 308 patients who had severe CAP (PSI classes IV and V) found that treatment with systemic steroids reduced mortality in the cohort of patients who had severe pneumonia (OR = 0.29; 95% CI, 0.11–0.73). The encouraging results of Confalonieri and colleagues[91] and Garcia-Vidal and colleagues[92] suggest that the effects of systemic steroid administration as immunomodulating agents in an immunocompetent host who has severe CAP can decrease mortality. Several ongoing randomized controlled trials may clarify this area of research in the near future.

Recombinant human activated protein C or drotrecogin alfa (activated)

CAP is the leading cause of severe sepsis.[93] Angus and colleagues[93] found that respiratory infections were 44% of severe sepsis cases in a cohort of 192,980 patients. In a recent study that included 1339 patients hospitalized for CAP, Dremsizov and colleagues[94] reported that severe sepsis developed in 48% of the patients. Activated protein C is an important modulator of inflammation and coagulation in sepsis. Bernard and colleagues[95] reported a randomized controlled trial of 1690 adult patients who had severe sepsis (at least one organ failing within the first 24 hours of evaluation) in whom drotrecogin alfa (activated) was evaluated for clinical efficacy and safety. They found a mortality rate of 24.7% with drotrecogin alfa (activated) compared with 30.8% in the placebo group (P = .005), with an absolute risk reduction of death of 6.1%.[95] Severe bleeding episodes (defined as intracranial hemorrhage, any life-threatening bleeding, any bleeding classified as serious by the investigator, or any bleeding that required the administration of at least three units of packed red blood cells on two consecutive days) occurred in 3.5% of patients receiving drotrecogin alfa (activated) compared with 2.0% of patients receiving placebo (P = .06). A post hoc analysis by the Food and Drug Administration (FDA) of data from this study suggested that the reduction in mortality was restricted to patients who had APACHE II scores of 25 or more.[96] In the PROWESS trial the lung was the most common site of infection (53.6%), and 73% of patients in the treatment group and 77% in the placebo group required mechanical ventilation.[95] Laterre and colleagues[97] in a secondary analysis of the severe CAP subgroup in the PROWESS trial found that 35.6% of the 1690 patients were classified as severe CAP. Of these, 26.1% had S pneumoniae infections. In patients who had severe CAP who received drotrecogin alfa (activated), there was a relative risk (RR) reduction in mortality of 28% (RR = 0.72; 95% CI, 0.55–0.94) at 28 days and 14% (RR = 0.86; 95% CI, 0.69–1.07) at 90 days. The survival benefit was most pronounced in patients who had severe CAP with S pneumoniae and in patients who had severe CAP at high risk for death as indicated by APACHE II score greater than 25, PSI score greater than 4, or CURB-65 score greater than 3.[97] These results, although not definitive, suggest that severe sepsis due to CAP may be responsive to drotrecogin alfa (activated) treatment, and might be considered on a case-by-case basis when treating patients who have severe sepsis resulting from CAP.[97] The administration of drotrecogin alfa (activated) in Early Stage Severe Sepsis (ADDRESS) trial, with patients who had less severe sepsis and a low risk for death (as defined by APACHE II scores < 25 or single-organ failure) show no impact on clinical effect with a similar rate of bleeding as a prior report.[98]

The IDSA/ATS CAP guidelines[24] and the new Surviving Sepsis Campaign guidelines[99] suggest that drotrecogin alfa (activated) should be considered for treatment of patients who have CAP within 24 hours of admission if they are in the subgroup of high risk for death: APACHE II scores of 25 or greater or multiple organ failure. Two randomized control trials were requested by the FDA to confirm these prior findings, however, and until the final results of these trials are available we recommend a case-by-case selection of patients who have severe sepsis who may benefit from this treatment.

Lung protective-ventilation strategy

CAP was the most common cause of ARDS in the ARDSNet trial.[100] Two randomized controlled trials[100,101] demonstrated that tidal volume (V_T) of 6 mL/kg predicted body weight (PBW) results in better outcomes than V_T of 12 mL/kg PBW in patients who have acute lung injury (ALI)/ARDS. The ARDSNet trial[100] showed that low V_T (6 mL/kg PBW) had a mortality of 31% when compared with higher V_T (12 mL/kg PBW) 40% mortality ($P = .007$). The absolute risk reduction for mortality in the pneumonia subgroup was 11%.[102] The IDSA/ATS guidelines recommend the use of a lung protective-ventilation strategy (with low V_T 6–8 mL/kg PBW and plateau pressure goal $\leq$ 30 cm H_2O) in patients who have ALI/ARDS, including those who have severe CAP.

COMMUNITY-ACQUIRED PNEUMONIA BUNDLE

The greatest opportunity to improve patient outcomes will probably come not from discovering new treatments but from the effective delivery of existing evidence-based therapies.[103] The bundle is a series of interventions or processes related to care of patients that, when implemented together, will achieve significantly better outcomes than when implemented individually. The components that make up the bundle have to be grounded by an extensive research base.[104] The components of the CAP bundle have shown an impact on clinical outcomes of patients who have CAP.[15,105] We concur with the experts[24,26] that an early CAP bundle should include a series of processes of care[15] in the management of CAP: (1) time to pulse oximetry monitoring (< 3 hours), (2) time to arterial blood gas sampling (in less than 3 hours from presentation), (3) time to blood culture sampling (before the first antibiotic dose), (4) time to first antibiotic dose within 4 to 8 hours (first 6 hours of presentation to the emergency department) of presentation or at least while still in the emergency room, (5) guideline-concordant antibiotic therapy, (6) collection of mortality data (PSI or CURB-65) for all patients who have CAP admitted, and (7) determination of what percentage of at-risk patients receive immunization for influenza or pneumococcal infection. This bundle allows the clinician to identify patients at risk for worst clinical outcomes in which an early and appropriate intervention will likely improve the outcomes of patients who have severe CAP.

SUMMARY

Severe CAP is a complex condition with significant morbidity, mortality, and health care cost. The use of risk stratification is important to better define which patients require a more intensive level of care and a more comprehensive approach. Appropriate antibiotic therapy with early initiation of combination therapy is an important component in the management of patients who have CAP in the ICU. Ideally, current approaches regarding the treatment of patients who have severe CAP are focused on combining conventional antibiotic therapy with early supportive non-antimicrobial therapies that may improve the outcomes of patients who have severe disease. Future research is needed in these areas, so that the risks for treatment failure, morbidity, mortality, and cost due to severe CAP may be minimized.

REFERENCES

1. Anon. Pneumonia and influenza death rates—United States, 1979–1994. MMWR Morb Mortal Wkly Rep 1995;44(28):535–7.

2. Marston BJ, Plouffe JF, File TM Jr, et al. Incidence of community-acquired pneumonia requiring hospitalization. Results of a population-based active surveillance study in Ohio. The community-based pneumonia incidence study group. Arch Intern Med 1997;157(15):1709–18.

3. Leeper KV Jr. Severe community-acquired pneumonia. Semin Respir Infect 1996;11(2):96–108.

4. National Center for Health Statistics. Health Statistics, 2006. Available at: http://www.cdc.gov/nchs/fastats. Accessed June 17, 2009.

5. Grossman RF, Rotschafer JC, Tan JS. Antimicrobial treatment of lower respiratory tract infections in the hospital setting. Am J Med 2005;118(Suppl 7A):29S–38S.

6. Angus DC, Marrie TJ, Obrosky DS, et al. Severe community-acquired pneumonia: use of intensive care services and evaluation of American and British Thoracic Society diagnostic criteria. Am J Respir Crit Care Med 2002;166(5):717–23.

7. Rodriguez A, Mendia A, Sirvent JM, et al. Combination antibiotic therapy improves survival in patients with community-acquired pneumonia and shock. Crit Care Med 2007;35(6):1493–8.

8. Fine MJ, Auble TE, Yealy DM, et al. A prediction rule to identify low-risk patients with community-acquired pneumonia. N Engl J Med 1997;336(4):243–50.

9. Restrepo MI, Mortensen EM, Velez JA, et al. A comparative study of community-acquired pneumonia patients admitted to the ward and the ICU. Chest 2008;133(3):610–7.

10. Fine MJ, Smith MA, Carson CA, et al. Prognosis and outcomes of patients with community-acquired pneumonia. A meta-analysis. JAMA 1996;275(2):134–41.

11. Tejerina E, Frutos V, Restrepo MI, et al. Prognosis factors and outcome of community-acquired pneumonia needing mechanical ventilation. J Crit Care 2005;20(3):56–65.

12. Marrie TJ, Carriere KC, Jin Y, et al. Factors associated with death among adults <55 years of age hospitalized for community-acquired pneumonia. Clin Infect Dis 2003;36(4):413–21.

13. Pascual FE, Matthay MA, Bacchetti P, et al. Assessment of prognosis in patients with community-acquired pneumonia who require mechanical ventilation. Chest 2000;117(2):503–12.

14. Mehta R, Groth M. Clinical application of a prognostic model for severe community-acquired pneumonia. Chest 2001;119(1):312–3.

15. Meehan TP, Fine MJ, Krumholz HM, et al. Quality of care, process, and outcomes in elderly patients with pneumonia. JAMA 1997;278(23):2080–4.

16. Mortensen EM, Coley CM, Singer DE, et al. Causes of death for patients with community-acquired pneumonia: results from the Pneumonia Patient Outcomes Research Team cohort study. Arch Intern Med 2002;162(9):1059–64.

17. Kozak LJ, Hall MJ, Owings MF. National Hospital Discharge Survey: 2000 annual summary with detailed diagnosis and procedure data. Data From the National Health Survey. Vital Health Stat 13 2002;(153):1–194.

18. Niederman MS, McCombs JS, Unger AN, et al. The cost of treating community-acquired pneumonia. Clin Ther 1998;20(4):820–37.

19. Mandell LA, Wunderink RG, Anzueto A, et al. Guidelines for the management of adults with hospital-acquired, ventilator-associated, and healthcare-associated pneumonia. Am J Respir Crit Care Med 2005;171(4):388–416.

20. Rello J, Rodriguez A, Torres A, et al. Implications of COPD in patients admitted to the intensive care unit by community-acquired pneumonia. Eur Respir J 2006;27(6):1210–6.

21. Restrepo MI, Mortensen EM, Pugh JA, et al. COPD is associated with increased mortality in patients with community-acquired pneumonia. Eur Respir J 2006; 28(2):346–51.
22. Feldman C, Viljoen E, Morar R, et al. Prognostic factors in severe community-acquired pneumonia in patients without co-morbid illness. Respirology 2001; 6(4):323–30.
23. File TM Jr, Tan JS, Plouffe JF. The role of atypical pathogens: Mycoplasma pneumoniae, Chlamydia pneumoniae, and Legionella pneumophila in respiratory infection. Infect Dis Clin North Am 1998;12(3):569–92, vii.
24. Mandell LA, Wunderink RG, Anzueto A, et al. Infectious Diseases Society of America/American Thoracic Society Consensus Guidelines on the Management of Community-Acquired Pneumonia in Adults. Clin Infect Dis 2007;44(S2): S27–72.
25. Woodhead M, Blasi F, Ewig S, et al. Guidelines for the management of adult lower respiratory tract infections. Eur Respir J 2005;26(6):1138–80.
26. Bartlett JG, Dowell SF, Mandell LA, et al. Practice guidelines for the management of community-acquired pneumonia in adults. Infectious Diseases Society of America. Clin Infect Dis 2000;31(2):347–82.
27. Mandell LA, Bartlett JG, Dowell SF, et al. Update of practice guidelines for the management of community-acquired pneumonia in immunocompetent adults. Clin Infect Dis 2003;37(11):1405–33.
28. Mandell LA, Marrie TJ, Grossman RF, et al. Canadian guidelines for the initial management of community-acquired pneumonia: an evidence-based update by the Canadian Infectious Diseases Society and the Canadian Thoracic Society. The Canadian Community-Acquired Pneumonia Working Group. Clin Infect Dis 2000;31(2):383–421.
29. Niederman MS, Mandell LA, Anzueto A, et al. Guidelines for the management of adults with community-acquired pneumonia. Diagnosis, assessment of severity, antimicrobial therapy, and prevention. Am J Respir Crit Care Med 2001;163(7):1730–54.
30. Lieberman D, Schlaeffer F, Boldur I, et al. Multiple pathogens in adult patients admitted with community-acquired pneumonia: a one year prospective study of 346 consecutive patients. Thorax 1996;51(2):179–84.
31. Neill AM, Martin IR, Weir R, et al. Community acquired pneumonia: aetiology and usefulness of severity criteria on admission. Thorax 1996;51(10):1010–6.
32. Ruiz M, Ewig S, Marcos MA, et al. Etiology of community-acquired pneumonia: impact of age, comorbidity, and severity. Am J Respir Crit Care Med 1999; 160(2):397–405.
33. Francis JS, Doherty MC, Lopatin U, et al. Severe community-onset pneumonia in healthy adults caused by methicillin-resistant Staphylococcus aureus carrying the Panton-Valentine leukocidin genes. Clin Infect Dis 2005;40(1):100–7.
34. Hageman JC, Uyeki TM, Francis JS, et al. Severe community-acquired pneumonia due to Staphylococcus aureus, 2003–2004 influenza season. Emerg Infect Dis 2006;12(6):894–9.
35. Arancibia F, Bauer TT, Ewig S, et al. Community-acquired pneumonia due to gram-negative bacteria and pseudomonas aeruginosa: incidence, risk, and prognosis. Arch Intern Med 2002;162(16):1849–58.
36. Hatchette TF, Gupta R, Marrie TJ. Pseudomonas aeruginosa community-acquired pneumonia in previously healthy adults: case report and review of the literature. Clin Infect Dis 2000;31(6):1349–56.
37. Cordero E, Pachon J, Rivero A, et al. Community-acquired bacterial pneumonia in human immunodeficiency virus-infected patients: validation of severity

criteria. The Grupo Andaluz para el Estudio de las Enfermedades Infecciosas. Am J Respir Crit Care Med 2000;162(6):2063–8.

38. Luna CM, Famiglietti A, Absi R, et al. Community-acquired pneumonia: etiology, epidemiology, and outcome at a teaching hospital in Argentina. Chest 2000; 118(5):1344–54.

39. Mira J-P, Max A, Burgel P-R. The role of biomarkers in community-acquired pneumonia: predicting mortality and response to adjunctive therapy. Crit Care 2008;12(Suppl 6):S5.

40. Lim WS, Lewis S, Macfarlane JT. Severity prediction rules in community acquired pneumonia: a validation study. Thorax 2000;55(3):219–23.

41. Lim WS, van der Eerden MM, Laing R, et al. Defining community acquired pneumonia severity on presentation to hospital: an international derivation and validation study. Thorax 2003;58(5):377–82.

42. Ewig S, de Roux A, Bauer T, et al. Validation of predictive rules and indices of severity for community acquired pneumonia. Thorax 2004;59(5):421–7.

43. Ewig S, Ruiz M, Mensa J, et al. Severe community-acquired pneumonia. Assessment of severity criteria. Am J Respir Crit Care Med 1998;158(4):1102–8.

44. Capelastegui A, Espana PP, Quintana JM, et al. Validation of a predictive rule for the management of community-acquired pneumonia. Eur Respir J 2006;27(1):151–7.

45. Ewig S, Kleinfeld T, Bauer T, et al. Comparative validation of prognostic rules for community-acquired pneumonia in an elderly population. Eur Respir J 1999; 14(2):370–5.

46. Riley PD, Aronsky D, Dean NC. Validation of the 2001 American Thoracic Society criteria for severe community-acquired pneumonia. Crit Care Med 2004;32(12): 2398–402.

47. Metlay JP, Fine MJ. Testing strategies in the initial management of patients with community-acquired pneumonia. Ann Intern Med 2003;138(2):109–18.

48. España PP, Capelastegui A, Gorordo I, et al. Development and validation of a clinical prediction rule for severe community-acquired pneumonia. Am J Respir Crit Care Med 2006;174(11):1249–56.

49. Charles PG, Wolfe R, Whitby M, et al. SMART-COP: a tool for predicting the need for intensive respiratory or vasopressor support in community-acquired pneumonia. Clin Infect Dis 2008;47(3):375–84.

50. Rello J, Rodriguez A, Lisboa T, et al. PIRO score for community-acquired pneumonia: a new prediction rule for assessment of severity in intensive care unit patients with community-acquired pneumonia. Crit Care Med 2009;37(2):456–62.

51. Heffelfinger JD, Dowell SF, Jorgensen JH, et al. Management of community-acquired pneumonia in the era of pneumococcal resistance: a report from the drug-resistant Streptococcus pneumoniae Therapeutic Working Group. Arch Intern Med 2000;160(10):1399–408.

52. Shefet D, Robenshtok E, Paul M, et al. Empirical atypical coverage for inpatients with community-acquired pneumonia: systematic review of randomized controlled trials. Arch Intern Med 2005;165(17):1992–2000.

53. Leroy O, Santre C, Beuscart C, et al. A five-year study of severe community-acquired pneumonia with emphasis on prognosis in patients admitted to an intensive care unit. Intensive Care Med 1995;21(1):24–31.

54. Moine P, Vercken JB, Chevret S, et al. Severe community-acquired pneumonia. Etiology, epidemiology, and prognosis factors. French study group for community-acquired pneumonia in the intensive care unit. Chest 1994;105(5):1487–95.

55. Fogarty C, Siami G, Kholer R, et al. Multicenter, open label, randomized study to compare the safety and efficacy of levofloxacin versus ceftriaxone sodium and

erythromycin followed by clarithromycin and amoxicillin-clavulanate in the treatment of serious community-acquired pneumonia in adults. Clin Infect Dis 2004; 38(S1):S16–23.

56. Leroy O, Saux P, Bedos JP, et al. Comparison of levofloxacin and cefotaxime combined with ofloxacin for ICU patients with community-acquired pneumonia who do not require vasopressors. Chest 2005;128(1):172–83.

57. Waterer GW, Somes GW, Wunderink RG. Monotherapy may be suboptimal for severe bacteremic pneumococcal pneumonia. Arch Intern Med 2001;161(15): 1837–42.

58. Baddour LM, Yu VL, Klugman KP, et al. Combination antibiotic therapy lowers mortality among severely ill patients with pneumococcal bacteremia. Am J Respir Crit Care Med 2004;170(4):440–4.

59. Martinez JA, Horcajada JP, Almela M, et al. Addition of a macrolide to a beta-lactam-based empirical antibiotic regimen is associated with lower in-hospital mortality for patients with bacteremic pneumococcal pneumonia. Clin Infect Dis 2003;36(4):389–95.

60. Giamarellos-Bourboulis EJ, Baziaka F, Antonopoulou A, et al. Clarithromycin co-administered with amikacin attenuates systemic inflammation in experimental sepsis with Escherichia coli. Int J Antimicrob Agents 2005;25(2):168–72.

61. Giamarellos-Bourboulis EJ. Immunomodulatory therapies for sepsis: unexpected effects with macrolides. Int J Antimicrob Agents 2008;32(Suppl 1):S39–43.

62. Metersky ML, Ma A, Houck PM, et al. Antibiotics for bacteremic pneumonia: improved outcomes with macrolides but not fluoroquinolones. Chest 2007; 131(2):466–73.

63. Lujan M, Gallego M, Fontanals D, et al. Prospective observational study of bacteremic pneumococcal pneumonia: effect of discordant therapy on mortality. Crit Care Med 2004;32(3):625–31.

64. Waterer GW, Baselski VS, Wunderink RG. Legionella and community-acquired pneumonia: a review of current diagnostic tests from a clinician's viewpoint. Am J Med 2001;110(1):41–8.

65. Mufson MA. Pneumococcal pneumonia. Curr Infect Dis Rep 1999;1(1):57–64.

66. Restrepo MI, Mortensen EM, Waterer GW, et al. Impact of macrolide therapy on mortality for patients with severe sepsis due to pneumonia. Eur Respir J 2009; 33(1):153–9.

67. Giamarellos-Bourboulis EJ, Pechere JC, Routsi C, et al. Effect of clarithromycin in patients with sepsis and ventilator-associated pneumonia. Clin Infect Dis 2008;46(8):1157–64.

68. Giamarellos-Bourboulis E, Adamis T, Sabracos L, et al. Clarithromycin: immunomodulatory therapy of experimental sepsis and acute pyelonephritis by Escherichia coli. Scand J Infect Dis 2005;37(1):48–54.

69. Cazzola, Matera MG, Pezzuto G. Inflammation—a new therapeutic target in pneumonia. Respiration 2005;72(2):117–26.

70. Bodi M, Rodriguez A, Sole-Violan J, et al. Antibiotic prescription for community-acquired pneumonia in the intensive care unit: impact of Adherence to Infectious Diseases Society of America Guidelines on Survival. Clin Infect Dis 2005;41(12): 1709–16.

71. Dean NC, Silver MP, Bateman KA, et al. Decreased mortality after implementation of a treatment guideline for community-acquired pneumonia. Am J Med 2001;110(6):451–7.

72. Garcia Vazquez E, Mensa J, Martinez JA, et al. Lower mortality among patients with community-acquired pneumonia treated with a macrolide plus a

beta-lactam agent versus a beta-lactam agent alone. Eur J Clin Microbiol Infect Dis 2005;24(3):190–5.

73. Mortensen EM, Restrepo M, Anzueto A, et al. Effects of guideline-concordant antimicrobial therapy on mortality among patients with community-acquired pneumonia. Am J Med 2004;117(10):726–31.

74. Restrepo MI, Mortensen EM, Anzueto A, et al. Mortality in monotherapy versus combination therapy in severe community-acquired pneumonia: a systematic review. Chest 2003;124(4S):190S.

75. Menendez R, Torres A, Zalacain R, et al. Guidelines for the treatment of community-acquired pneumonia: predictors of adherence and outcome. Am J Respir Crit Care Med 2005;172(6):757–62.

76. Simpson SH, Marrie TJ, Majumdar SR. Do guidelines guide pneumonia practice? A systematic review of interventions and barriers to best practice in the management of community-acquired pneumonia. Respir Care Clin N Am 2005;11(1):1–13.

77. Dresser LD, Niederman MS, Paladino JA. Cost-effectiveness of gatifloxacin versus ceftriaxone with a macrolide for the treatment of community-acquired pneumonia. Chest 2001;119(5):1439–48.

78. Halley HJ. Approaches to drug therapy, formulary, and pathway management in a large community hospital. Am J Health Syst Pharm 2000;57(Suppl 3)):S17–21.

79. Yost NP, Bloom SL, Richey SD, et al. An appraisal of treatment guidelines for antepartum community-acquired pneumonia. Am J Obstet Gynecol 2000;183(1):131–5.

80. Palmer CS, Zhan C, Elixhauser A, et al. Economic assessment of the community-acquired pneumonia intervention trial employing levofloxacin. Clin Ther 2000; 22(2):250–64.

81. Fogarty CM, Greenberg RN, Dunbar L, et al. Effectiveness of levofloxacin for adult community-acquired pneumonia caused by macrolide-resistant Streptococcus pneumoniae: integrated results from four open-label, multicenter, phase III clinical trials. Clin Ther 2001;23(3):425–39.

82. Clark LC, Davis CW. Experiences at a large teaching hospital with levofloxacin for the treatment of community-acquired pneumonia. Am J Health Syst Pharm 2000;57(Suppl 3):S10–3.

83. Capelastegui A, Espana PP, Quintana JM, et al. Improvement of process-of-care and outcomes after implementing a guideline for the management of community-acquired pneumonia: a controlled before-and-after design study. Clin Infect Dis 2004;39(7):955–63.

84. Benenson R, Magalski A, Cavanaugh S, et al. Effects of a pneumonia clinical pathway on time to antibiotic treatment, length of stay, and mortality. Acad Emerg Med 1999;6(12):1243–8.

85. Suchyta MR, Dean NC, Narus S, et al. Effects of a practice guideline for community-acquired pneumonia in an outpatient setting. Am J Med 2001;110(4):306–9.

86. Mandell LA, File TM Jr. Short-course treatment of community-acquired pneumonia. Clin Infect Dis 2003;37(6):761–3.

87. Puren AJ, Feldman C, Savage N, et al. Patterns of cytokine expression in community-acquired pneumonia. Chest 1995;107(5):1342–9.

88. Monton C, Ewig S, Torres A, et al. Role of glucocorticoids on inflammatory response in nonimmunosuppressed patients with pneumonia: a pilot study. Eur Respir J 1999;14(1):218–20.

89. Fernandez-Serrano S, Dorca J, Coromines M, et al. Molecular inflammatory responses measured in blood of patients with severe community-acquired pneumonia. Clin Diagn Lab Immunol 2003;10(5):813–20.

90. Monton C, Torres A, El-Ebiary M, et al. Cytokine expression in severe pneumonia: a bronchoalveolar lavage study. Crit Care Med 1999;27(9):1745–53.
91. Confalonieri M, Urbino R, Potena A, et al. Hydrocortisone infusion for severe community-acquired pneumonia: a preliminary randomized study. Am J Respir Crit Care Med 2005;171(3):242–8.
92. Garcia-Vidal C, Calbo E, Pascual V, et al. Effects of systemic steroids in patients with severe community-acquired pneumonia. Eur Respir J 2007;30(5):951–6.
93. Angus DC, Linde-Zwirble WT, Lidicker J, et al. Epidemiology of severe sepsis in the United States: analysis of incidence, outcome, and associated costs of care. Crit Care Med 2001;29(7):1303–10.
94. Dremsizov T, Clermont G, Kellum JA, et al. Severe sepsis in community-acquired pneumonia: when does it happen, and do systemic inflammatory response syndrome criteria help predict course? Chest 2006;129(4):968–78.
95. Bernard GR, Vincent JL, Laterre PF, et al. Efficacy and safety of recombinant human activated protein C for severe sepsis. N Engl J Med 2001;344(10):699–709.
96. Administration UFaD. Xigris: drotrecogin alfa (activated): PV 3420 AMP. 2001.
97. Laterre PF, Garber G, Levy H, et al. Severe community-acquired pneumonia as a cause of severe sepsis: data from the PROWESS study. Crit Care Med 2005; 33(5):952–61.
98. Abraham E, Laterre PF, Garg R, et al. Drotrecogin alfa (activated) for adults with severe sepsis and a low risk of death. N Engl J Med 2005;353(13):1332–41.
99. Dellinger RP, Levy MM, Carlet JM, et al. Surviving sepsis campaign: international guidelines for management of severe sepsis and septic shock: 2008. Crit Care Med 2008;36(1):296–327.
100. The Acute Respiratory Distress Syndrome Network: Ventilation with lower tidal volumes as compared with traditional tidal volumes for acute lung injury and the acute respiratory distress syndrome. N Engl J Med 2000;342:1301–8.
101. Amato MB, Barbas CS, Medeiros DM, et al. Effect of a protective-ventilation strategy on mortality in the acute respiratory distress syndrome. N Engl J Med 1998;338(6):347–54.
102. Eisner MD, Thompson T, Hudson LD, et al. Efficacy of low tidal volume ventilation in patients with different clinical risk factors for acute lung injury and the acute respiratory distress syndrome. Am J Respir Crit Care Med 2001;164(2):231–6.
103. Pronovost PJ, Rinke ML, Emery K, et al. Interventions to reduce mortality among patients treated in intensive care units. J Crit Care 2004;19(3):158–64.
104. Ihi. Institute for healthcare improvement: bundle up for safety. Available at: http://www.ihi.org/IHI/Topics/CriticalCare/IntensiveCare/ImprovementStories/ BundleUpforSafety.htm. Accessed May 22, 2009.
105. Blot SI, Rodriguez A, Solé-Violán J, et al. Community-Acquired Pneumonia Intensive Care Units (CAPUCI) Study Investigators. Effects of delayed oxygenation assessment on time to antibiotic delivery and mortality in patients with severe community-acquired pneumonia. Crit Care Med 2007;35(11).

Management of Ventilator-Associated Pneumonia

Emili Diaz, MD, PhD*, Marta Ulldemolins, DPharm,
Thiago Lisboa, MD, Jordi Rello, MD, PhD

KEYWORDS

- Ventilator-associated pneumonia • ICU • Management
- Antibiotic • Treatment

Ventilator-associated pneumonia (VAP) management depends on the interaction between the infective agent, the host response, and the antimicrobial drug used. After the pathogen reaches the lungs, two outcomes are possible: either the microorganisms are eliminated by the host immune system, or they overcome the immune system and cause pulmonary infection. In some infectious diseases, a close relationship has been established between the outcome and the time when antibiotic therapy is started.[1-3]

When a patient is thought to have VAP, two steps are strongly recommended: etiologic diagnostic testing and the immediate initiation of antibiotics. Initial empiric antibiotic therapy should be based on risk factors for specific microorganisms and local epidemiology, and should then be adapted when microbiological findings are available.[1,4]

The microbiological results may also help physicians to narrow the spectrum of empiric antibiotics. Identification of a causative pathogen and its antibiotic susceptibility pattern allows de-escalation, that is, the strategy of starting with broad-spectrum antibiotics after obtaining microbiological tests followed by clinical and lab assessment.[5] De-escalation involves three steps: (1) the collection of microbiological samples; (2) the start of empiric antibiotic therapy, bearing in mind local epidemiology and risk factors; and (3) the adaptation of the final antibiotic therapy in the light of the clinical evolution and microbiological data.

ETIOLOGIC DIAGNOSTIC TESTS

The choice of the best diagnostic test is a matter of debate. The most specific tests involved bronchoscopic samples (protected specimen brush, bronchoalveolar lavage) but nonbronchoscopic techniques, mainly tracheal aspirate, are cheaper.

Supported in part by CIBERES 06/06/0036 and AGAUR 05/SGR/920.

Critical Care Department, Joan XXIII University Hospital, University Rovira i Virgili, IISPV, CIBER Enfermedades Respiratorias (CIBERES), Carrer Mallafre Guasch 4, 43007 Tarragona, Spain
* Corresponding author.
E-mail address: emilio.diaz.santos@gmail.com (E. Diaz).

Infect Dis Clin N Am 23 (2009) 521–533
doi:10.1016/j.idc.2009.04.004
id.theclinics.com

Physicians' ability to diagnose VAP is often poor, as several pulmonary diseases may present with similar clinical signs. The presence of clinical signs of pneumonia in intensive care unit (ICU) patients (fever, pulmonary infiltrates and purulent pulmonary secretion) is caused by VAP in only 30%–40% of cases.[6–8] The use of quantitative cultures of respiratory samples has been advocated as a way to improve the accuracy of VAP diagnosis; however, studies to date have not demonstrated any effect on reducing antibiotic use or rates of superinfection, or any improvement in outcomes. Culture of pulmonary secretions may help to refine physicians' clinical suspicion[9] but must not be used alone to confirm or reject it. Microbiologic findings may help to tailor antibiotic spectra in selected patients, but they should be considered in conjunction with a reassessment of clinical response within 48–72 hours of pneumonia onset.[9]

One currently accepted approach involves the use of the diagnostic technique available at each site and the prompt initiation of antibiotic therapy.[1] However, when a multidrug resistant microorganism is suspected, or in case of treatment failure, a bronchoscopic approach is highly recommended. In a multinational study of 27 ICUs across Europe, Koulenti and colleagues[10] reported that VAP diagnosis is mainly based on noninvasive procedures: from a total of 465 VAP episodes, the etiologic diagnoses were based on bronchoscopic samples in only 85 (18.3%). Diagnostic samples can help physicians with the initial empiric antibiotic treatment if Gram stain is performed;[4] they can guide antibiotic changes[4,5,11] and can provide the final etiology and susceptibility patterns within 24 hours.[12]

APPROPRIATE INITIAL EMPIRIC ANTIBIOTIC TREATMENT

Inappropriate initial antibiotic therapy has been demonstrated to be a risk factor for mortality in nosocomial infections.[13] Although it seems that changing antibiotics can improve the outcome, mortality remains higher than with initial adequate therapy.[4,11] De-escalation is a potentially useful strategy for avoiding a high rate of inappropriate initial antibiotic therapy. Starting with broad-spectrum antibiotic coverage leads to a higher probability of correct pathogen coverage and adapting to a narrow spectrum antibiotic allows lower selection pressure.

Sandiumenge and colleagues[14] analyzed four different antibiotic prescription strategies for VAP in a 44-month study. This study demonstrated that prescription strategies for VAP promoting antibiotic diversity were associated with a lower risk of multidrug resistant pathogen selection.

In addition to considering the effect of diversity on ecology, the initial antibiotic therapy should be based on local epidemiology and risk factors predisposing to certain agents. Soo Hoo and colleagues[15] compared two periods in which different approaches were used to treat HAP. Based on their local epidemiology, those authors implemented a new treatment protocol emphasizing the role of empiric treatment, microbiological samples, and de-escalation. These changes achieved a higher rate of appropriate antibiotic therapy and lower mortality at 14 days, without increasing the presence of multidrug resistant microorganisms. As local susceptibility patterns may show changes over time, surveillance reports should be updated periodically, at least once a year.

Since initial empiric antibiotic treatment is a major influence on mortality, the assessment of risk factors for multidrug resistant organisms is a key point in therapy. At this point, a two-step evaluation approach should be considered. First, for early-onset VAP, it should be established whether the patient has a previous risk of presenting a multidrug resistant microorganism. Risk factors for prior acquisition of multidrug resistant (MDR) microorganisms have been described for health care associated pneumonia,[16] and for patients with VAP (**Table 1**);[17] patient-dependent characteristics for MDR colonization differ according to the causative organism. Second, if no risk factors are present, MDR should be considered if the patient has been treated with antibiotics in the last 90 days[16] or if VAP is diagnosed after 5 days of hospitalization. The cut-off point for considering a patient to be at risk for MDR is between 5[16] and 7 days[18] after admission. However, early-onset VAP due to MDR has also been reported in certain hospitals,[19] highlighting once again the critical relevance of local epidemiology.

Another issue to be considered is MDR colonization pressure. In a prospective two-year study, Merrer and colleagues[20] demonstrated that colonization pressure was the most important factor for MRSA acquisition: the higher the MRSA colonization rate in the ICU, the higher risk of MRSA acquisition by the other patients. In that study, the risk of MRSA acquisition increased fivefold when the ratio MRSA-carrier patient-days versus. the total number of patient-days was above 30%.

PRESCRIPTION OF ANTIBIOTICS AT THE BEDSIDE
Combination or Monotherapy in Ventilator-Associated Pneumonia

Empiric antimicrobial treatment choice should be patient-specific, based on risk factors and comorbidities, and individualized, considering local microbiologic

Table 1
Risk factors for VAP due to antibiotic-resistant bacteria
Health care associated methicillin-resistant *Staphylococcus aureus* (HA-MRSA)
COPD
Steroid therapy
Longer duration of mechanical ventilation
Prior antibiotic therapy
Prior bronchoscopy
MRSA colonization
Community-acquired methicillin-resistant *Staphylococcus aureus* (CA-MRSA) (low predictive value)
Skin trauma
Cosmetic body shaving
Incarceration
Pseudomonas aeruginosa
COPD
Steroid therapy
Longer duration of mechanical ventilation
Prior antibiotic therapy
Acinetobacter baumannii
ARDS
Head trauma
Neurosurgery
Gross aspiration
Prior cephalosporin therapy

Data from Diaz E, Muñoz E, Agbaht K, et al. Management of ventilator-associated pneumonia caused by multiresistant bacteria. Curr Opin Crit Care 2007;13:2548.

data.[17,21] Antibiotic selection in early-onset VAP without risk factors for multidrug resistant pathogens includes mostly a single narrow-spectrum agent, while in late-onset episodes the possibility of multidrug resistant organisms, and as a result a broad-spectrum treatment strategy, should be considered.

Some authors argue that a combination regimen increases the likelihood of therapeutic success through wider coverage in monomicrobial episodes of VAP and especially in polymicrobial episodes. However, some studies suggest that combination therapy may be more expensive and may be associated with greater toxicity and the emergence of multiresistant microorganisms.[22]

Recently, Heyland and colleagues[23] reported a randomized clinical trial comparing combination therapy (meropenem plus ciprofloxacin) versus monotherapy (only meropenem) with broad-spectrum antibiotics for suspected late VAP. They found no differences in 28-day mortality between combination and monotherapy groups, or between ICU and hospital length of stay, clinical and microbiological treatment response, or emergence of antibiotic-resistant bacteria. However, when evaluating a subgroup of patients with multidrug resistant Gram-negative bacteria, microbiological eradication of infecting organisms was significantly higher in the combination therapy group, though there were no differences in clinical outcomes. This finding may be explained by the statistically significant difference between the groups in terms of antibiotic adequacy (combination = 84.2% versus monotherapy = 18.8%). The authors' group[24] described similar findings in a multicenter study comparing the use of monotherapy versus combination as empiric therapy for monomicrobial VAP episodes due to *Pseudomonas aeruginosa*. In that study, use of combination therapy was less likely to be inappropriate than monotherapy (9.5% versus 43.3%). Nevertheless, when only appropriate therapy was considered, there was no difference in outcomes between the two treatment groups. A recent meta-analysis[25] demonstrated that monotherapy is not inferior to combination therapy for the empiric treatment of VAP. However, the heterogeneity of the studies conducted so far limits the data quality, and further studies are necessary to clarify the issue.

In clinical practice, the choice of combination therapy in patients with a high susceptibility to multidrug-resistant pathogens such as *Pseudomonas aeruginosa* should take account of local microbiological data to ensure that appropriate empiric therapy is given. This approach is the key determinant of mortality risk in these patients.[1]

Choosing the Regimen

After considering the above arguments, the physician must decide whether to start an antibiotic alone or in combination. Unless the patient is immunocompromised, antifungal therapy should be not prescribed. In early-onset VAP in patients without risk factors for MDR pathogens, therapy should be active against core pathogens (*Haemophilus influenzae*, *Streptococcus pneumoniae* and methicillin-sensitive *Staphylococcus aureus*). However, in patients who have VAP caused by *Pseudomonas* spp, *Acinetobacter baumannii* or extended-spectrum beta-lactamase (ESBL) producing Enterobacteriaceae, the appropriateness of initial antibiotic regimen is higher with combination therapy.[23] Options for empiric antibiotic therapy are detailed in **Table 2**. In patients at risk of MDR, a three-step approach is recommended (**Fig. 1**).

First, if there is a risk of methicillian-resistant *Staphylococcus aures* (MRSA) colonization, the authors suggest linezolid as part of empiric therapy (**Fig. 2**).[26] Vancomycin has been the anti-MRSA drug of choice for several years, but the mortality rate for patients with MRSA VAP treated with vancomycin has been reported to be as high as 50%.[27] Vancomycin's poor tissue penetration in the lung limits its ability to

Table 2
Final recommendation for antibiotic treatment in patients with VAP

Patient Category	Antibiotic Treatment
No risk factors for MDR organisms	Amoxicillin-clavulanate
	Ampicillin-sulbactam
	Ertapenem
	Ceftriaxone
At risk for: Pseudomonas aeruginosa	Initial empiric antibiotic treatment
	Imipenem/cilastatin: 2 h infusion
	Meropenem: 3 h infusion
	Doripenem: 4 h infusion
	Piperacillin-tazobactam: 4 infusion
	Ceftazidime/cefepime: continuous infusion
	Combination with
	Ciprofloxacin
MRSA	Linezolid
	Vancomycin: continuous infusion to
	trough levels of 15–20 microg/mL
Acinetobacter baumannii	Carbapenem
	Sulbactam
	Colistin
Previously treated with antibiotic:	
Previous	Recommendation
β-lactam	Carbapenem
Ciprofloxacin	Avoid imipenem
Carbapenem	Piperacillin-tazobactam
Aminoglycoside	Ciprofloxacin or change aminoglycoside type

optimally treat VAP episodes in spite of its in vitro appropriateness. Although no random controlled trial (RCT) comparing vancomycin versus linezolid has been designed in patients with VAP, the pooled results of two studies showed better outcomes for patients treated with linezolid compared with those treated with vancomycin. Other

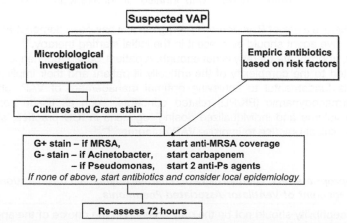

Fig. 1. Treatment decision tree for ventilator-associated pneumonia. *Modified from* Rello J, Diaz E. Pneumonia in the intensive care unit. Crit Care Med 2003;31:2548; with permission.

THERAPEUTIC MANAGEMENT of VAP- When S. aureus is a consideration

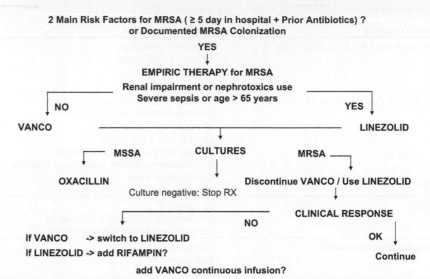

Fig. 2. Management of ventilator-associated pneumonia in patients at risk for methicillin-resistant *Staphylococcus aureus*. *Modified from* Lisboa T, Rello J. Nosocomial pneumonia due to Gram-positive microorganism. Enferm Infecc Microbiol Clin 2007;25(Suppl 4):58; with permission.

new agents with anti-MRSA activity, such as telavancin, iclaprim, ceftaroline or PZ-601, are being investigated in ongoing clinical trials. Unfortunately, most new agents (eg, daptomycin, tigecycline) have been approved for nonpulmonary indications such as abdominal or skin and soft tissue infections.

Second, if there is a risk of *Acinetobacter baumannii* colonization, carbapenem should be considered. In a case control study, patients who had VAP caused by *Acinetobacter baumannii* treated with carbapenem showed no differences in mortality compared with control patients with similar severity scores.[28] In patients who had carbapenem-resistant strains, therapy with inhaled or intravenous colistin has been tested.[29]

Third, if there is a risk of *Pseudomonas aeruginosa,* it has been demonstrated that at least one active agent should be present in the initial starting therapy.[24]

However, appropriate therapy is not enough. A patient-based regimen, considering issues related to the complexity of the critically ill patient and their implications for treatment is fundamental to achieving optimal management of VAP. pharmacokinetic/pharmacodynamic (PK/PD) related concepts, such as tissue penetration, distribution volume and individualized dosing regimens in ICU practice, should be included in clinical practice to improve VAP outcome.[30–32]

Beyond Appropriateness: Pharmacokinetic-Pharmacodynamic Considerations in the Management of Ventilator-Associated Pneumonia

In vitro susceptibility should not be the only criterion in the choice of the appropriate antibiotic. Treatment failure with an antibiotic to which the pathogen was sensitive in vitro is not uncommon.

Host factors

Critically ill patients are subject to physiologic changes that may affect the concentration achieved in both blood and peripheral tissues. Situations such as sepsis are known to increase patients' distribution volume, producing an effect known as "third spacing,"[32] which leads to a decrease in the blood concentration of hydrophilic drugs. This development is especially relevant in the case of antibiotics, because of the resulting probability of achieving lower concentrations than expected, thus leading to underdosing.

Moreover, renal failure is also frequent in the ICU, as the use of nephrotoxic medicaments such as iodine contrast or situations of hypovolemia or myocardial depression is relatively common. A decrease in the kidney filtration rate produces an inversely proportional increase in the half-life of drugs that are mainly excreted renally, leading to higher than expected drug concentrations in both plasma and peripheral tissue.[32]

Furthermore, ventilated patients with shock usually receive fluidotherapy and/or inotropic agents as therapy to reverse the situation. The extra volume and the increase in the cardiac output[31,33] leads to higher values of renal preload, which raises filtration rates and shortens drug half-life.[32]

Albumin levels are also important, as the incidence of hypoalbuminemia is relatively high in critically ill patients. Domínguez de Villota and colleagues[34] reported that 64% of the patients admitted to their ICU had low albumin levels. Its immediate consequence is a decrease in the colloid osmotic pressure, which in physiologic terms leads to a movement of liquid to the extravascular space, producing edema and lower than expected blood drug concentrations. Moreover, drugs can bind to plasmatic proteins in a variable percentage depending on their physicochemistry, and it is known that the unbound fraction is cleared faster. Hypoalbuminemia leads to higher free drug concentrations and may decrease drug half-life.[35]

Antibiotic factors

An antibiotic drug's structure has implications for its distribution, metabolism and excretion, making each antibiotic suitable for certain types of infection. Consequently, the quantitative evaluation of lung penetration is a cornerstone in the selection of the most appropriate antibiotic for treating VAP.

Time-dependent antibiotics exhibit better profiles of activity when administered in prolonged-infusion multiple-daily dosing rather than in once-daily bolus dosing. Beta-lactams, carbapenems and glycopeptides are included in this group. In contrast, concentration-dependent antibiotics, such as fluoroquinolones, aminoglycosides and macrolides, achieve better outcomes when administered in high doses once daily.

As time-dependent antibiotics, beta-lactams and carbapenems require a certain time >minimum inhibitory concentration (MIC) between doses which usually ranges between 40% and 50% in penicillins; 50%–70% in cephalosporins; and 30%–40% in carbapenems.[36,37] Fast regrowth of causative bacteria has been reported.[38–40] To examine this point, several studies have compared bolus administration versus prolonged infusion, concluding that long infusions achieve better outcomes.[41–45] Piperacillin-tazobactam in extended-infusion has been administered in critically ill patients infected with *Pseudomonas aeruginosa*, more than half of respiratory origin.[46] In this study, 14-day mortality was lower for patients treated with extended-infusion of piperacillin-tazobactam compared with intravenous administration for 30 min every 4 or 6 hours. Doripenem, a carbapenem approved for treatment of patients with VAP, has been tested in extended-infusion. A 4-hour infusion of doripenem was not inferior to a 30- or 60-minute infusion of imipenem and exhibited better results for patients with higher severity as measured by APACHE II score and older age.[47] Some reports suggest that vancomycin should be administered in continuous infusion with a trough level of 15–20 microg/mL.[27]

Linezolid seems to follow a time-dependent profile of activity in animal models; however, in humans the best outcomes were obtained with t>MIC of 85% and AUC/MIC of 100, suggesting that its behavior is mixed.[48]

The best outcomes with fluoroquinolones are achieved with high-dose, once-daily administrations. The study by Benko and colleagues showed that levofloxacin given to treat VAP in a schedule of 500 mg twice daily as loading dose and 500 mg once daily until the end of therapy achieved the recommended pharmacodynamic values of maximum concentration (Cmax)/MIC >10 and AUC/MIC = 100 - 150.[49,50] Similar results have been reported for ciprofloxacin, confirming the dose- dependence of fluoroquinolones.[51]

EVALUATION OF CLINICAL RESPONSE AND ADJUSTMENT OF EMPIRIC REGIMEN
Clinical Resolution

In 2003, a decision tree algorithm giving full follow-up for patients with a VAP episode was published (**Fig. 3**).[1] One of the key points was the clinical resolution assessment. In a clinical study of patients without acute respiratory distress syndrome (ARDS), the time to evaluate the clinical response was defined to be adequate at 48–72 hours, when around 75% of patients with good resolution exhibited an improvement in hypoxemia and fever.[52] Clinical resolution was assessed based on the evaluation of fever, hypoxemia (measured as PaO2/FiO2 ratio), leukocyte count in peripheral blood, clearance of tracheal secretions, and opacities in chest radiograph. The most important finding was that fever and hypoxemia resolved within the first 72 hours of evolution in more than 70% of patients. The etiology comprised mainly non-difficult to treat bacteria (18.8% of *Pseudomonas aeruginosa*, *Acinetobacter baumannii* or MRSA). A new study by the same group, focusing on the influence of microorganisms on VAP resolution, showed that the resolution of VAP by methicillin-sensitive *Staphylococcus aureus*, *Haemophilus influenzae*, and *Pseudomonas aeruginosa* was similar;

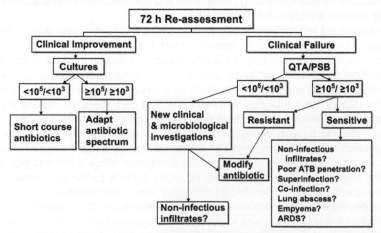

Fig. 3. Follow-up for patients having ventilator-associated pneumonia according to microbiological results and clinical assessment. *Modified from* Rello J, Diaz E. Pneumonia in the intensive care unit. Crit Care Med 2003;31:2544–51; with permission. ATB, antibiotic therapy; ARDS, acute respiratory distress syndrome.

however, when the VAP episode was caused by MRSA the median time to resolution was 10 days.[53]

In addition to clinical parameters, biomarkers have been investigated in patients who have VAP. Procalcitonin[54,55] and C-reactive protein (CRP) have proved to be useful tools to assess prognosis in VAP patients.[54] Moreover, a dynamic reassessment of CRP levels at day four of VAP was a marker of appropriateness and clinical response to antibiotic therapy.[56]

Changing the Empiric Regimen

There are three ways of changing a previously prescribed antibiotic therapy: escalation to another regimen, de-escalation, or continuation of the initial antibiotic regimen. In de-escalation, treatment starts with a broad-spectrum antibiotic therapy, providing maximum coverage and minimizing the risk of inappropriate empiric treatment. When a positive culture is available, de-escalation allows the treatment to be changed to a narrow-spectrum specific therapy, minimizing the risk of emergence of resistance as the exposure to broad-spectrum agents decreases.[5] Another study[57] found that de-escalation was performed in 22% of VAP episodes. The mortality rate was lower among patients in whom therapy was de-escalated compared with those without changes in therapy. The combination of clinical resolution and antibiotic susceptibility of causative microorganisms gives clinicians four options (**Table 3**). Without microbiological data, de-escalation is impossible by definition, because adjustment to a low antibiotic class does not guarantee correct coverage. In this situation, a) if clinical resolution is achieved, the first option is to maintain the initial antibiotic regimen. However, b) if clinical resolution of VAP is poor, the physician should consider escalating the therapy, with coverage of uncovered pathogens, and with special attention to multidrug resistant microorganisms. However, c) if microbiological results are available and VAP is likely to resolve the treatment can be modified according to the results, either maintaining the current therapy or, if possible, de-escalating. And, d) if microbiological data are present and the patient's condition is deteriorating, the antibiotic should be modified with escalation to a broad spectrum agent, or one that covers the untreated pathogens. Finally, the entire schedule should be seen as a dynamic process in which the information is constantly updated and which considers other diagnoses such as pleural empyema, and wrong initial diagnosis. In addition, the clinical resolution pattern may differ between patients with or without ARDS.

Antibiotic Duration

The optimal duration of antibiotic therapy is not known. In a multicenter study performed to define the duration of antibiotic treatment, Chastre and colleagues compared 8 to 15 days of antibiotic treatment for VAP and found no difference in intent-to-treat (ITT) analysis. However, patients had longer treatment than that indicated in the protocol (17 days versus 12.5 days). In this study of patients with VAP

Table 3
2 X 2 table according to empiric antibiotic therapy and availability of microbiological results

	Clinical Resolution	
Microbiological Results	**Positive**	**Negative**
Available	Continue or de-escalate	Escalate
Not available	Continue	Escalate

caused by nonfermentative Gram-negative bacilli, higher recurrence was seen in the group of shorter duration.[58] This higher recurrence was not observed in a retrospective study focusing only on patients with nonfermentative bacilli.[59] Other tools to decrease the antibiotic time duration are not widely applied, although repeating bronchoalveolar lavage has proved useful in trauma patients.[60]

A customized, patient-specific approach based on clinical response to antibiotic treatment, using dynamic clinical variables and biomarkers such as CRP and procalaitonin (PCT), may help to optimize treatment duration. Nonetheless, this strategy is still to be validated in prospective clinical trials.

SUMMARY

The daily management of VAP remains a challenge for physicians in the ICU. In recent years, a more dynamic approach has evolved, updating local epidemiology, evaluating VAP and diagnostic tools every day, and assessing host response using clinical and biochemical parameters. In this situation, PK/PD properties have emerged as an important element in antibiotic therapy.

REFERENCES

1. Rello J, Diaz E. Pneumonia in the intensive care unit. Crit Care Med 2003;31: 2544–51.
2. Roberts JA, Paratz JD, Lipman J. Continuous infusion of beta-lactams in the intensive care unit–best way to hit the target? Crit Care Med 2008;36:1663–4.
3. Houck PM, Bratzler DW, Nsa W, et al. Timing of antibiotic administration and outcomes for Medicare patients hospitalized with community-acquired pneumonia. Arch Intern Med 2004;164:637–44.
4. Rello J, Gallego M, Mariscal D, et al. The value of routine microbial investigation in ventilator-associated pneumonia. Am J Respir Crit Care Med 1997;156:196–200.
5. Rello J, Vidaur L, Sandiumenge A, et al. De-escalation therapy in ventilator-associated pneumonia. Crit Care Med 2004;32:2183–90.
6. Lisboa T, Craven DE, Rello J. Safety in critical care and pulmonary medicine: should ventilator-associated pneumonia be a quality indicator for patient safety? Clin Pulm Med 2009;16:28–32.
7. Klompas M, Kulldorff M, Platt R. Risk of misleading ventilator-associated pneumonia rates with use of standard clinical and microbiological criteria. Clin Infect Dis 2008;46:1443–6.
8. Uçkay I, Ahmed QA, Sax H, et al. Ventilator-associated pneumonia as a quality indicator for patient safety? Clin Infect Dis 2008;46:557–63.
9. Klompas M. Does this patient have ventilator-associated pneumonia? JAMA 2007;297:1583–93.
10. Koulenti D, Lisboa T, Brun-Buisson C, et al, for EU-VAP/CAP Study Group. The spectrum of practice in the diagnosis of nosocomial pneumonia in patients requiring mechanical ventilation in European ICUs. Crit Care Med, in press.
11. Luna CM, Vujacich P, Niederman MS, et al. Impact of BAL data on the therapy and outcome of ventilator-associated pneumonia. Chest 1997;111:676–85.
12. Cercenado E, Cercenado S, Marin M, et al. Evaluation of direct E-test on lower respiratory tract samples: a rapid and accurate procedure for antimicrobial susceptibility testing. Diagn Microbiol Infect Dis 2007;58:211–6.
13. Ibrahim EH, Sherman G, Ward S, et al. The influence of inadequate antimicrobial treatment of bloodstream infections on patient outcomes in the ICU setting. Chest 2000;118:146–55.

14. Sandiumenge A, Diaz E, Rodriguez A, et al. Impact of diversity of antibiotic use on the development of antimicrobial resistance. J Antimicrob Chemother 2006; 57:1197–204.
15. Soo Hoo GW, Wen YE, Nguyen TV, et al. Impact of clinical guidelines in the management of severe hospital-acquired pneumonia. Chest 2005;128: 2778–87.
16. American Thorac Society. Infectious diseases of America. Guidelines for the management of adults with hospital-acquired, ventilator-associated, and health-care-associated pneumonia. Am J Respir Crit Care Med 2005;171:388–416.
17. Diaz E, Muñoz E, Agbaht K, et al. Management of ventilator-associated pneumonia caused by multiresistant bacteria. Curr Opin Crit Care 2007;13:45–50.
18. Trouillet JL, Chastre J, Vuagnat A, et al. Ventilator-associated pneumonia caused by potentially drug-resistant bacteria. Am J Respir Crit Care Med 1998;157: 531–9.
19. Akça O, Koltka K, Uzel S, et al. Risk factors for early-onset, ventilator-associated pneumonia in critical care patients: selected multirresistant versus nonresistant bacteria. Anesthesiology 2000;93:638–45.
20. Merrer J, Santoli F, Appere de Vecchi C, et al. "Colonization pressure" and risk of acquisition of methicillin-resistant Staphylococcus aureus in a medical intensive care unit. Infect Control Hosp Epidemiol 2000;21:718–23.
21. Vidaur L, Sirgo G, Rodríguez AH, et al. Clinical approach to the patient with suspected ventilator-associated pneumonia. Respir Care 2005;50:965–74.
22. Wolff M. Role of aminoglycosides in the treatment VAP. Clin Pulm Med 2000;7: 120–7.
23. Heyland DK, Dodek P, Muscedere J, et al. Canadian Critical Care Trials Group. Randomized trial of combination versus monotherapy for the empiric treatment of suspected ventilator-associated pneumonia. Crit Care Med 2008;36:737–44.
24. Garnacho-Montero J, Sa-Borges M, Sole-Violan J, et al. Optimal management therapy for Pseudomonas aeruginosa ventilator-associated pneumonia: an observational, multicenter study comparing monotherapy with combination antibiotic therapy. Crit Care Med 2007;35:1888–95.
25. Aarts MA, Hancock JN, Heyland D, et al. Empiric antibiotic therapy for suspected ventilator-associated pneumonia: a systematic review and meta-analysis of randomized trials. Crit Care Med 2008;36:108–17.
26. Lisboa T, Rello J. Nosocomial pneumonia due to Gram-positive microorganism. Enferm Infecc Microbiol Clin 2007;25(Suppl 4):53–60.
27. Rello J, Sole-Violan J, Sa-Borges M, et al. Pneumonia caused by oxacillin-resistant Staphylococcus aureus treated with glycopeptides. Crit Care Med 2005; 33:1983–7.
28. Garnacho J, Sole-Violan J, Sa-Borges M, et al. Clinical impact of pneumonia caused by Acinetobacter baumannii in intubated patients: a matched cohort study. Crit Care Med 2003;31:2478–82.
29. Garnacho-Montero J, Ortiz-Leyba C, Jiménez-Jiménez FJ, et al. Treatment of multidrug-resistant Acinetobacter baumannii ventilador-associated pneumoniae (VAP) with intravenous colistin: a comparison with imipenem-susceptible VAP. Clin Infect Dis 2003;36:1111–8.
30. Roberts JA, Lipman J, Blot S, et al. Better outcomes through continuous infusion of time-dependent antibiotics to critically ill patients? Curr Opin Crit Care 2008; 14:390–6.
31. Roberts JA, Lipman J. Pharmacokinetic issues for antibiotics in the critically ill patient. Crit Care Med 2009;37:840–51.

32. Roberts J, Lipman J. Antibacterial dosing in intensive care. Pharmacokinetics, degree of disease and pharmacodynamics of sepsis. Clin Pharmacokinet 2006;45:755–73.
33. Kumar A, Schupp E, Bunnell E, et al. Cardiovascular response to dobutamine stress predicts outcome in severe sepsis and septic shock. Crit Care 2008;12: R35.
34. Domínguez de Villota E, Mosquera JM, Rubio JJ, et al. Assotiation of a low serum albumin with infection and increasedmortality in critically ill patients. Intensive Care Med 1980;7:19–22.
35. Burkhardt O, Kumar V, Katterwe D, et al. Ertapenem in critically ill patients with early- onset ventilator- associated pneumonia: pharmacokinetics with special consideration of free- drug concentration. J Antimicrob Chemother 2007;59: 277–84.
36. Craig WA. Interrelationship between pharmacokinetics and pharmacodynamics in determining dosage regimens for broad- spectrum cephalosporins. Diagn Microbiol Infect Dis 1995;22:89–96.
37. Craig WA. Pharmacokinetic/pharmacodynamic parameters: rationale for bacterial dosing of mice and man. Clin Infect Dis 1998;26:1–10 [quiz 11–2].
38. Craig WA. Pharmacokinetic and experimental data on beta- lactam antibiotics in the treatment of patients. Eur J Clin Microbiol Infect Dis 1984;3:575–8.
39. Vogelman B, Craig WA. Postantibiotic effects. J Antimicrob Chemother 1985; 15(Suppl A):37–46.
40. Moulton JW, Vinks AA, Punt NC. Pharmacokinetic- pharmacodynamic modeling of activity of ceftazimide during continuous and intermittent infusion. Antimicrobial Agents Chemother 1997;41:733–8.
41. Moulton JW, Vinks AA. Is continuous infusion of beta- lactam antibiotics worthwhile? - efficacy and pharmacokinetic considerations. J Antimicrob Chemother 1996;38:5–15.
42. Tam VH, Louie A, Lomaestro BM, et al. Integration of population pharmacokinetics, a pharmacodynamic target and microbiologic surveillance data to generate a rational empiric dosing strategy for cefepime against Pseudomonas aeruginosa. Pharmacotherapy 2003;23:291–5.
43. Roberts JA, Lipman J. Optimizing use of beta- lactam antibiotics in the critically ill. Semin Respir Crit Care Med 2007;28:579–85.
44. Roberts JA, Boots R, Rickard CM, et al. Is continuous infusion ceftriaxone better than once- a- day dosing in intensive care? A randomized controlled pilot study. J Antimicrob Chemother 2007;59:285–91.
45. Roberts JA, Paratz J, Paratz E, et al. Continuous infusion of β- lactam antibiotics in severe infections: a review of its role. Int J Antimicrob Agents 2007;30:11–8.
46. Lodise TP, Lomaestro B, Drusano GL. Piperacillin-tazobactam for Pseudomonas aeruginosa infection: clinical implications o fan extended-infusion doping strategy. Clin Infect Dis 2007;44:357–63.
47. Chastre J, Wunderink R, Prokocimer P, et al. Efficacy and safety of intravenous infusión of doripenem versus imipenem in ventilador-associated pneumonia: a multicenter, randomized study. Crit Care Med 2008;36:1089–96.
48. MacGowan AP. Pharmacokinetic and pharmacodynamic profile of linezolid in healthy volunteers and patients with gram- positive infections. J Antimicrob Chemother 2003;51:ii17–25.
49. Benko R, Matuz M, Doro P, et al. Pharmacokinetics and pharmacodynamics of levofloxacin in critically ill patients with ventilator- associated pneumonia. Int J Antimicrob Agents 2007;30:162–8.

50. Preston SL, Drusanl GL, Berman AL, et al. Pharmacodynamics of levofloxacin; a new paradigm for early clinical trials. JAMA 1998;279:125–9.
51. Forrest A, Nix DE, Ballow CH, et al. Pharmacodynamics of intravenous ciprofloxacin in seriously ill patients. Antimicrobial Agents Chemother 1993;37:1073–81.
52. Vidaur L, Gualis B, Rodriguez A, et al. Clinical resolution in patients with suspicion of ventilator-associated pneumonia: a cohort study comparing patients with and without acute respiratory distress syndrome. Crit Care Med 2005;33:1248–53.
53. Vidaur L, Planas K, Sierra R, et al. Ventilator-associated pneumonia: impact of organisms on clinical resolution and medical resources utilization. Chest 2008; 133:625–32.
54. Seligman R, Meisner M, Lisboa TC, et al. Decreases in procalcitonin and C-reactive protein are strong predictors of survival in ventilator-associated pneumonia. Crit Care 2006;10:R125 doi:10.1186/cc5036.
55. Pelosi P, Barassi A, Severgnini P, et al. Prognostic role of clinical and laboratory criteria to identify early ventilator-associated pneumonia in brain injury. Chest 2008;134:101–8.
56. Lisboa T, Seligman R, Diaz E, et al. C-reactive protein correlates with bacterial load and appropriate antibiotic therapy in suspected ventilator-associated pneumonia. Crit Care Med 2008;36:166–71.
57. Kollef MH, Morrow LE, Niederman MS, et al. Clinical characteristics and treatment patterns among patients with ventilator-associated pneumonia. Chest 2006;129:1210–8.
58. Chastre J, Wolff M, Fagon JY, et al. PneumATrial Group. Comparison of 8 versus 15 days of antibiotic therapy for ventilator-associated pneumonia in adults: a randomized trial. JAMA 2003;290:2588–98.
59. Hedrick TL, McElearney ST, Smith RL, et al. Duration of antibiotic therapy for ventilator-associated pneumonia caused by non-fermentative gram-negative bacilli. Surg Infect (Larchmt) 2007;8:589–97.
60. Mueller EW, Croce MA, Boucher BA, et al. Repeat bronchoalveolar lavage to guide antibiotic duration of ventilator-associated pneumonia. J Trauma 2007;63: 1329–37.

Approach to the Immunocompromised Host with Infection in the Intensive Care Unit

Peter K. Linden, MD[a,b,*]

KEYWORDS

- Immunocompromised • Immunosuppression
- Opportunistic infection • Nosocomial infection
- Organ transplantation • HIV • Neutropenia

The frequency of community and hospitalized patients with compromised host defenses has increased dramatically over recent decades such that it is common for medical and surgical ICU physicians to routinely encounter immunocompromised hosts. The origin of this trend is multifactorial and includes: (1) the appearance of HIV-1–related illness since the early 1980s; (2) the greater use of solid and hematologic transplantation strategies for otherwise untreatable, underlying conditions; (3) patients with cancer treated with conventional chemotherapy and immunotherapy; and (4) the introduction of novel monoclonal antibody therapy (eg, anti-tumor necrosis factor [TNF]) for common conditions, such as Crohn's disease, rheumatoid arthritis, and other native conditions which can be successfully controlled with iatrogenic immunosuppression. Improved survival among patients with HIV-1 caused by highly active antiretroviral therapy and refinements in immunosuppression among organ transplant recipients has not only increased the numbers of immunocompromised patients, but also modified the incidence, timing, severity, and composition of opportunistic infection among such patients.[1,2]

Despite significant advances in the prevention, diagnosis, and treatment of infection in the immunocompromised host it remains a major cause of morbidity, increased length of stay, increased total costs, and of course mortality. Intensive care mortality rates are significantly higher among immunocompromised hosts caused in part by the higher incidence of infection severity. The superimposition of the compromised host

[a] Department of Critical Care Medicine, University of Pittsburgh Medical Center, Room 602A, Scaife Hall, 3550 Terrace Street, Pittsburgh, PA 15261, USA
[b] Abdominal Organ Transplant ICU, University of Pittsburgh Medical Center, Montefiore Hospital, 5th Floor, 3459 5th Avenue, Pittsburgh, PA 15213, USA
* Department of Critical Care Medicine, University of Pittsburgh Medical Center, Room 602A, Scaife Hall, 3550 Terrace Street, Pittsburgh, PA 15261.
E-mail address: plinden@wpahs.org

Infect Dis Clin N Am 23 (2009) 535–556
doi:10.1016/j.idc.2009.04.014
0891-5520/09/$ – see front matter © 2009 Elsevier Inc. All rights reserved.

defenses and critical illness make the detection and management of infections in such patients more difficult, but crucial toward salvaging patient outcome. Moreover, while there is a rapidly increasing evidence base in intensive care medicine, many interventional trials for the management of severe sepsis (activated protein C, adjunctive corticosteroids, goal based resuscitation), acute lung injury (low stretch ventilation), and other organ failures have excluded immunocompromised hosts.[3–6]

GENERAL TRUTHS ABOUT INFECTION IN THE IMMUNOCOMPROMISED HOST
Altered Clinical Expression

Because of diminished or absent inflammatory responses, the expected local clinical and radiographic signs of infection may not be present. In patients who are critically ill there are other confounders which may camouflage symptom and sign detection, such as iatrogenic sedation, and multiple processes (fluid overload, atelectasis), which produce pulmonary radiographic changes unrelated to infection. Detectable but atypical presentations caused by opportunistic pathogens are also more prevalent (eg, multidermatomal *Herpes zoster*, *P jiroveci*) presenting with discrete nodules in patients infected with HIV-1.

Broader Spectrum of Pathogen

A more diverse range of pathogens even in the nosocomial setting is expected. Also there is some specificity related to the category of immunocompromise. For example, *M avium-complex* infections are much more associated with late stages of HIV-1 infection than in solid organ, hematologic transplant, or patients treated with corticosteroid. Similarly, CT enhancing discrete brain lesions in patients with HIV-1 usually represent toxoplasmosis or central nervous system (CNS) lymphoma while such lesions are predominantly caused by mycelia (eg, *Aspergillus*) in solid organ recipients.

Susceptibility to the Environment

Immunocompromised hosts are exquisitely vulnerable to perturbations in their environment which may produce exposure to pathogens not problematic to immunocompetent hosts. Many such exposures are partly unavoidable in the community but can be controlled in the nosocomial and ICU settings. Thus, geographic- or temporal-clustering pathogen patterns need to be promptly recognized to control the source of the outbreak and are best avoided by having quality assured oversight of all environmental manipulations in the hospital setting. Routine isolation of all immunocompromised hosts is not indicated and may produce impediments to care.

Timing of Infection

There are characteristic time windows in which the likelihood of infection with some pathogens becomes greater. Classic examples are *Herpes simplex virus* (HSV) mucocutaneous infection during the early posttransplant period (weeks 1-4), and cytomegalovirus (CMV) -related illness peaking during the middle posttransplant period (months 1–6). Infections occurring during unanticipated times may be caused by the effects of heavier than usual immunosuppression, environmental hazards, or the use of antiinfective prophylaxis which can delay, but not prevent, an infection.

Aggressive Diagnostic Methods

The broader list of potential pathogens, which can produce the same clinical syndrome, coupled with the high potential for rapid deterioration without appropriate therapy favors a prompt and aggressive diagnostic methodology. Tissue biopsy, if done with appropriate safeguards, is often the quickest method to establish the diagnosis of infection and to avoid unnecessary and potentially toxic antiinfective treatments.

Early Appropriate Therapy

Delays in antimicrobial administration and source control are poorly tolerated in immunocompromised hosts with critical illness. Early empiric therapy needs to be tailored to the available clinical and epidemiologic evidence and should never be delayed for a pending diagnostic study.

INITIAL ASSESSMENT OF THE IMMUNOCOMPROMISED PATIENT

A pathogen-based discussion does not accurately emulate real clinical practice where the clinician initially only has knowledge of the type of immune defects and the patient's signs and symptoms suggestive of infection. There is a common ethic to the diagnostic assessment of the diverse population who meet the definition of immunocompromised host. The specific types of natural or acquired immune compromise predisposes such hosts to infection with a spectrum of pathogens which can be further differentiated based upon duration and severity of immunocompromise, or the net state of immunosuppression, prior community, nosocomial and latent epidemiologic exposures, including potentially selective antiinfective therapy, and the dominant clinical features **(Fig. 1)**. Prompt assessment of these factors can refine the clinician's differential diagnosis and direct the subsequent diagnostic workup, and if indicated, the choice of empiric treatment and isolation needs. Although the differential diagnosis may be more diverse than immunocompetent patients automatic triggering of broad microbiologic, serologic, and other specialized laboratory testing, which is not tailored to the specific host and clinical presentation is ineffective on a clinical and cost basis. The net state of immunosuppression includes prior iatrogenic and native immunosuppression, aggravating metabolic conditions, anatomic disruptions and foreign bodies, and other miscellaneous contributors **(Box 1)**. Certain easily measurable real-time indicators, such as the absolute neutrophil count and T-helper lymphocyte count, provide important information regarding risk level and probable pathogens in chemotherapy, induced neutropenia and HIV-1 infection respectively; however, the duration and etiology of neutropenia and lymphopenia is also integral to this determination. Thus, a solid organ recipient just rendered neutropenic from

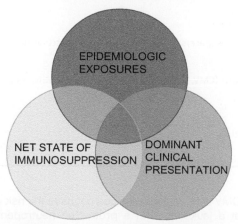

Fig. 1. Major clue categories in suspected infection in patients who are immunocompromised.

Box 1
Assessing the net state of immunosuppression

Iatrogenic immunosuppression (timing, dose, duration)

Corticosteroid (dose and duration)

Myelosuppressive chemotherapy

Calcineurin inhibitors

TNF-antagonists

Antimetabolite

Monoclonal, polyclonal anti-lymphocyte therapy

Radiation

Native immunosuppression

Human immunodeficiency virus

Lymphoma, leukemia, myeloma

Hypogammaglobulinemia

Other humoral deficiency states

Postsplenectomy state or functional asplenia

Autoimmune disease

Metabolic conditions

Diabetes mellitus

Hepatic insufficiency or frank cirrhosis

Renal failure

Iron overload states

Malnutrition

Anatomic barrier disruptions

Temporary or long term vascular access

Bladder catheterization

Peritoneal dialysis access

Surgical drains

Wounds or decubitus ulcers

Permanent foreign bodies (pacers, prosthetic joints, endovascular graft, valves)

Miscellaneous

Immunomodulatory virus (CMV, Epstein-Barr virus [EBV], hepatitis B,C)

Recent blood products

Solid tumors

Total parenteral nutrition

Pregnancy

---

recent treatment of CMV with ganciclovir does not have the risk exposure for opportunistic infection that a leukemic with a protracted neutropenic nadir caused by myelosuppressive and mucolytic chemotherapy. The epidemiologic history entails the exposure history of the host to potential microbial pathogens (**Box 2**). An

---

Box 2
Major data elements in assessing the epidemiologic exposure of the immunocompromised host

Community exposure

Influenza outbreak

Known exposure to transmissible source patient (M. tuberculosis, varicella)

Pet or other animal, rodent exposure

Travel to tropical or subtropical areas

Origin from geography with endemic infection

Food borne illness outbreaks

Mosquito, tick, or other insect vectors

Nosocomial exposure

Surveillance cultures (nasal swabs – methicillin-resistant *S aureus*[MRSA], rectal swabs-vancomycin-resistant enterococci [VRE])

Cultures from clinical sites

Endemic pattern of resistant bacteria

Recent epidemic outbreaks (eg, Legionella)

Exposure to antimicrobials selective for multidrug resistant (MDR) organisms

Recent construction

Latent or dormant pathogens

Serology (T pallidum, Herpesviruses, toxoplasmosis, Coccioides immitis, Histoplasma capsulatum, Blastomyces dermatitidis, Cryptococcus neoformans)

Skin testing (M tuberculosis [ppd], C immitis)

Saprophytic colonization (Aspergillus spp)

Other important exposures

Donor organ or nonvisceral tissue

Blood products

Antimicrobial exposure for treatment or prophylaxis

---

immunocompromised host may develop an infection with a specific pathogen but prior exposure to the pathogen is an obligate requirement for such infection to develop. Evidence of prior contact or harboring of a pathogen may be inferred from the history and prior available testing; however, often this cannot be discerned particularly for ubiquitous nongeographic pathogens, such as *Cryptococcus neoformans*, *Nocardia, P jiroveci, Aspergillus* spp or other saprophytic commensals with low intrinsic virulence. Depending upon the clinical presentation of the immunocompromised host, only certain data elements are needed to develop a differential diagnosis, diagnostic plan, and treatment regimen. Moreover, some information may not be obtainable because of limitations of obtaining a history or retrieving serologic testing results from the distant past. Medical centers with large immunocompromised cohorts, such as bone marrow or solid organ transplantation recipients increasingly maintain the relevant epidemiologic history in a retrievable database format which expedites the determination of distant epidemiologic exposure. Establishing the location or locations of an infection requires a meticulous history taking with particular attention to exposures and the rapidity of onset for the clinical syndrome (ie, acute, subacute, chronic, relapsing). Physical examination should devote close attention to the skin and mucosa, lymph nodes, catheter-entry sites, surgical incisions and wounds, and subtle neurologic signs.

COMMON CLINICAL PRESENTATIONS

Although there is a diverse number of opportunistic pathogens which may cause invasive disease in the immunocompromised host, there are a finite number of stereotypical presentations or syndromes (**Box 3**). Systemic signs of infection coupled with respiratory insufficiency/failure and radiographic infiltrates, altered sensorium with

---

Box 3
Common clinical syndromes caused by opportunistic infection in the immunocompromised host

Fever with or without localizing signs/symptoms

Sepsis with or without localizing signs/symptoms

Respiratory tract infection

- focal cavitary or noncavitary lesion(s)
- diffuse interstitial or alveolar infiltrates
- tracheobronchitis

Mucocutaneous

- stomatitis, esophagitis
- diffuse rash
- discrete skin lesions

Central nervous system

- encephalitis
- meningitis
- meningoencephalitis
- focal signs (seizure)

Gastrointestinal

- diarrhea
- obstruction
- perforation
- hemorrhage

Disseminated syndromes ($\geq$2 tissues)

- lymphatic
- mucocutaneous
- lung
- gastrointestinal tract
- central nervous system
- bone marrow

or without focal neurologic signs and fever/sepsis of unknown origin are two characteristic presentations which usually culminate in ICU admission and merit discussion herein. In addition, disseminated presentations include pulmonary, central nervous system (*Nocardia*, aspergillosis and other mycelia, cryptococcosis), pulmonary and mucocutaneous lesions (histoplasmosis, aspergillosis), lymphatic-visceral disease (EBV mediated posttransplant lymphoproliferative disease), and candidiasis, which can present with cutaneous, joint, bone, ocular, and hepatosplenic invasion. It is especially important to realize that patients who present with a single organ involvement, such as a pulmonary lesion, may be in the incipient stages of dissemination to noncontiguous extrapulmonary organs, which only manifests with time and may alter the diagnostic plan.

Respiratory Insufficiency/Failure and Pulmonary Infiltrates

The patient who is immunocompromised and requiring ICU care for respiratory compromise and pulmonary infiltrates is a common complication and associated with high mortality rates of 30% to 90%.[7–11] Although noninfectious causes (radiation, chemotherapy, sirolimus, diffuse alveolar hemorrhage, idiopathic pneumonitis, acute respiratory distress syndrome, pulmonary edema, pulmonary emboli, or rejection in the lung recipient) are not uncommon, infectious etiologies remain the prime concern and require primary diagnostic and empiric treatment considerations. The differential of infectious etiologies based upon host category and radiographic pattern is summarized in **Table 1**. However, no radiographic pattern is pathognomic for a specific pathogen in any host category. Plain-chest films are useful as screening tests but too

Table 1
Likely respiratory pathogens in specific immunocompromised- host categories based upon presenting radiographic pattern

	Diffuse Interstitial-Alveolar	Lobar-Segmental	Reticulonodular	Discrete Nodule
Chemotherapy-induced granulocytopenia	CMV (ALL)	Bacterial	—	Bacterial Aspergillus Other mycelia
Bone marrow transplant	P jiroveci CMV RSV Influenzae Adenovirus	Bacterial Legionella RSV Influenzae	Nocardia	Aspergillus Other mycelia M tuberculosis Nocardia
Solid organ transplant	CMV Influenza, RSV, adenovirus, P jiroveci	Bacterial Legionella RSV Influenzae	Nocardia M tuberculosis Nontuberculous mycobacteria	Aspergillus Other mycelia M tuberculosis Nocardia PTLD (EBV)
HIV-1	P jiroveci CMV	Bacterial Rhodococcus equi Cryptococcus	P jiroveci Histoplasmosis Cryptococcus MAI	Bacterial M tuberculosis P jirovecii (rare) Cryptococcus Histoplasmosis Other endemic fungi

insensitive to rule out a pulmonary diagnosis. Studies with paired plain-chest films and chest CT scans (**Fig. 2**) revealed lesions not visualized on plain films in 50% of neutropenic and renal transplant recipients respectively.[12,13] Secondly, CT scans may guide subsequent semi-invasive or invasive pulmonary testing to a lung area with higher diagnostic yield. Fiber optic bronchoscopy with bronchoalveolar lavage (BAL) remains the procedure of choice with an excellent safety profile.[14] The sensitivity varies based upon the immunocompromised host category, pathogen, the infecting pathogen, and the postcollection microbiologic detection methods employed. Because of higher organism loads *P jiroveci* and mycobacterial infection are more easily detected with BAL in patients infected with HIV-1. The diagnostic sensitivity for *Aspergillus* and other fungi is lower but superior to the sensitivity of sputum or endotracheal aspirates.[15,16] Protected specimen brushing techniques have much lower diagnostic sensitivity than BAL and are associated with a higher hemorrhagic risk in coagulopathic patients.[14,17] Transbronchial biopsy may improve diagnostic sensitivity in patients with diffuse infiltrates that were negative by BAL, fungal and mycobacterial infection, and for the diagnosis of noninfectious causes of Pulmonary infiltrates (eg, lung rejection, post

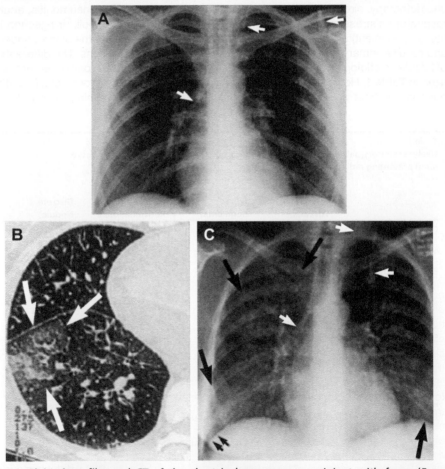

Fig. 2. Plain chest film and CT of the chest in bone marrow recipient with fever. (*From* Heussel CP, Kauczor HU, Heussel G, et al. Early detection of pneumonia in febrile neutropenic patients: Use of thin-section CT. AJR 1997;169:1347–53; with permission.)

engraftment syndrome, idiopathic pneumonitis, graft versus host disease, and bronchiolitis obliterans). Focal lesions for which BAL was nondiagnostic may best be approached with either CT guided needle. For enigmatic cases, open lung biopsy may be performed, however its use needs to be tempered by the high-complication rate particularly in neutropenic and bone marrow transplant recipients and the overall low rate of significant alterations in management and outcome.[18,19] Visual-assisted thorascopic biopsy may be a safer alternative in patients with pleural, subpleural lesions, or diffuse lung infiltrates[20] Nonpulmonary adjunctive tests can include blood cultures, isolator (centrifugation-lysis) tube for mycobacteria and fungi, urine legionella RIA, blood CMV, polymerase chain reaction (PCR) or antigenemia, serum galactomannan assay, serum cryptococcal antigen latex agglutination and histoplasmosis mycelial phase antigen.

Central Nervous System

In critically ill immunocompromised hosts, neurologic changes may be an accompanying finding of sepsis from non-CNS infection. stroke, metabolic (hypoxemia, hypercapnia, hyponatremia, hypernatremia, uremia, hypoglycemia, hyperglycemia), or drug-related side effects. Unless a clear etiology can be rapidly established, appropriate CNS diagnostics, and in certain cases empiric antiinfective coverage, are indicated.[21] Noncontrast head CT imaging can be done quickly and is adequately sensitive to rule out hemorrhage, cerebral edema, subdural processes and mass effect which would otherwise contraindicate lumbar puncture. Gadolinium-enhanced MR imaging is superior to contrast-enhanced brain CT scans for the detection of small abscesses, white matter lesions, meningeal changes consistent with infection or inflammation, and evaluation of the brainstem and vertebral column spinal-cord anatomy.[22,23] Cerebrospinal fluid must be obtained for appropriate stains (eg, Gram's, India ink, acid-fast), cultures, antigen detection for C neoformans, and PCR for HSV, CMV, human herpesvirus(HHV)-6. Other diagnostic tools include electroencephalogram to evaluate for seizures or temporal localization consistent with HSV encephalitis, serology for CNS pathogens (cryptococcal antigen, histoplasmosis antigen, CMV and HHV-6 PCR) and blood cultures (L monotytogenes, S pneumoniae, Cryptococcus neoformans). The likely pathogens related to host category and clinical presentation are summarized in **Table 2**. Nuchal rigidity, focal neurologic deficits (seizures, paresis, or paralysis), diminished level of consciousness, bizarre personality changes, progressive cognitive decline, visual changes, and headache or localized back pain, are all indicative of possible CNS infection or inflammation. An acute presentation with frank meningismus and a clear sensorium should be considered a pyogenic meningitis (N meningitides, S pneumnoniae, H influenzae) in any host, but among patients who are immunocompromised, it is most associated with markedly impaired humoral immunity. Listeria must be considered for any acute or subacute meningoencephalitic presentation in cancer, solid organ and hematologic transplant recipients, or other patients with cell-mediated immunodeficiency.[24] The incidence of listeriosis has fallen over the past two decades, which has been attributed to the uniform use of trimethoprim/sulfa (tmp/smx), however it is not established that tmp/smx offers complete protection against this sporadic infection. Thus, ampicillin needs to be included in any empiric regimen when this pathogen is a consideration. Most cerebral abscesses occur in the gray or gray-white matter territory, are ring enhancing, and usually present as a new focal deficit, seizure, or a meningoencephalitis. Although the differential is broad, it can be narrowed based upon the host category. Fungal etiologies (Aspergillus, other mycelia) predominate in organ recipients while Toxoplasma gondii continues to be the predominant pathogen in HIV-1 disease

Table 2
Likely central nervous system pathogens in specific immunocompromised-host categories based upon presentation

	Meningitis	Meningoencephalitis	Encephalitis	Mass Lesion
Chemotherapy-induced granulocytopenia	S pneumoniae S aureus E coli P aeruginosa S aureus	L monocytogenes	HSV	Aspergillus Nocardia Cryptococcus Pyogenic bacteria
Bone marrow transplant	—	L monocytogenes C neoformans S stercoralis HHV-6	HSV CMV Varicella zoster virus (VZV) West Nile virus JC virus	Aspergillus Zygomycetes P boydii, other mycelia Nocardia Endemic mycoses M tuberculosis T gondii
Solid organ transplant	—	L monocytogenes C neoformans S stercoralis HHV-6	HSV CMV VZV West Nile virus JC virus	Aspergillus P boydii, other mycelia Nocardia Endemic mycoses M tuberculosis PTLD
HIV-1	S pneumoniae	T gondii	JC virus	T gondii M tuberculosis Endemic mycoses C neoformans
B-lymphocyte defects	S pneumoniae H influenzae N meningitides	—	—	—

even with highly active antiretroviral therapy (HAART) exposure. Cryptococcal meningitis is seen in both populations but cryptococcomas are much more frequent in the latter. Cerebral abscesses usually do not produce cerebrospinal fluid (CSF) changes unless the lesion communicates with the ventricular or subarachnoid spaces. Discrete white matter lesions have a narrower differential including calcineurin-induced demyelination usually in the posterior territory and progressive multifocal leukoencephalopathy (*JC papova* virus) which is characteristically nonenhancing and without mass effect. Thus, CT-guided stereotactic biopsy is required for approachable discrete lesions to obtain tissue histology and cultures, if a diagnosis cannot be established with other methods.

Considerations for specific immunocompromised host categories

Cancer and chemotherapy-associated neutropenia Although the duration and severity of neutropenia remains the most easily measured and dominant immune defect, oncologic patients requiring ICU care are usually a composite of multiple-compromised host defenses including anatomic breeches, cell-mediated, and humoral immunodeficiencies, which may alter diagnostic and empiric management strategy. Antiinfective prophylaxis and early initiation of broad spectrum antimicrobial therapy in the febrile neutropenic has resulted in shorter febrile duration, fewer culture-documented bloodstream and nonbloodstream infections, and lowered mortality in the culture negative and culture positive subsets. There remain residual controversies and variations in practice across oncology centers in the United States and Europe. A recent meta-analysis of 46 trials (7642 subjects) comparing combination therapy to monotherapy (mostly a third generation cephalosporin or carbapenem) in febrile neutropenia showed comparable survival, however there was a significantly lower incidence of adverse events in the monotherapy group primarily caused by a lower incidence of nephrotoxicity.[25] A second meta-analysis of 33 trials which only examined monotherapy showed improved survival and fewer treatment modifications with carbapenem monotherapy compared with third generation cephalosporins but an increased rate of pseudomembranous colitis in the carbapenem groups.[26] Thus although such large scale data favors monotherapy and perhaps carbapenem monotherapy, the choice of empiric febrile coverage in the neutropenic continues to be governed by local sensitivity data and perceived efficacy and tolerance issues. However most of this important data has not analyzed patients who resided in the ICU at the onset of fever or required ICU admission in the follow-up period. Such patients remain a subset for which standardized evidence-based recommendations are lacking. For instance, the empiric inclusion of vancomycin as part of the initial empiric fever coverage regimen has clearly been shown not to confer improved survival.[27] However, empiric addition of vancomycin is quite prudent in a neutropenic patient admitted to the ICU with sepsis of unknown origin, new infiltrates, or a suspected catheter-related infection. Several other important considerations need to be entertained including breakthrough bloodstream or nonbloodstream infection with a multidrug bacteria not covered by a quinolone prophylactic regimen (S viridans, enterococci, MRSA), the empiric regimen (ESBL, P aeruginosa, A baumanii, MRSA, VRE), a yeast or mycelial infection, or a discrete anatomic focus (retained central venous catheter, typhlitis, perirectal abscess). Thus a neutropenic patient on a third generation cephalosporin with de novo septic shock might require initiation of an antipseudomonal carbapenem and an aminoglycoside, and addition of vancomycin (if MRSA colonized or suspected), linezolid or daptomycin (if VRE colonized or suspected based upon the endemic pattern) and *Candida* coverage with a glucan synthetase inhibitor or polyene.

Nontunneled central vascular catheters in place for more than 3 days should be considered for removal in frankly septic patients without an obvious other source of infection as the absence of local signs and symptoms are notoriously insensitive in the neutropenic host. In patients with cancer with candidemia, the likelihood that fungemia is secondary to a non-catheter source is higher particularly in patients with prior chemotherapy or corticosteroids in the prior month.[28] Removal of a tunneled long-term vascular catheter may be considered in the presence of local changes, frank sepsis and bacteremia with the exception of low grade virulent organism such as coagulase-negative staphylococci where antibiotic lock therapy or systemic therapy may be tried. Abdominal distension and tenderness should prompt suspicion of either typhlitis (ileocecitis) or C difficile colitis even in the absence of frank diarrhea. Suspected typhlitis (ileocecitis) should be confirmed with CT imaging and covered with the addition of metronidazole and antifungal therapy for Candida coverage.

Hematologic transplant recipients Before the 1990s the reported outcome of hematologic transplant recipients who required ICU admission for either infectious or noninfectious posttransplant complications was dismal with hospital survival of only 13% to 23% and survival less than 3% to 7% in the subset requiring mechanical ventilation.[29,30] In more recent years, refinements in pretransplant conditioning, post bone-marrow prophylaxis and preemptive antiinfective strategies for CMV and fungi, improved management of graft-versus-host disease (GVHD), and the advent of peripheral and umbilical cord stem-cell transplantation coupled with advances in critical-care management have resulted in still low, but improved, hospital survival up to 44%.[31] Although severe infection is a common reason for ICU admission, there are a diverse number of reasons why such transplant recipients require intensive care support other than infection including respiratory disease pulmonary edema, diffuse alveolar hemorrhage, idiopathic pneumonitis, cardiogenic or hemorrhagic shock, venoocclusive disease and GVHD (**Fig. 3**).[32] The usual temporal pattern of expected pathogens during the neutropenic-preengraftment phase (2-4 weeks), early postengraftment (4 weeks–3 months) where cell mediated and humoral deficiencies predominate and late postengraftment phase (>3 months) and beyond 6 months where chronic GVHD and severe community acquired infections are more common. Preengraftment period risks for infections are dominated by protracted neutropenia, mucocutaneous barrier disruptions and respiratory failure leading to nosocomial infection. Bone-marrow recipients requiring ICU admission are highly impacted by the local MDR microflora, which are flora with organisms that breakthrough, or are selected for, ongoing or prior antimicrobials exposure. A trend favoring gram-positive bloodstream infection established in the 1990s has begun to change toward gram-negative organisms in recent years.[33,34]

Coverage for methicillin-resistant Staphylococcus aureus with vancomycin and multidrug resistance Enterobactericae, P aeuriginosa usually with a carbapenem and aminoglycoside is indicated in recipients with sepsis of unknown origin. Prior colonization with VRE or an endemic pattern of VRE indicate the need for coverage with linezolid although use of this agent for greater than 7 to 10 days could prolong the duration of myelosuppression. Alternatives include daptomycin, except for suspected pulmonary infection, and tigecycline, although there is very limited efficacy data at present. Streptococcal sepsis caused by S viridans has become more common in such patients receiving quinolone or ampicillin prophylaxis after either autologous or allogeneic transplantation.[35,36] Vancomycin is the empiric and definitive therapy of choice, however this syndrome carries a significant mortality rate if complicated by protracted

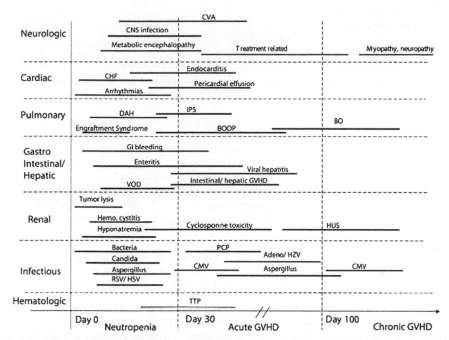

Fig. 3. Temporal relationship of stem-cell transplantation with complications that can result in critical illness. (*From* Soubani AO. Critical care considerations of hematopoietic stem-cell transplantation. Crit Care Med 2006;34(Suppl):S251–67; with permission.)

neutropenia. Candidemia may occur in up to 10% to 15% of recipients and is most common during the neutropenic period. Although fluconazole prophylaxis has lowered the incidence of deep and superficial candidiasis the clinician must consider using a polyene or glucan synthetase inhibitor in patients who are azole-exposed patients empirically before speciation and susceptibilities are available.[37,38] Nonbacterial major respiratory tract infections include aspergillosis and other mycelia and viruses (CMV, respiratory syncytial virus (RSV), influenzae and parainfluenzae). *Aspergillus* has two peak periods: during the neutropenic period affecting allogeneic and autologous recipients and during the postengraftment period in patients who are allogeneic. Risk factors among allogeneic recipients include a positive pretransplant CMV serology and delayed engraftment. Nodular densities or a halo-sign on CT chest scan are sufficient evidence to initiate empiric therapy for *Aspergillus* with voriconazole although a mycologic diagnosis is still needed to rule out a non-Aspergillus mycelium or nonfungal pathogen (eg, *P aeruginosa, S aureus, Nocardia, Mycobacteria*). Broad combination antifungal therapy, which includes an amphotericin compound, seems to be a rationale approach which includes in the unstable patient with a clinical and radiologic picture compatible with fungal infection. Recent retrospective data has shown improved outcomes with combination of voriconazole and caspofungin in refractory aspergillosis cases, however this approach has not yet been validated with a prospective trial.[39]

Solid organ transplant recipients Infection following solid organ transplantation is still best characterized by discrete but potentially overlapping posttransplant time intervals during which the need for intensive care support is not uncommon (**Fig. 4**).[40] Early

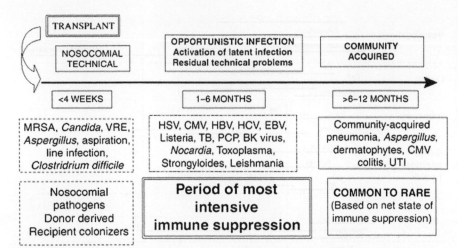

Fig. 4. Timeline of posttransplant infections following solid organ transplantation. (*From* Gabrielli A, Layon AJ, Mihae Y. Civetta, Taylor and Kirby's Critical Care. 4th edition. Philadelphia: Lippincott Williams & Wilkins; 2009; with permission.)

postoperative infections are predominantly related to the anatomic breeches from the transplant surgery itself (wound, vascular, excretory and other donor-recipient anastomoses) and from invasive access devices (bladder drainage, vascular access catheters, and ventilator or hospital-associated respiratory tract infection). There is a strong predisposition for serious infections to be localized to the allograft or periallograft caused by either normally expected dysfunction of the graft or technical complications (**Table 3**). For instance, among solid organ recipients, pulmonary infections are most common after lung transplantation, because of allograft contact with the airborne environment, impaired lymphatic drainage and mucociliary clearance, diminished cough reflex, and organisms in the donor-lung flora which are transmitted with transplantation.[41] *Staphylococcus aureus, P aeruginosa* and *Enterobactericiae* are most

Table 3
Early infections related to technical allograft complications following solid organ transplantation

Type Transplant	Complication
Kidney	Ureteral anastomotic leak
	Ureteral stenosis
	Perinephric collection
	Vascular anastomotic leak
Pancreas	Leak at enteric anastomosis
	Ischemic pancreatitis
Liver	Biliary leak
	Hepatic artery stenosis/thrombus
	Infected hematoma
Intestinal	Obstruction
	Leak at proximal or distal anastomosis
	Severe translocation caused by ischemia
Heart	Mediastinitis
	Sternal wound infection
Lung	Tracheal or bronchial dehiscence
	Pleural collection

common although early pneumonia caused by *Burkholderia cepacia* and *Aspergillus* are well described in patients with cystic fibrosis who may have pretransplant respiratory-tract colonization with these organisms.[42] Bronchoscopic techniques are needed to enhance diagnostic sensitivity but also to examine the tracheal or bronchial anastomotic sites and perform transbronchial biopsy to assess for rejection.

In all solid organ transplant types, allograft dysfunction coupled with either local or systemic signs of infection are the most common presentation which should raise suspicion of a technical allograft complication (**Box 4**) with post preservation injury and early allograft rejection also in the differential. Management requires prompt surgical correction or in some cases radiologic-assisted drainage or decompression and appropriate antimicrobial therapy. The microbial pathogens in the early period originate from the recipient's endogenous or modified endogenous flora caused by the effects of antimicrobial exposure and contacts with the health-care environment. Thus, the endemic pattern of resistance at the transplant center and the recipient's recent antimicrobial exposures should be factored when making empiric treatment decisions in the febrile or septic solid organ patient. Increasingly, transplant centers are performing admission and weekly surveillance cultures for problematic multidrug-resistant bacteria (MRSA, VRE, ESBL, and MDR *P aeruginosa* or *Acinetobacter)* principally to direct enhanced isolation precautions, however such data can also guide empiric coverage when clinical site cultures are not yet available. Less commonly documented are occult incubating infection before the transplant that may become manifest in the early posttransplant period particularly with the introduction of high doses of induction chemotherapy. Rarely, bloodstream and nonbloodstream infections which were present in the ante mortem donor can be transmitted, although usually notification

---

Box 4
Specific infectious disease considerations for solid organ transplant recipients

Lung Transplant

Highest risk for pneumonia

Highest risk for aspergillosis

Longest risk period for CMV and P jiroveci

Burkholderia cepacia more frequent in patients with cystic fibrosis

Infections at the tracheal or bronchial anastomosis

Liver transplant

Highest incidence of Candida infection

VRE infections common in endemic centers

Intra-abdominal sepsis

Kidney transplant

BK polyoma virus causing ureteral stenosis, hemorrhagic cystitis, interstitial nephritis

Lowest overall incidence of infection

Heart transplant

T. gondii myocarditis in seronegative recipients of seropositive donors

Intestinal transplants

Highest incident of post-transplant lymphoproliferative disease

Translocation-induced sepsis syndrome with concurrent rejection/ischemia

of the transplant center is made so tailored preemptive treatment can be initiated.[43] Thus, it is important for the transplant coordinator or organ procurement agency to retrieve such information from the center where the organ was harvested.

Beyond the first posttransplant month the aggregate effects of iatrogenic immunosuppression coupled with the distant and recent epidemiologic exposures of the recipient shifts the pathogen spectrum although residual early infections may persist in patients with poor allograft function who remained hospitalized for a prolonged period. Although there are many similarities across different organ transplant types, there remain organ-specific patterns which are summarized in **Table 2**. Despite prophylactic and preemptive antiviral strategies with either ganciclovir or valganciclovir, CMV still remains a dominant pathogen during the middle posttransplant period with effects ranging from invasive disease, allograft dysfunction and rejection, and superinfection with other pathogens.[44–47] Mismatched donor-recipient CMV pairing resulting in primary CMV infection carries the highest risk of serious invasive disease and relapse.[48,49] CMV reactivation has also been associated with concurrent critical illness from non-CMV disease and appears to be mediated by proinflammatory cytokines and subsequent immune downregulation.[50,51] Hepatitis, pneumonitis, and gastroenteritis remain the most common sites, which can be confirmed with biopsy and histology, although increasingly rapidly elevating serum markers (antigenemia, PCR) are the earliest virologic prompt for anti-CMV treatment. The immunosuppressive burden and CMV history closely predicts the incidence and severity of other infections including fungal, bacterial, and other viral pathogens.[40] Diagnostic workup and empiric coverage in the critically ill recipient depend upon the specifics of the clinical presentation and immunosuppressive-epidemiologic history.

HIV-1 infection Respiratory failure caused by respiratory tract infection secondary to *P jiroveci* was the leading cause of admission to the ICU from the first appearance of HIV-1 in 1981 until the advent of HAART in the mid 1990s coupled with universal chemoprophylaxis for pneumocystosis.[1] A recent survey of 281 patients with HIV-1 requiring ICU admission from 2000 to 2004 at San Francisco General Hospital showed a decline in the incidence of respiratory failure from 52% (2000) to 34% (2004) and a parallel decline in the incidence of *P jiroveci*.[2] Although the incidence of *P jiroveci* pneumonitis was reduced with HAART, there was no influence on hospital survival indicative of the absence of short-term benefits in critical illness. Greater likelihood of *P jiroveci* is also associated with antiretroviral resistance, lower T-helper lymphocyte counts, and noncompliance with chemoprophylaxis. Thus, the contemporaneous assessment of the patient with HIV-1 who requires ICU admission for respiratory failure and suspected respiratory infection must include whether the patient is receiving HAART and chemoprophylaxis, although whether this influences early diagnostic and empiric therapy strategies is unclear. Pulmonary radiographic patterns are notably less specific for particular pathogens in HIV-1– related illness as there is a higher frequency of variant or atypical presentations. These include diffuse opacities *(P jiroveci,* bacterial pneumonia, *M tuberculosis,* nontuberculous mycobacteria, Kaposi's sarcoma, fungal, CMV), nodular densities (*M tuberculosis* and atypical mycobacteria, Kaposi's sarcoma, *P jiroveci,* and fungi, and cavitary lesions *M tuberculosis, P jiroveci, P aeruginosa, Rhodococcus equi* and fungi). The development of a pneumothorax is strongly suggestive of *P jiroveci* infection unless a recent transbronchial biopsy was performed. Bacterial pneumonia either caused by community or nosocomial pathogens is another prominent consideration in the patient with HIV-1 with a respiratory picture suggestive of infection.[52,53] Health care-associated pathogens are more likely caused by the long-term exposure of patients with HIV to the health-care environment and antimicrobials. Thus, empiric coverage of the rapidly deteriorating patient with HIV-1 with respiratory compromise requires combination antimicrobial coverage for health care-associated bacteria including *P aeruginosa* and *Enterobactericiae* and *P jiroveci* in patients who are at risk until adequate diagnostics are performed and stains and cultures are available.

Immune reconstitution inflammatory syndrome (IRIS) occurring weeks after the initiation of HAART may occasionally be severe enough to precipitate respiratory failure although it can also indicate latent or incipient mycobacterial disease.[54,55] Consideration of IRIS still requires BAL and transbronchial biopsy to rule out occult infections. Management of IRIS is usually with a tapering course of corticosteroids. Finally, despite longer term benefits, initiating HAART in patients who are critically ill recovering from serious infection is problematic because of its interaction with multiple other medications, unpredictable gastrointestinal absorption, and the potential to precipitate an IRIS syndrome with recent infection.[1]

MANAGEMENT OF IATROGENIC IMMUNOSUPPRESSION

Withdrawal or rapid tapering of iatrogenic immunosuppression, particularly corticosteroids, is a well-described option particularly in organ transplant recipients with rapid deterioration caused by life-threatening infection or posttransplant lymphoproliferative disease.[56,57] However there are several mitigating factors which need to be considered on a case-by-case basis:

Is allograft rejection already occurring? Unexplained allograft dysfunction should be investigated with a biopsy to rule out active acute or chronic rejection which might require even enhanced immunosuppression.

What has been the allograft tolerance of the recipient? Patients with relapsing episodes of rejection may be put on alternative antirejection therapy in lieu of corticosteroids.

Can the allograft be sacrificed with fallback on an artificial support? Examples include pancreas (insulin therapy), renal transplant (dialysis) and small bowel transplant (parenteral nutrition).

Will withdrawal of corticosteroids culminate in adrenal insufficiency? Induction doses of corticosteroids and only short-term maintenance periods predictably suppress pituitary corticotropin secretion and adrenal responsiveness quite early. Abrupt withdrawal of iatrogenic steroids may precipitate or aggravate an absolute or relative state of adrenal insufficiency well described in critically ill septic patients. Random cortisol or corticotropin stimulation tests may not help identify patients who could benefit from adjunctive steroid therapy. Thus, clinical discrimination focused on the pressor requirements to maintain hemodynamic stability in the patient who has been volume-resuscitated is the most rationale cue as to the need for adjunctive steroids or allowance for tapering or withdrawing steroid therapy.

Are corticosteroids separately indicated to manage inflammatory mediated changes (moderate to severe *P jiroveci* pneumonitis or immune reconstitution syndrome), or localized, but clinically significant edema (cerebral toxoplasmosis) mediated caused by the original infection.

PROTECTIVE ISOLATION AND SPECIAL PRECAUTIONS

Despite the higher prevalence of multidrug resistant bacteria in the ICU, more severe illness of the immunocompromised host requiring ICU care, the vast majority of immunocompromised hosts requiring intensive care do not routinely require protective or reverse isolation. The intent of protective isolation is to prevent the acquisition of exogenous organisms by maintaining them in a single room, with a closed door to limit entry, coupled with ambient positive pressure. Such practices have usually been limited to neutropenic patients and pre-engraftment bone-marrow transplant recipients. However the majority of infections in these hosts arise from their endogenous colonizing microflora. Thus, although reverse isolation remains a common and traditional practice even in the ICU, its use is not based upon a strong evidence level.[58] Airborne mycelia spores, particularly *Aspergillus*, are a notable exception; however, only laminar-flow rooms with high-efficiency particular-air filtration filters have been shown to reduce the incidence of aspergillosis in patients with hematologic-oncologic/bone-marrow transplant.[59] Most ICU do have such dedicated technology.

Conversely, special isolation precautions however are frequently indicated in immunocompromised hosts both on an empiric basis and for definitive isolation of specific organisms potentially transmissible to other patients. Negatively pressurized ICU rooms with an ante-room are required for suspected or documented infections transmissible through air including *M tuberculosis, influenzae* and *varicella-zoster*. Delayed respiratory isolation has resulted in catastrophic spread of *M tuberculosis,* particularly source patients infected with HIV-1.[60]

EMERGING TRENDS AMONG IMMUNOCOMPROMISED HOSTS RELEVANT TO ICU PRACTICE

Multidrug-resistant bacteria, particularly from the nosocomial setting, have become more prevalent among immunocompromised hosts because of their greater time exposure to the health-care environment and selective pressure from prophylactic and therapeutic anti-infective exposure. Since the 1990s, VRE has become a prominent pathogen in oncologic and liver-transplant recipients although its clinical impact has diminished somewhat with the use of linezolid therapy. Early reports of linezolid-resistant enterococci occurred predominantly in immunocompromised hosts who resided in an ICU.[61,62] Severe *C difficile* colitis has increased in recent years related to fluoroquinolone use across all patient categories, but it manifests higher severity and relapse rates among immunocompromised hosts.[63] Long-term exposure to fluconazole may favor the emergence of *Candida* species which exhibit either dose-dependent susceptibility (*C glabrata*) or resistance (*C glabrata, C krusei*). Thus, *Candida* speciation and azole susceptibility testing are advised in such settings. Breakthrough infection with *Zygomycoses* has been reported among hematologic-transplant recipients receiving voriconazole prophylaxis, although the net benefit of voriconazole still appears favorable.[64,65] Despite the monolithic use of ganciclovir for CMV-related illness, reports of CMV-resistant strains have been mostly limited to long-term usage in patients with HIV-1 and lung recipients receiving protracted courses for recurrent pneumonitis.[66,67]

REFERENCES

1. Rosen MJ, Narasimhan M. Critical care of immunocompromised patients: human immunodeficiency virus. Crit Care Med 2006;34(Suppl):S245–50.
2. Powell K, Davis JL, Morris AM, et al. Survival for patients with HIV admitted to the ICU continues to improve in the current era of combination antiretroviral therapy. Chest 2009;135:11–7.
3. Bernard GR, Vincent JL, Laterre PF, et al. Efficacy and safety of recombinant human activated protein C for severe sepsis. N Engl J Med 2001;344:699–709.

4. Annane D, Sebille V, Charpentier C, et al. Effect of treatment with low doses of hydrocortisone and fludrocortisone on mortality in patients with septic shock. JAMA 2002;288:862–71.
5. Rivers E, Nguyen B, Havstad S, et al. Early goal directed therapy in the treatment of severe sepsis and septic shock. N Engl J Med 2001;345:1368–77.
6. The Acute Respiratory Distress Syndrome Network. Ventilation with lower tidal volumes as compared with traditional tidal volumes for acute lung injury and the acute respiratory distress syndrome. N Engl J Med 2000;342: 1301–8.
7. Shorr AF, Sulsa GM, O'Grady NP. Pulmonary infiltrates in the non-HIV infected immunocompromised patient. Etiologies, diagnostic strategies and outcomes. Chest 2004;125:260–71.
8. Shorr AF, Moores LK, Edenfield WJ, et al. Mechanical ventilation in hematopoietic stem cell transplantation: can we effectively predict outcomes? Chest 1999;116: 1012–8.
9. Hilbert G, Gruson D, Varges F, et al. Non-invasive ventilation in immunosuppressed patients with pulmonary infiltrates, fever and acute respiratory failure. N Engl J Med 2001;344:481–7.
10. Duran FG, Piqueras B, Romero M, et al. Pulmonary complications following orthotopic liver transplant. Transpl Int 1998;11(Suppl 1):S255–9.
11. Kotloff RM, Ahya VN, Crawford SW. Pulmonary complications of solid organ and hematopoietic stem cell transplantation. Am J Respir Crit Care Med 2004;170: 22–48.
12. Heussel CP, Kauczor HU, Heussel G, et al. Early detection of pneumonia in febrile neutropenic patients: use of thin-section CT. AJR Am J Roentgenol 1997;169: 1347–53.
13. Barloon JT, Galvin JR, Mori M, et al. High-resolution ultrafast chest CT in the management of febrile bone marrow transplant patients with normal or nonspecific chest roentgenograms. Chest 1991;99:928–33.
14. Jain P, Sandur S, Meli Y, et al. Role of fiber optic bronchoscopy in immunocompromised patients with lung infiltrates. Chest 2004;125:712–22.
15. Paterson DL, Singh N. Invasive aspergillosis in transplant recipients. Medicine 1999;78:128–38.
16. Paterson TF, Kirkpatrick WR, White M, et al. Invasive aspergillosis: disease spectrum, treatment practices, and outcomes. Medicine 2000;79:250–60.
17. Rano A, Agusti C, Jimenez P, et al. Pulmonary infiltrates in non-HIV immunocompromised patients; a diagnostic approach using non invasive and bronchoscopic procedures. Thorax 2001;56:379–87.
18. White DA, Wong PW, Downey R. The utility of open lung biopsy in patients with hematologic malignancies. Am J Respir Crit Care Med 2002;161:723–9.
19. Weill D, McGriffin DC, Zorn GL, et al. The utility of open lung biopsy following lung transplantation. J Heart Lung Transplant 2000;19:852–7.
20. Feins RH. The role of thoracoscopy in the AIDS/immunocompromised patient. Ann Thorac Surg 1993;56:649–50.
21. Cunha BA. Central nervous system infections in the compromised host: a diagnostic approach. Infect Dis Clin North Am 2001;15:567–90.
22. Coley SC, Jagar HR, Szydlo RM, et al. CT and MRI manifestations of central nervous system infection following allogeneic bone marrow transplantation. Clin Radiol 1999;54:390–7.
23. Foerster BR, Thurnher MM, Malani PN, et al. Intracranial infections: clinical and imaging characteristics. Acta Radiol 2007;48:875–93.

24. Mylonakis E, Hohmann EL, Calderwood SB. Central nervous system infection with *Listeria monocytogenes*; 33 years of experience from a general hospital and review of 776 cases from the literature. Medicine 1998;77:313–36.

25. Paul M, Soares-Weiser K, Leibovici L. Beta lactam monotherapy versus beta lactam-aminoglycoside combination therapy for fever with neutropenia: systematic review and meta-analysis. BMJ 2003;326:1111–26.

26. Paul M, Yahav D, Fraser A, et al. Empirical antibiotic monotherapy for febrile neutropenia: systematic review and meta-analysis of randomized controlled trials. J Antimicrob Chemother 2006;57:176–89.

27. Raad I, Hanna H, Boktour M, et al. Management of central venous catheters in patients with cancer and candidemia. Clin Infect Dis 2004;38:1119–27.

28. Raad I, Hanna H, Boktour M, et al. Management of central venous catheters in patients with cancer and candidemia. Clin Infect Dis 2004;38:1119–27.

29. Alessa B, Tefferi A, Hoagland HC, et al. Outcome of recipients of bone marrow transplants who require intensive-care unit support. Mayo Clin Proc 1992;67: 117–22.

30. Paz HL, Crilley P, Weinar M, et al. Outcome of patients requiring medical ICU admission following bone marrow transplantation. Chest 1993;104:527–31.

31. Afessa T, Tefferi A, Dunn WF, et al. Intensive care unit support and acute physiology and chronic health evaluation III performance in hematopoietic stem cell transplant recipients. Crit Care Med 2003;31:1715–21.

32. Soubani AO. Critical care considerations of hematopoietic stem cell transplantation. Crit Care Med 2006;34(Suppl):S251–67.

33. Colin BA, Leather HL, Wingard JR, et al. Evolution, incidence and susceptibility of bacterial bloodstream isolates from 519 bone marrow transplant patients. Clin Infect Dis 2001;33:947–53.

34. Mossad SB, Longworth DL, Goormastic M, et al. Early infectious complications in autologous bone marrow transplantation: a review of 219 patients. Bone Marrow Transplant 1996;18:265–71.

35. Bilgrami S, Feingold JM, Dorsky D, et al. *Streptococcus viridans*, bacteremia following autologous peripheral blood stem cell transplantation. Bone Marrow Transplant 1998;21:591–5.

36. Bochud PY, Calandra T, Francioli P. Bacteremia due to viridans streptococci in neutropenic patients: a review. Am J Med 1994;97:256–64.

37. Marr KA, Siedel K, Slavin MA, et al. Prolonged fluconazole prophylaxis is associated with persistent protection against candidiasis-related death in allogeneic marrow transplant recipients: long term follow-up of a randomized, placebo-controlled trial. Blood 2000;96:2055–61.

38. Bodey GP, Mardani M, Hanna HA, et al. The epidemiology of *Candida glabrata* and *Candida albicans* fungemia in immunocompromised patients with cancer. Am J Med 2002;112:380–5.

39. Marr KA, Boeckh M, Carter RA, et al. Combination therapy for invasive aspergillosis. Clin Infect Dis 2004;39:797–802.

40. Fishman JA. Infection in solid organ transplant recipients. N Engl J Med 2007; 357:2601–14.

41. Avery RK. Infections after lung transplantation. Semin Respir Crit Care Med 2006; 27:544–51.

42. Hadjiliadis D. Special considerations for patients undergoing lung transplantation for cystic fibrosis. Chest 2007;131:1224–31.

43. Freeman RB, Giatras I, Falagas ME, et al. Outcome of transplantation of organs procured from bacteremic donors. Transplantation 1999;68:1107–11.

44. Rubin RH. The indirect effects of *cytomegalovirus* infection on the outcome of organ transplantation. JAMA 1989;261:3607–9.
45. Snydman DR. The case for cytomegalovirus prophylaxis in solid organ transplantation. Rev Med Virol 2006;16:289–95.
46. Kalil AC, Levitsky J, Lyden E, et al. Meta-analysis: the efficacy of strategies to prevent organ disease by cytomegalovirus in solid organ transplant recipients. Ann Intern Med 2005;143:870–80.
47. Hodson EM, Jones CA, Webster AC, et al. Antiviral medications to prevent cytomegalovirus disease and early death in recipients of solid organ transplants: a systematic review of randomised controlled trials. Lancet 2005;365:2105–15.
48. Falagas ME, Snydman DR, Griffith J, et al. Clinical and epidemiological predictors of recurrent cytomegalovirus disease in orthotopic liver transplant recipients. Boston Center for Liver Transplantation CMVIG Study Group. Clin Infect Dis 1997; 25:314–7.
49. Bonatti H, Tab relli W, Ruttmann E, et al. Impact of cytomegalovirus match on survival after cardiac and lung transplantation. Am Surg 2004;70:710–4.
50. Mutimer D, Mirza D, shaw J, et al. Enhanced *cytomegalovirus* viral replication associated with septic bacterial complications in liver transplant recipients. Transplantation 1997;63:1411–5.
51. Humar A, St Louis P, Mazzulli T, et al. Elevated serum cytokines are assoicated with *cytomegalovirus* infection and disease in bone marrow transplant recipients. J Infect Dis 1999;179:484–8.
52. Wolff AJ, O'Donnell AE. Pulmonary manifestations of HIV infection in the era of highly active antiretroviral therapy. Chest 2001;120:1888–93.
53. Allen SH, Brennan P, Nelson M, et al. Pneumonia due to antibiotic resistant *Streptococcus pneumoniae* and *Pseudomonas aeruginosa* in the HAART era. Postgrad Med J 2003;79:691–4.
54. Wislez M, Bergot E, Antoine M, et al. Acute respiratory failure following HAART introduction in patients treated for *Pneumocystis carinii* pneumonia. Am J Respir Crit Care Med 2001;164:847–51.
55. Narita M, Ashkin D, Hollender ES, et al. Paradoxical worsening of tuberculosis following antiretroviral therapy in patients with AIDS. Am J Respir Crit Care Med 1998;158:157–61.
56. Manez R, Kusne S, Linden P, et al. Temporary withdrawal of immunosuppression for life-threatening infections after liver transplantation. Transplantation 1994;57: 149–51.
57. Swinnen LJ. Organ transplant related lymphoma. Curr Treat Options Oncol 2001; 2:301–8.
58. Srividyalakshmi S, Baumann MA. Reverse isolation for neutropenic patients. Community Oncol 2008;5:628–32.
59. Hahn T, Cummings KM, Michalek AM, et al. Efficacy of high efficiency particulate air filtration in preventing aspergillosis in immunocompromised patients with hematologic malignancies. Infect Control Hosp Epidemiol 2002;23:525–31.
60. Fischl MA, Uttamchandani Rb, Dalkos GL, et al. An outbreak of tuberculosis caused by multiple drug resistant tubercle bacilli among patients with HIV infection. Ann Intern Med 1992;117:177–83.
61. Herrero IA, Issa NC, Patel R. Nosocomial spread of linezolid-resistant, vancomycin-resistant *Enterococcus faecium*. N Engl J Med 2002;346:867–9.
62. Poque JM, Paterson DL, Pasculle AW, et al. Determination of risk factors associated with isolation of linezolid-resistant strains of vancomycin-resistant *Enterococcus*. Infect Control Hosp Epidemiol 2007;28:1382–8.

63. Schaier M, Wendt C, Zaier M, et al. *Clostridium difficile* diarrhea in the immuno-suppressed patient. Update on prevention and therapy. Nephrol Dial Transplant 2004;19:2432-6.
64. Trifilio S, Singhal S, Williams S, et al. Breakthrough fungal infections after alloge-neic hematopoietic stem cell transplantation in patients on prophylactic voricona-zole. Bone Marrow Transplant 2007;40:451-6.
65. Siwek GT, Dodgson KJ, de Magalhaes-Silverman M, et al. Invasive zygomycosis in hematopoietic stem cell transplant recipients receiving voriconazole prophy-laxis. Clin Infect Dis 2004;39:584-7.
66. Limaye AP, Raghu G, Koelle DM, et al. High incidence of ganciclovir-resistant *cytomegalovirus* infection among lung transplant recipients receiving preemptive therapy. J Infect Dis 2002;185:20-7.
67. Martin BK, Ricks MO, Forman MS, et al. Change over time in incidence of ganci-clovir resistance in patients with *cytomegalovirus* retinitis. Clin Infect Dis 2007;44: 1001-8.

Bloodstream Infection in the ICU

Jordi Vallés, MD, PhD*, Ricard Ferrer, MD

KEYWORDS

- Bloodstream infection • Bacteremia
- Critically ill patients • ICU • Hospital-acquired infection

Hospital-acquired infections (HAI) occur in 5%–10% of patients admitted to hospitals in the Unites States, and HAIs remain a leading cause of morbidity and mortality.[1] The endemic rates of HAI vary markedly between hospitals and between areas of the same hospital. Patients in intensive care units (ICUs), representing 8% to 15% of hospital admissions, suffer a disproportionately high percentage of HAI compared with patients in noncritical care areas.[2–8] Patients admitted to ICUs account for 45% of all hospital-acquired pneumonias and bloodstream infections (BSIs), although critical care units comprise only 5% to 10% of all hospital beds.[3] The severity of underlying disease, invasive diagnostic and therapeutic procedures that breach normal host defenses, contaminated life-support equipment, and the prevalence of resistant microorganisms are critical factors in the high rate of infection in the ICUs.[9]

On admission to the ICU, 40% of patients have community-acquired infections, and 17% of these have BSI.[10] The rate of patients with community-acquired BSI admitted to general ICUs is about 9–10 episodes per 1000 admissions,[11,12] and represent 30%–40% of all episodes of BSI diagnosed in a general ICU (**Fig. 1**).

This article discusses the clinical importance of BSI, including hospital- and community-acquired episodes in the ICU.

DEFINITIONS

Infections have traditionally been classified as either nosocomial or community-acquired. Nosocomial BSI in the ICU is defined as a clinically significant positive blood culture for a bacterium or fungus obtained more than 72 hours after admission to the ICU; positive blood cultures obtained within 72 hours after admission are also considered nosocomial BSI when they are directly related to invasive manipulation on ICU admission (eg, urinary catheterization or insertion of an intravenous line). In contrast, a community-acquired BSI is defined as an infection that develops in a patient before hospital and ICU admission or within the first 48 hours of hospital and ICU admission when it is not be associated with any procedures performed after admission.

Critical Care Center, Hospital Sabadell, Institut Universitari Parc Taulí. UAB, CIBER Enfermedades Respiratorias, Parc Taulí s/n, 08208 Sabadell, Spain
* Corresponding author.
E-mail address: jvalles@tauli.cat (J. Vallés).

Infect Dis Clin N Am 23 (2009) 557–569
doi:10.1016/j.idc.2009.04.005
0891-5520/09/$ – see front matter © 2009 Elsevier Inc. All rights reserved.

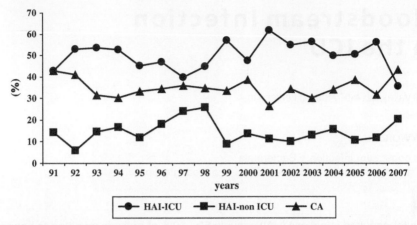

Fig. 1. Distribution of bloodstream infections in the medical-surgical ICU of Hospital Sabadell (1991–2007). HAI-ICU: Bloodstream infections acquired in the ICU, HAI-non ICU: Bloodstream infections acquired in wards, CA: Community-acquired bloodstream infections.

According to these definitions from the Centers for Disease Control and Prevention (CDC) all infections that are not nosocomial infections are community-acquired by default.[13] However, patients residing in the community who are receiving care at home, living in nursing homes or rehabilitation centers, receiving chronic dialysis, or receiving chemotherapy in physicians' offices may present BSIs. Because these BSIs do not fit the definition for nosocomial infection, they are categorized as community-acquired BSI under traditional classification schemes. However, these patients are exposed to risks and pathogens that are clearly different from those that affect healthy individuals living in the community; thus, some investigators proposed a new class of "health care–associated" infections, distinct from both community-acquired and hospital-acquired infections.[14,15]

Health care–associated BSI is defined as a positive blood culture obtained at the time of hospital admission or within 48 hours of admission from a patient fulfilling any of the following criteria: (1) Received intravenous therapy at home, received wound care or specialized nursing care, or had self-administered intravenous medical therapy; (2) attended a hospital hemodialysis clinic or received intravenous chemotherapy; (3) was hospitalized in an acute care hospital for 2 or more days in the 90 days before the bloodstream infection; or (4) resided in a nursing home or long-term care facility.[15]

HOSPITAL-ACQUIRED BLOODSTREAM INFECTIONS IN THE ICU
Epidemiology

Patients in the ICU not only have higher endemic rates of hospital-acquired infections than patients in general wards, but the distribution of their infections also differs. The two most common hospital-acquired infections in general wards are urinary tract infections and surgical wound infections, whereas in the ICU, lower respiratory tract infections and BSI are the most frequent.[16] This distribution is related to the widespread use of mechanical ventilation and intravenous catheters. Data compiled through the CDC's National Nosocomial Infections Surveillance System revealed that BSIs accounted for almost 20% of hospital-acquired infections in ICU patients, and 87% of these were associated with a central line.[17] A recent nationwide surveillance study in 49 United States hospitals (SCOPE) reported that 51% of hospital-acquired BSIs occurred in ICUs.[18]

The studies conducted in critically ill patients show that the incidence of nosocomial BSIs in the ICU ranges from 27 to 68 episodes per 1000 admissions (**Table 1**),[19–23] depending on the type of ICU (surgical or medical or coronary care unit), the severity of patient's condition, the use of invasive devices and the length of ICU stay. These infection rates among ICU patients are as much as 5–10 times higher than those recorded for patients admitted to general wards.

Risk Factors

Factors that predispose an individual to BSI include not only the host's underlying conditions but therapeutic, microbial and environmental factors as well. Diseases associated with an increased risk of BSI include: hematologic and nonhematologic malignancies; diabetes mellitus; renal failure requiring dialysis; chronic hepatic failure; immune deficiency syndromes; and conditions associated with the loss of normal skin barriers, such as serious burns and pressure ulcers. In the ICU, therapeutic maneuvers associated with an increased risk of hospital-acquired BSI include placement of intravascular and urinary catheters, endoscopic procedures, and drainage of intraabdominal infections.

Several risk factors have been associated with the acquisition of BSI by specific pathogens. Coagulase-negative staphylococci (CNS) are mainly associated with central venous line infection and with the use of intravenous lipid emulsions. *Candida* infections are related to exposure to multiple antibiotics, hemodialysis, isolation of *Candida* species from sites other than the blood, azotemia, and the use of indwelling catheters.[24] In an analysis of risk factors for hospital-acquired candidemia performed in the authors' ICU, the authors found that exposure to more than four antibiotics during the ICU stay (OR: 4.10), parenteral nutrition (OR: 3.37), previous surgery (OR: 2.60) and the presence of a solid malignancy (OR: 1.57) were independently associated with the development of *Candida* infection.[25]

Microbiology

The spectrum of microorganisms that invade the bloodstream in patients who have hospital-acquired infections during their stay in the ICU has been evaluated in several studies. Although almost any microorganism can produce BSI, staphylococci and Gram-negative bacilli account for the vast majority of cases. However, among the

Table 1
Rates of hospital-acquired bloodstream infections in the intensive care unit (ICU)

Year	Type of ICU	Episodes of Nosocomial Bloodstream Infection Per 1000 Admissions	Reference
1994	Medical-surgical ICU	67.2	Rello[19]
1994	Surgical ICU	26.7	Pittet[20]
1996	Adult ICUs Multicenter study	41	Brun-Buisson[21]
1997	Adult ICUs Multicenter study	36	Vallés[22]
2006	Adult ICUs Multicenter study	68	Garrouste-Orgas[23]

staphylococci, CNS has become the most common agent of BSI in the ICU.[19,22,26,27] The ascendance of this group of staphylococci has increased the interpretative difficulties for clinicians, because many CNS isolations represent contamination rather than true BSI. The increased incidence of BSI caused by CNS seems to be related to the increased use of multiple invasive devices in critically ill patients and to multiple antimicrobial therapy used for Gram-negative infections in ICU patients, which results in selection of Gram-positive microorganisms. The change in the spectrum of organisms causing hospital-acquired BSI in an adult ICU was confirmed by Edgeworth and colleagues,[28] who analyzed the evolution of hospital-acquired BSI in the same ICU over 25 years. Between 1971 and 1990, the frequency of isolation of individual organisms changed little, with S aureus, P aeruginosa, E coli, and K pneumoniae species predominating. However, between 1991 and 1995, the number of BSIs doubled, largely because of the increased isolation of CNS, Enterococus spp, and intrinsically antibiotic-resistant Gram-negative organisms, particularly P aeruginosa and Candida spp.

Currently, the leading pathogens among cases of hospital-acquired BSI in the ICU are Gram-positive microorganisms, representing nearly half of the organisms isolated (**Table 2**).[19,20,22,23,29] The most frequent Gram-positive bacteria in all studies are CNS, S aureus and enterococci; CNS is isolated in 20%–30% of all episodes of BSI. Gram-negative bacilli are responsible for 30%–40% of BSI episodes, and the remaining cases are mostly due to Candida spp. Polymicrobial episodes are relatively common, representing about 10%. Anaerobic bacteria are isolated in fewer than 5% of cases.

Among Gram-positive BSIs, the incidence of the pathogens is similar in different ICUs, CNS being the most frequently isolated organism, and S aureus the second in all studies. Only the incidence antibiotic-resistance strains, such as methicillin-resistant

Table 2
Microorganisms causing nosocomial bloodstream infection in adult ICUs

Reference	Gram-Positive Microorganisms	Gram-Negative Microorganisms	Fungi	Polymicrobial Episodes
Rello[19]	44.1% CNS S aureus Enterococci	40.5% P aeruginosa E coli Enterobacter spp.	5.4% Candida	9.9%
Pittet[20]	51.0% CNS S aureus Enterococci	39.0% Enterobacter spp Klebsiella spp S marcescens	4.8% Candida	21%
Vallés[22]	49.8% CNS S aureus Enterococci	32.6% P aeruginosa A baumannii K pneumoniae	4.4% Candida	12.7%
Jamal[29]	46.8% CNS S aureus Enterococci	36.6% Enterobacter spp S marcescens K pneumoniae	17.6% Candida	9.8%
Garrouste-Orgas[23]	52,5% CNS S aureus Enterococci	29,3% Enterobacteriaceae P aeruginosa Other	6,6% Candida	11.6%

Abbreviation: CNS, coagulase-negative staphylococci.

Staphylococcus aureus (MRSA) or vancomycin-resistant enterococci, differ substantially among individual institutions, depending on whether these microorganisms become established as endemic nosocomial pathogens in the ICU. However, the Gram-negative species isolated from hospital-acquired BSIs in the ICUs of different institutions show marked variability. The relative contribution of each Gram-negative species to the total number of isolates from blood varies from hospital to hospital and over time. The antibiotic policy of the institution may induce the appearance of highly resistant microorganisms and the emergence of endemic nosocomial pathogens, in particular *Pseudomonas* spp, *Acinetobacter* spp, and *Enterobacteriaceae* with extended-spectrum beta-lactamase (ESBL).

Sources

According to a recent analysis, 70% of nosocomial BSI in the ICU are secondary to other primary infection, including catheter-related infections, and the remaining 30% are of unknown origin. **Table 3** summarizes the sources of nosocomial bacteremias in the ICU in several series.[19,20,22,23,28] As shown, catheter-related infections and respiratory tract infections are the leading sources of secondary episodes.

The source of nosocomial BSI varies according to microorganism. CNS and *S aureus* commonly are associated with catheter-related infections, whereas Gram-negative bacilli are the main cause of BSI following respiratory tract, intraabdominal and urinary tract infections. Most BSIs of unknown origin are caused by Gram-positive microorganisms, mainly CNS, and they may also originate in device-related infections not diagnosed at the time of the development of the BSI.

Systemic Response

The host reaction to invading microbes involves a rapidly amplifying polyphony of signals and responses that may spread beyond the invaded tissue. Fever or hypothermia, chills, tachypnea, and tachycardia often herald the onset of the systemic inflammatory response to microbial invasion, also called sepsis. BSI have been simply defined as the presence of bacteria or fungi in blood cultures, and four stages of systemic response of increasing severity have been described: the systemic inflammatory response syndrome (SIRS), which is identified by a combination of simple and readily available clinical signs and symptoms (ie, fever or hypothermia, tachycardia, tachypnea, and changes in blood leukocyte count); sepsis, when the SIRS is caused by a documented infection; severe sepsis when patients have a dysfunction of the major organs; and septic shock, when patients have hypotension in addition

Table 3
Major sources of hospital-acquired bloodstream infection in the ICUs

Type of Infection	Rello[19] (%)	Pittet[20] (%)	Vallés[22] (%)	Edgewort[28] (%)	Garrouste-Orgas[23] (%)
Intravenous catheter	35	18	37.1	62	20.2
Respiratory tract	10	28	17.5	3	16.3
Intra-abdominal infection	9	NA	6.1	6.9	NA
Genitourinary tract	3.6	5.4	5.9	2.4	2.5
Surgical wound	8	8	2.4	3	9.9
Other	7	14.5	2.9	-	12.9
Unknown origin	27	20	28.1	22.4	32.7

to severe sepsis.[30] The presence of organisms in the blood is one of the most reliable criteria for characterizing a patient presenting with SIRS as having sepsis or one of its more severe presentations, such as severe sepsis or septic shock.

In a multicenter study, Brun-Buisson and colleagues[21] analyzed the relationship between BSI and severe sepsis in adults ICUs and general wards in 24 hospitals in France. In this study, of the 842 episodes of clinically significant BSI recorded, 162 (19%) occurred in patients hospitalized in ICUs; 377 episodes (45%) of BSI were hospital-acquired, and their incidence was 12 times greater in ICUs than in wards. The frequency of severe sepsis during BSI differed markedly between wards and ICUs (17% versus 65%, $P<.001$). The hospital-acquired episodes in the ICU represented an incidence rate of 41 episodes per 1000 admissions and the incidence of severe sepsis among patients with hospital-acquired BSI in the ICU was 24 episodes per 1000 admissions.

Another multicenter study reported by our group[22] analyzed 590 hospital-acquired BSIs in adult ICUs at 30 hospitals in Spain; patients' systemic response were classified as sepsis in 371 episodes (62.8%), severe sepsis in 109 episodes (18.5%), and septic shock in the remaining 110 (18.6%). Episodes of BSI associated with intravascular catheters showed the lowest rate of septic shock (12.8%), whereas episodes of BSI secondary to lower respiratory tract, intra-abdominal or genitourinary tract infections showed the highest incidence of severe sepsis and septic shock. Intravascular catheter-related BSI was also associated with a lower risk of severe sepsis in the study by Brun-Buisson and colleagues (OR = 0.2; 95% CI: 0.1 to 0.5; $P<.01$).[21]

The systemic response may differ according to the microorganism causing the episode of BSI. Gram-negative and *Candida* spp are associated with a higher incidence of severe sepsis and septic shock,[22] whereas CNS was the microorganism causing the lowest incidence of septic shock. In the French multicenter study, episodes caused by CNS were also associated with a reduced risk of severe sepsis (OR = 0.2; $P = .02$) compared with other microorganisms.[21]

Prognosis

Hospital-acquired BSIs remain a leading cause of morbidity and mortality in critically ill patients. The crude mortality related to hospital-acquired BSIs in ICU patients ranges from 20% to 60%, and the mortality directly attributable to the BSI ranges from 14% to 38%.[19–23] Although one-third of the deaths occur within the first 48 hours after the onset of symptoms, mortality can occur 14 or more days later. Late deaths are often caused by poorly controlled infection, complications during the ICU stay, or multiple organ failure. Bueno-Cavanillas and colleagues[31] analyzed the impact of hospital-acquired infection on the mortality rate in an ICU. In that study, compared with noninfected patients, the overall crude relative risk of mortality was 2.48 (95% CI = 1.47 to 4.16) in patients with a hospital-acquired infection and 4.13 (95% CI = 2.11 to 8.11) in patients with BSI. In a matched, risk-adjusted multicenter study in 12 ICUs, Garrouste-Orgas and colleagues[23] found that hospital-acquired BSI was associated with a three-fold increase in mortality.

A number of factors have been suspected as being associated with mortality in BSI. The most widely recognized prognostic factors are age, severity of the patient's underlying disease, and the appropriateness of antimicrobial therapy. Among other factors potentially related to the outcome of BSI, a multiple source of infection, secondary to other focus of infection, BSI caused by some difficult-to-treat organisms such as *Pseudomonas*, *Acinetobacter* or *Serratia* spp, polymicrobial BSI, and factors related to host response such as the occurrence of hypotension, shock, or organ failure have all been described as prognostically important.

COMMUNITY-ACQUIRED BLOODSTREAM INFECTIONS IN THE ICU
Epidemiology

Community-acquired infections are a common reason for admission to ICUs. Severe community-acquired pneumonia and intra-abdominal infections are the most frequent community-acquired infections that require admission to the ICU, and approximately a 20% of patients with these infections also present bacteremia. Few epidemiologic studies focusing solely on community-acquired BSI on admission to the ICU are available. Data from a recent multicenter study reported a community-acquired BSI rate of 10.2 episodes per 1000 ICU admissions.[32]

Microbiology

In community-acquired BSI patients admitted to the ICU, the incidence of Gram-positive bacteria is similar to that of Gram-negative bacteria and nearly 10% are polymicrobial episodes. E coli, S pneumoniae and S aureus are the leading pathogens, and the prevalence of these microorganisms is related to the main sources of BSI in these patients; urinary tract infections, pulmonary tract infections, and bacteremias of unknown origin (Table 4).[11,12,32]

Sources

Among community-acquired BSIs, lower respiratory tract, intra-abdominal, and genitourinary infections account for more than 80% of episodes of bacteremia admitted to the ICU (see Table 4). Approximately 20%–29% of episodes are of unknown origin; these include mainly meningococcal and staphylococcal infections.[11,12,32]

Systemic Response

The incidence of severe sepsis and septic shock in patients with community-acquired BSI is higher than in those with hospital-acquired episodes, in part because the severity of the systemic response is the motive for ICU admission. In the multicenter French study mentioned above, 74% of the community-acquired BSI episodes presented severe sepsis or septic shock at admission to the ICU.[21] In a multicenter Spanish study performed in 30 ICUs, the incidence of severe sepsis and septic shock was 75%. In this study, Gram-negative microorganisms and urinary tract infections and intarabdominal infections were more frequently associated with septic shock.[32]

Table 4		
Microorganisms and sources of community-acquired bloodstream infections admitted to the ICU		
Reference	**Sources**	**Microorganisms**
Forgacs[11]	Pulmonary 38.5%	S pneumoniae 32.3%
	Genitourinary 23.0%	E coli 27.2%
	Endocarditis 8.0%	S aureus 13.5%
	Biliary tract 5.9%	Other GNB 14.2%
	Other 11.1%	Other GPC 8.2%
	Unknown origin 20.0%	Other 14.2%
Vallés[32]	Pulmonary 20.0%	E.coli 28.1%
	Abdominal 20.1%	S.pneumoniae 17.9%
	Genitourinary 19.8%	S.aureus 14.9%
	Other 10.3%	Other GNB 18.6%
	Unknown origin 29.2%	Other GPC 9.5%
		Other 11.07%

Abbreviations: GNB, Gram-negative bacilli; GPC, Gram-positive cocci.

Prognosis

Patients admitted to the ICU with community-acquired BSI present a crude mortality of nearly 40%, compared with a mortality of 18% in patients admitted to general wards.[12,32,33] This elevated mortality is partly caused by the severity of the systemic response that leads to admission to the ICU.[12,32] In addition to the severity of the systemic response (severe sepsis and septic shock) and associated complications, the most important variable influencing the outcome of these patients is the appropriateness of empiric antimicrobial treatment.[12,32] In two studies, the incidence of inappropriate antibiotic treatment in community-acquired BSIs admitted to the ICU ranged between 15% and 20% and the mortality among patients with inappropriate empiric antibiotic treatment was more than 70%.[32,34]

HEALTH CARE–ASSOCIATED BLOODSTREAM INFECTIONS IN THE ICU
Epidemiology

A new classification scheme for BSIs was proposed to distinguish among infections occurring among outpatients having recurrent or recent contact with the health care system, true community-acquired infections and hospital-acquired infections. According to this classification, approximately 40% to 50% of patients admitted to the hospital with BSI (traditionally defined as community-acquired BSI) should be classified as health care–associated BSI.[14,15] More recently, in a large United States' database, health care–associated BSI accounted for more than half of all BSIs admitted to the hospital. In this study, if the patients with health care–associated BSI were included in the community-acquired BSI category according to the traditional classification scheme, they would account for approximately 60% of community-acquired BSI patients who needed hospitalization.[35]

No studies about the importance of health care–associated BSI in ICU patients are available; however, recent studies suggest that health care–associated BSI are less frequent than hospital-acquired and community-acquired BSI in critically ill patients. In a multicenter study of 1157 episodes of BSI in three hospitals in Spain, 50% were classified as community-acquired, 26% hospital-acquired, and 24% health care–associated BSI.[36] The distribution of BSI in patients admitted to the ICU was different; 60% of BSI episodes were hospital-acquired, 30% were community-acquired, and only 10% were classified as health care–associated. More recently the authors performed a multicenter study in 28 ICUs in Spain (data not published) analyzing 1590 episodes of BSI; the results confirm the low incidence of health care–associated BSI in ICU patients compared with patients admitted to conventional wards. Most BSIs (77%) were hospital-acquired, followed by community-acquired BSIs (21%), and only 8% were health care–associated BSI. Compared with patients with community-acquired episodes, patients with health care–associated BSI are older and more likely to have severe comorbidities, such as congestive heart failure, peripheral vascular disease, chronic renal disease, and cancer. Poor baseline condition leading to orders to withhold treatment may be responsible for lower rates of ICU admission in these patients.

Microbiology

The pathogens responsible for health care-associated BSI and their susceptibility patterns are similar to those that cause hospital-acquired infections. In a prospective observational study of 504 patients with BSIs, Friedman and colleagues[15] found that S aureus was the most common pathogen in patients with both health care–associated and hospital-acquired BSI; MRSA was present in 19% of health care–associated

BSI and in 20% in hospital-acquired episodes. Moreover, resistance to ampicillin-sulbactam and ciprofloxacin occurred with similar frequency in Enterobacteriaceae isolated from patients with health care–associated BSI and those with hospital-acquired BSI. Another multicenter study in the United States found similar results in the frequency of S aureus and MRSA in health care–associated and hospital-acquired BSIs.[35] However, the distribution of pathogens in both groups was not identical. Whereas E coli and Proteus were identified more frequently in patients with health care–associated infections, fungal organisms were more prevalent in patients with hospital-acquired BSI. In the authors' experience,[36] the distribution of pathogens seen in health care-associated BSI is more similar to that seen in hospital-acquired BSI than in community-acquired BSI (**Table 5**). In addition, episodes of health care–associated BSI had a higher prevalence of MRSA infections (5%) than community-acquired episodes (0.2%) (OR, 30.4; 95% CI, 3.9–232.4; P<.001) or hospital-acquired episodes (0.7%) (OR, 7.7; 95% CI, 1.7–34.1; P = .001). A recently published study performed in Spain found a high prevalence of MRSA among residents in community long-term care facilities; the prevalence of MRSA was 16.8% (95% CI 14.9–18.8) and it was isolated from 15.5% of nasal swabs and from 59% of decubitus ulcers.[37]

Sources

Urinary tract infection, intravascular-device-related BSI, gastrointestinal-related bacteremia, and respiratory tract infections are the most frequent sources of health care-associated BSIs.[15,36] Intravascular-device-related bacteremia occurs with similar frequencies in patients with health care–associated BSI and in those with hospital-acquired BSI.

Systemic Response

In a recent multicenter study performed in ICUs in Spain, from 50% to 60% of patients with health care–associated BSI admitted to ICUs presented septic shock. The frequency of severe sepsis and septic shock was similar in patients with

Table 5
Pathogens most frequently found in bloodstream infections by epidemiologic type of infection in a Spanish multicenter study

Pathogen	Total n = 1157 (%)	CBSI n = 581 (%)	HBSI n = 295 (%)	HCBSI n = 281 (%)	P Value
Escherichia coli	472 (40.8)	308 (53)	61 (20.7)	103 (36.7)	<0.001
Methicillin-susceptible S aureus	86 (7.4)	25 (4.3)	31 (10.5)	30 (10.6)	<0.001
Coagulase-negative staphylococci	62 (5.3)	4 (0.7)	49 (16.6)	9 (3.2)	<0.001
Streptococcus pneumoniae	80 (6.9)	64 (11)	5 (1.7)	11 (3.9)	<0.001
Pseudomonas aeruginosa	63 (5.4)	9 (1.5)	27 (9.2)	27 (9.6)	<0.001
Klebsiella pneumoniae	41 (3.5)	23 (4)	9 (3.1)	9 (3.2)	NS
Candida spp	12 (1)	0 (0)	11 (3.7)	1 (0.3)	<0.001
Polymicrobial	72 (6.2)	23 (3.9)	26 (8.8)	23 (8.1)	0.01

Abbreviations: CBSI, community-acquired bloodstream infection; HBSI, hospital-acquired bloodstream infection; HCBSI, health care–associated bloodstream infection.
From Vallés J, Calbo E, Anoro E, et al. Bloodstream infections in adults: importance of health care-associated infections. J Infect 2008;56:27–34; with permission.

community-acquired BSI and in those with hospital-acquired BSI originating in conventional wards because in all cases BSI or its consequences (severe systemic response) was the main reason for admission to the ICU (data not published).

Prognosis

A few studies have analyzed prognosis in patients with health care-associated BSI. Friedman and colleagues[15] found higher mortality at follow-up in patients with health care-associated BSI (29% versus 16%; P = .019) or hospital-acquired BSI (37% versus. 16%; $P<.001$) than in patients with community-acquired infection. Shorr and colleagues[35] found similar results, with a significantly higher risk of death for BSI acquired in the hospital or associated with previous health care exposure. Consistent with these reports, the authors also found significantly higher mortality at follow up in hospital-acquired BSI (27.3%) and health care–associated BSI (27.5%) than in community-acquired BSI (10.4%) ($P<.001$). Among patients with community-acquired and health care–associated BSI, a multivariate analysis, adjusted for age and comorbidities, found health care–associated BSI (OR, 2.4; 95% CI, 1.5–3.7; $P<.001$) was independently associated with mortality.[36]

TREATMENT

Bloodstream infections are among the most serious infections causing severe sepsis or septic shock in patients requiring intensive care. The mainstay of therapy for patients with bacteremia remains antimicrobial therapy, together with optimal management of its consequences (eg, shock or metastatic suppurative complications) and surgical treatment, (eg, debridement, abscess drainage, or removal of intravascular devices) when necessary.[38] Appropriate antimicrobial therapy reduces mortality among patients with bacteremia and, when initiated early, improves outcome in critically ill patients.[35] The initial antimicrobial therapy is necessarily empiric, targeting the most likely etiologic pathogens. However, inappropriate empiric treatment is applied in up to 30% of cases; it is more frequent in the following circumstances: hospital-acquired infection, health care–associated infection, prior administration of antibiotics, and presence of multidrug-resistant pathogens.

The distribution of the pathogens associated with community-acquired BSI is relatively uniform. However, an increase in the incidence of infections caused by antibiotic-resistant microorganisms, such as community-acquired MRSA and infections caused by ESBL-producing E $coli$ or K $pneumoniae$, has been reported in most countries, and these circumstaces should be taken into account when initiating empiric antibiotic treatment. Hospital-acquired and health care–associated BSIs are associated with increased incidence of resistant microorganisms, such as MRSA, ESBL-producing $Enterobacteriaceae$, A $baumannii$, and P $aeruginosa$. In these cases, it is more difficult for empiric treatment to be appropriate, especially in patients admitted in the ICU with a major incidence of multidrug-resistant microorganims. In these cases, in addition to the recommendations in the guidelines, it is indispensable to know the local flora predominant in each area before initiating empiric antibiotic treatment.

SUMMARY

Bloodstream infections are among the most serious infections causing severe sepsis or septic shock acquired by hospitalized patients requiring intensive care. Hospital-acquired BSI accounted for almost 20% of hospital-acquired infections in critically ill patients, and more than 80% of these are associated with a central line. Infection rates among ICU patients are as much as 5–10 times higher than those recorded for patients admitted to general wards. Also, community-acquired infections represent an important reason for admission to ICUs. Severe community-acquired pneumonia, urinary tract infections, and intra-abdominal infections are the most frequent community-acquired infections that require admission to the ICU; approximately 20% of patients with these infections will also present bacteremia, associated with a high incidence of severe sepsis and septic shock. Recently, a new classification scheme for BSIs was proposed to distinguish between infections occurring among outpatients having recurrent or recent contact with the health care system and patients with true community-acquired infections. According to this classification, approximately 40% to 50% of patients admitted to the hospital with BSI traditionally defined as community-acquired should be classified as health care–associated BSI. However, the importance of healthcare-associated BSI among critically ill patients seems to be lesser than among patients admitted to conventional wards. BSIs in critically ill patients are associated with greater hospital mortality and clinical efforts should be aimed at reducing the incidence of inappropriate antimicrobial treatment and at preventing episodes associated with intravascular devices.

REFERENCES

1. Wenzel RP. Organization for infection control. In: Mandell GL, Douglas RG Jr, Bennett JE, editors. Principles and practice of infectious diseases. 3rd edition. New York: Churchill Livingstone; 1990. p. 2176–80.
2. Weinstein RA. Epidemiology and control of nosocomial infections in adult intensive care units. Am J Med 1991;91(Suppl 3B):179S–84S.
3. Wenzel RP, Thompson RL, Landry SM, et al. Hospital-acquired infections in intensive care unit patients: an overview with emphasis on epidemics. Infect Control 1983;4:371–5.
4. Maki DG. Risk factors for nosocomial infection in intensive care: "devices vs nature" and goals for the next decade. Arch Intern Med 1989;149:30–5.
5. Donowitz LG, Wenzel RP, Hoyt JW. High risk of hospital-acquired infection in the ICU patient. Crit Care Med 1982;10:355–7.
6. Brown RB, Hosmer D, Chen HC, et al. A comparison of infections in the different ICUs within the same hospital. Crit Care Med 1985;13:472–6.
7. Daschner F. Nosocomial infections in intensive care units. Intensive Care Med 1985;11:284–7.
8. Trilla A, Gatell JM, Mensa J, et al. Risk factors for nosocomial bacteremia in a large Spanish teaching hospital: a case-control study. Infect Control Hosp Epidemiol 1991;12:150–6.
9. Massanari RM, Hierholzer WJ Jr. The intensive care unit. In: Bennett JV, Brachman PS, editors. Hospital infections. 2nd edition. Boston: Little, Brown and Company; 1986. p. 285–98.
10. Ponce de León-Rosales S, Molinar-Ramos F, Domínguez-Cherit G, et al. Prevalence of infections in intensive care units in Mexico: a multicenter study. Crit Care Med 2000;28:1316–21.
11. Forgacs IC, Eykyn SJ, Bradley RD. Serious infection in the intensive therapy unit: a 15-year study of bacteraemia. Q J Med 1986;60:773–9.
12. Vallés J, Ochagavía A, Rué M, et al. Critically ill patients with community-acquired bacteremia: characteristics and prognosis. Intensive Care Med 2000;26(Suppl 3): S222.

13. Garner JS, Jarvis WR, Emori TG, et al. CDC definitions for nosocomial infections. Am J Infect Control 1988;16:128–40.
14. Siegman-Igra Y, Fourer B, Orni-Wasserkauf R, et al. Reappraisal of community-acquired bacteremia: a proposal of a new classification for the spectrum of acquisition of bacteremia. Clin Infect Dis 2002;34:1431–9.
15. Friedman ND, Kaye KS, Stout JE, et al. Health care-associated bloodstream infections in adults: a reason to change the accepted definition of community-acquired infections. Ann Intern Med 2002;137:791–7.
16. Trilla A. Epidemiology of nosocomial infections in adult intensive care units. Intensive Care Med 1994;20:S1–4.
17. Richards MJ, Edwards JR, Culver DH, et al. Nosocomial infections in medical intensive care units in the United States. Crit Care Med 1999;27:887–92.
18. Wisplinghoff H, Bischoff T, Tallent SM, et al. Nosocomial bloodstream infections in US Hospitals: analysis of 24,179 cases from a prospective nationwide surveillance study. Clin Infect Dis 2004;39:309–17.
19. Rello J, Ricart M, Mirelis B, et al. Nosocomial bacteremia in a medical-surgical intensive care unit: epidemiologic characteristics and factors influencing mortality in 111 episodes. Intensive Care Med 1994;20:94–8.
20. Pittet D, Tarara D, Wenzel RP. Nosocomial bloodstream infection in critically ill patients. Excess length of stay, extra costs, and attributable mortality. JAMA 1994;271:1598–601.
21. Brun-Buisson C, Doyon F, Carlet J, et al. Bacteremia and severe sepsis in adults: a multicenter prospective survey in ICUs and wards of 24 hospitals. Am J Respir Crit Care Med 1996;154:617–24.
22. Vallés J, León C, Alvarez-Lerma F, et al. Nosocomial bacteremia in critically ill patients: a multicenter study evaluating epidemiology and prognosis. Clin Infect Dis 1997;24:387–95.
23. Garrouste-Orgeas M, Timsit JF, Tafflet M, et al. Excess risk of death from intensive care unit-acquired nosocomial bloodstream infections: a reappraisal. Clin Infect Dis 2006;42:1118–26.
24. Wenzel RP. Isolation of *Candida* species from sites other than the blood. Clin Infect Dis 1995;20:1531–4.
25. Díaz E, Villagrá A, Martínez M, et al. Nosocomial candidemia risk factors. Intensive Care Med 1998;24(Suppl 1):S143.
26. Towns ML, Quartey SM, Weinstein MP, et al. The clinical significance of positive blood cultures: a prospective, multicenter evaluation, abstr. C-232. In: Abstracts of the 93rd General Meeting of the American Society for Microbiology 1993. American Society for Microbiology, Washington, DC. Atlanta, GA; May 8–13, 1993.
27. Weinstein MP, Towns ML, Quartey SM, et al. The clinical significance of positive blood cultures in the 1990s: a prospective comprehensive evaluation of the microbiology, epidemiology, and outcome of bacteremia and fungemia in adults. Clin Infect Dis 1997;24:584–602.
28. Edgeworth JD, Treacher DF, Eykyn SJ. A 25-year study of nosocomial bacteremia in an adult intensive care unit. Crit Care Med 1999;27:1421–8.
29. Jamal WY, El-Din K, Rotimi VO, et al. An analysis of hospital-acquired bacteraemia in intensive care unit patients in a university hospital in Kuwait. J Hosp Infect 1999;43:49–56.
30. Levy MM, Fink MP, Marshall JC, et al. 2001 SCCM/ESICM/ACCP/ATS/SIS International sepsis definitions conference. Intensive Care Med 2003;29:530–8.

31. Bueno-Cavanillas A, Delgado-Rodríguez M, López-Luque A, et al. Influence of nosocomial infection on mortality rate in an intensive care unit. Crit Care Med 1994;22:55–60.
32. Vallés J, Rello J, Ochagavía A, et al. Community-acquired bloodstream infection in critically ill adult patients: impact of shock and inappropriate antibiotic therapy on survival. Chest 2003;123:1615–24.
33. Cartón JA, García-Velasco G, Maradona JA, et al. Non-hospital acquired bacteremia in adults. Prospective analysis of 333 episodes. Spanish. Med Clin (Barc) 1988;90:525–30.
34. Ibrahim EH, Sherman G, Ward S, et al. The influence of inadequate antimicrobial treatment of bloodstream infections on patient outcomes in the ICU setting. Chest 2000;118:146–55.
35. Shorr AF, Tabak YP, Killian AD, et al. Healthcare-associated bloodstream infection: a distinct entity? Insights from a large U.S. database. Crit Care Med 2006; 34:2588–95.
36. Vallés J, Calbo E, Anoro E, et al. Bloodstream infections in adults: importance of healthcare-associated infections. J Infect 2008;56:27–34.
37. Manzur A, Gavalda L, Ruiz de Gopegui E, et al. Prevalence of methicillin-resistant *Staphylococcus aureus* and factors associated with colonization among residents in community long-term-care facilities in Spain. Clin Microbiol Infect 2008;14:867–72.
38. Dellinger RP, Levy MM, Carlet JM, et al. Surviving sepsis campaign: international guidelines for management of severe sepsis and septic shock. Crit Care Med 2008;36:296–327.

Severe Soft Tissue Infections

Lena M. Napolitano, MD, FACS, FCCP, FCCM

KEYWORDS

- Skin infections • Soft tissue infections
- Necrotizing soft tissue infections • Abscess
- Drainage • Debridement • Methicillin-resistant *S aureus*
- Antimicrobial therapy

Skin and soft tissue infections (SSTIs) span a spectrum of clinical entities from limited cellulitis to rapidly progressive necrotizing fasciitis, which may be associated with septic shock or toxic shock syndrome.[1,2] These SSTIs may result in critical illness and require management in the ICU.[3] The complex interplay of environment, host, and pathogen is important to consider when evaluating SSTIs and planning therapy. The key to a successful outcome in caring for patients who have severe SSTIs is:

Early diagnosis and differentiation of necrotizing versus non-necrotizing SSTI
Early initiation of appropriate empiric broad-spectrum antimicrobial therapy with consideration of risk factors for specific pathogens and mandatory coverage for methicillin-resistant *Staphylococcus aureus* (MRSA).
Source control of early SSTI (ie, early aggressive surgical intervention for drainage of abscesses and debridement of necrotizing soft tissue infections)
Pathogen identification and appropriate de-escalation of antimicrobial therapy

In addition, appropriate critical care management, including fluid resuscitation, organ support, and nutritional support are necessary components of treatment of severe SSTIs.

EARLY DIAGNOSIS AND DIFFERENTIATION OF NECROTIZING VERSUS NON-NECROTIZING SKIN AND SOFT TISSUE INFECTIONS
Classification of Skin and Soft Tissue Infections

The US Food and Drug Administration (FDA) classifies SSTIs into two broad categories for the purpose of clinical trials evaluating new antimicrobials for the treatment of SSTIs: uncomplicated and complicated (**Box 1**). Uncomplicated SSTIs include superficial infections such as cellulitis, simple abscesses, impetigo, and furuncles. These infections can be treated by antibiotics or surgical incision for drainage of

Division of Acute Care Surgery, (Trauma, Burns, Critical Care, Emergency Surgery), Department of Surgery, University of Michigan Health System, Room 1C340A-UH, 1500 E. Medical Center Drive, SPC 5033, Ann Arbor, MI 48109-5033, USA
E-mail address: lenan@umich.edu

Infect Dis Clin N Am 23 (2009) 571–591
doi:10.1016/j.idc.2009.04.006
0891-5520/09/$ – see front matter © 2009 Published by Elsevier Inc.

> **Box 1**
> **Classification of severe skin and soft tissue infections by the US Food and Drug Administration**
>
> *Uncomplicated*
>
> Superficial infections, such as:
>
>   Simple abscesses
>
>   Impetiginous lesions
>
>   Furuncles
>
>   Cellulitis
>
>   Can be treated by surgical incision alone
>
> *Complicated*
>
> Deep soft tissue, requires significant surgical intervention
>
>   Infected ulcers
>
>   Infected burns
>
>   Major abscesses
>
>   Significant underlying disease state that complicates response to treatment
>
> *Data from* http://www.fda.gov/ohrms/dockets/98fr/2566dft.pdf. Accessed April 17, 2009.

abscess alone. In contrast, complicated sSTIs include deep soft tissue infections that require significant surgical intervention, such as infected ulcers, infected burns, and major abscesses, Additionally, these patients also have significant underlying comorbidities (ie, disease states that complicate [and usually delay] response to treatment). Complicated SSTIs are a significant clinical problem, in part related to the increasing resistance of infecting bacteria to current antibiotic therapies.

Uncomplicated SSTIs are associated with *low* risk for life- or limb-threatening infection. Patients who have uncomplicated SSTIs can be treated with empiric antibiotic therapy according to likely pathogen and local resistance patterns.

Complicated SSTIs are associated with *high* risk for life- or limb-threatening infection. In patients who have complicated SSTIs, it is of paramount importance to initiate appropriate and adequate broad-spectrum initial empiric antimicrobial therapy with coverage for MRSA and to consider the need for surgical intervention for abscess drainage or debridement.

Patients who have complicated SSTIs require hospitalization for treatment. Specific circumstances that warrant hospitalization include the presence of tissue necrosis, sepsis, severe pain, altered mental status, immunocompromised state, and organ failure (respiratory, renal, hepatic). SSTIs can lead to serious potentially life-threatening local and systemic complications. The infections can progress rapidly, and early recognition and proper medical and surgical management are the cornerstones of therapy.

Another classification for SSTIs that is used commonly is the differentiation of **necrotizing soft tissue infections (NSTIs)** from **non-necrotizing infections**. This differentiation is critical, because necrotizing infections warrant prompt aggressive surgical debridement. Clinical clues to the diagnosis of NSTIs are listed in **Box 2**. The differentiation of necrotizing infections from non-necrotizing infections is critical to achieving adequate surgical therapy.[4] A clear approach to these infections must allow rapid identification and treatment of NSTIs, because they are limb- and life-threatening.

When "hard clinical signs" (bullae, crepitus, gas on radiograph, hypotension with systolic blood pressure less than 90 mm Hg, or skin necrosis) of NSTI are present,

---

Box 2
Clinical clues to the diagnosis of necrotizing soft tissue infections

Skin findings

Erythema

Tense edema

Gray or discolored wound drainage

Vesicles or bullae

Skin necrosis

Ulcers

Crepitus

Systemic features

Severe pain out of proportion to physical findings

Pain that extends past margin of apparent skin infection

Fever

Tachycardia, tachypnea

Diaphoresis

Delirium

---

establishing the diagnosis of NSTI is not difficult. Hard signs of NSTIs, however, are often absent on presentation, thus potentially delaying diagnosis and surgical intervention. Studies have documented that less than 50% of patients who had a definitive diagnosis of NSTI presented with hard clinical signs of NSTI.[5] Admission white blood cell count greater than $15,400 \times 10^9$/L or serum sodium less than 135 mEq/L was documented to help differentiate NSTI from non-NSTI and aided in early diagnosis.[6,7] The Laboratory Risk Indicator for Necrotizing Fasciitis (LRINEC) score is also helpful as a laboratory aid in distinguishing necrotizing from non-necrotizing SSTIs.

If there is any question regarding the possible diagnosis of an NSTI, it is imperative to proceed with surgical intervention and to be certain that the surgical incision is continued down to the fascial and muscle level to make a definitive diagnosis.

EARLY INITIATION OF APPROPRIATE EMPIRIC BROAD-SPECTRUM ANTIMICROBIAL THERAPY WITH CONSIDERATION OF RISK FACTORS FOR SPECIFIC PATHOGENS AND MANDATORY COVERAGE FOR METHICILLIN-RESISTANT *STAPHYLOCOCCUS AUREUS* (MRSA)

Antimicrobial therapy is an essential element for managing severe SSTIs. As in all serious life-threatening infections, it is important to initiate **early** and **appropriate** empiric antimicrobial therapy. It has been established that prompt appropriate treatment of hospitalized infections reduces mortality.[8] Similar findings were reported in studies of patients with ventilator-associated pneumonia[9] and sepsis.[10] A study of ICU patients found that the higher mortality rate associated with inappropriate initial therapy was still observed when antibiotics were switched from an inappropriate to an appropriate treatment.[11]

Furthermore, appropriate and timely antibiotic therapy improves treatment outcomes for SSTIs caused by MRSA.[12] In a study of 492 patients who had community-onset MRSA SSTIs, 95% of episodes treated with an active antibiotic within 48 hours were treated successfully, compared with an 87% rate of successful treatment in patients who did not receive an active antibiotic ($P = .001$). In logistic regression analysis, failure to initiate active antimicrobial therapy within 48 hours of presentation was the only independent predictor of treatment failure (adjusted odds ratio [OR], 2.80; 95% CI, 1.26 to 6.22; $P = .011$). Similarly, in a study of patients admitted to the hospital with MRSA sterile-site infection, multivariate analysis found inappropriate antimicrobial treatment to be an independent risk factor for hospital mortality (adjusted OR, 1.92; 95% CI, 1.48 to 2.50; $P = .013$).[13]

An empiric treatment algorithm for SSTI directed against community-associated (CA-MRSA) in the emergency[14] department (ED) that promotes both the use of antibiotics likely active against CA-MRSA and early incision and drainage of abscesses was examined. Clinical failure occurred in only 3% of cases treated according to the algorithm, compared with 62% of those not treated according to the algorithm ($P < .001$). Furthermore, among cases that underwent immediate incision and drainage, initial treatment with antibiotics active in vitro against the MRSA isolate was associated with a decreased clinical failure rate when compared with those treated with inactive antibiotics (0% versus 67%, $P < .001$).

Empiric antibiotic therapy should be initiated in **all** patients who have complicated SSTIs (cSSTIs). Intravenous broad-spectrum antimicrobial therapy should be initiated:

When an infection is severe or progresses rapidly
When there are signs of systemic illness
When the patient has comorbidities or is immunosuppressed
For very old or young patients
When an abscess cannot be completely drained
When the infection does not respond to incision and drainage[15]

Timely initiation of antimicrobial therapy is also important for treating severe SSTIs, particularly if associated with septic shock. In a study of 2731 adult patients who had septic shock, a strong relationship between the delay in effective antimicrobial initiation and in-hospital mortality was noted (adjusted OR 1.119 [per hour delay], 95% CI 1.103 to 1.136, $P < .0001$).[16] Administration of an antimicrobial effective for isolated or suspected pathogens within the first hour of documented hypotension was associated with a survival rate of 79.9%. Each hour of delay in antimicrobial administration over the ensuing 6 hours was associated with an average decrease in survival of 7.6%. By the second hour after onset of persistent/recurrent hypotension, the in-hospital mortality rate was increased significantly relative to receiving therapy within the first hour (OR 1.67; 95% CI, 1.12 to 2.48). In multivariate analysis (including Acute Physiology and Chronic Health Evaluation II score and therapeutic variables), time to initiation of effective antimicrobial therapy was the single strongest predictor of outcome. Interestingly, only 50% of septic shock patients received effective antimicrobial therapy within 6 hours of documented hypotension.

Epidemiology and Microbiology of Skin and Soft Tissue Infections

An understanding of the changing epidemiology and microbiology of all SSTIs is required for diagnosing and selecting appropriate empiric antibiotic therapy. Staphylococci and streptococci long have been the leading microbiologic causes of cSSTIs.[17] In recent years, however, *S aureus* has emerged as the most common cause of SSTIs. In addition to Group A streptococci and *S aureus*, the indigenous aerobic and anaerobic cutaneous and mucous membranes' local microflora usually are responsible for polymicrobial infections, such as NSTIs and diabetic foot infections. Severe SSTIs also can be caused by *Clostridium spp*, microorganisms associated with water sources (*Vibrio spp*, *Aeromonas*), and polymicrobial/mixed infections.

CA-MRSA infections have risen rapidly in the last decade, and SSTIs are the predominant site of infection, accounting for 74% of all CA-MRSA infections in one study.[18] A 15-year study of the changing epidemiology of MRSA infections from military medical facilities in San Diego from 1990 to 2004 documented that 65% of MRSA infections were community-acquired, with SSTIs as the major site of infection in 95% of cases.[19]

MRSA was the most common identifiable cause of SSTI presenting to EDs in a recent prospective multicenter United States study. *S aureus* was isolated from 320 (76%) of 422 patients who had SSTIs. The prevalence of MRSA was 59% overall and ranged from 15% to 74% by ED. Pulsed-field type USA300 accounted for 97% of MRSA isolates; 72% of these were a single indistinguishable strain (USA300-0114). SCCmec type IV and the Panton-Valentine leukocidin (PVL) toxin gene each were detected in 98% of MRSA isolates. Among methicillin-susceptible *S aureus* (MSSA) isolates, 31% were USA300, and 42% contained PVL genes.[20] The spectrum of skin infections caused by CA-MRSA is wide and can range from simple cutaneous abscesses to large abscesses, severe pyomyositis, and fulminant necrotizing soft tissue infections.[21] Other studies have confirmed similar findings.[22,23]

MRSA also has been identified as the most common cause of severe SSTIs requiring surgical drainage and debridement in a single-center 7-year study from Houston.[24] From 2000 to 2006, 288 patients who had SSTIs that required operative debridement were identified. The most common microorganism retrieved from intraoperative cultures was *S aureus*, 70% of which were MRSA. *Streptococcus* species accounted only for 15% of microbes isolated. Monomicrobial etiology was identified in 67% of patients, and MRSA was also the predominant microbe isolated from such cultures (68%). The frequency of MRSA isolates increased significantly during the study, from 34% in 2000 to 77% in 2006 (*P*<.001) **Fig. 1**. Interestingly, the examination of vancomycin minimum inhibitory concentration (MIC) demonstrated a shift for MRSA isolates over this time period, with 38% of the isolates having an MIC greater than or equal to 1 μg/mL, with 31% of isolates with an MIC of 2 μg/mL. This is concerning given recent reports documenting high treatment failure rates for MRSA infections with increased MIC.[25,26]

In a study of 12,506 hospitalized patients who had culture-proven skin, soft tissue, bone, or joint infection, *S aureus* caused infection in 54.6% of patients, and 28.0% of

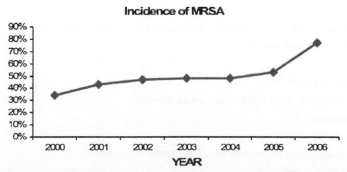

Fig. 1. Incidence of methicillin-resistant *Staphylococcus aureus* isolated from patients presenting with severe skin and soft tissue infections and requiring surgical intervention over 7 years (2000 through 2006). (*From* Awad SS, Elhabash SI, Lee L, et al. Increasing incidence of methicillin-resistant *Staphylococcus aureus* skin and soft tissue infections: reconsideration of empiric antimicrobial therapy. Am J Surg 2007;194:606–10; with permission.)

the *S aureus* isolates recovered were methicillin-resistant. Health care-associated infections and complicated SSTIs were associated with significantly higher mortality rates and longer and more costly length of hospital stay.[27]

Based on this change in microbiologic etiology of SSTIs, all patients who present with severe cSSTIs should be treated with broad-spectrum antimicrobial therapy, including mandatory coverage for MRSA. Patients who present to the hospital with severe infection or infection progressing despite antibiotic therapy should be treated aggressively. In these cases, if *S aureus* is cultured, the clinician should assume the organism may be resistant and should treat with agents effective against MRSA, such as vancomycin, linezolid, or daptomycin.[28] Although risk factors for MRSA SSTIs have been identified, in patients who have severe SSTIs, one should not rely solely on the use risk factors for MRSA in the decision making regarding whether empiric anti-MRSA antimicrobials should be used (**Box 3**).

Choice of empiric antimicrobial therapy for SSTIs is guided by several factors. For patients who have severe SSTIs that are surgical site infections (SSIs), it is important to choose an empiric antimicrobial agent that is different than the class of antibiotics that was used for SSI prophylaxis at the time of the initial surgery. In the case of SSI, the type and site of operation dictate which pathogens are suspected. Infections following operations in the gastrointestinal or genitourinary tract may be monomicrobial or mixed, and may be caused by gram-positive or gram-negative bacteria. In contrast, infections following clean operations in other parts of the body typically are caused by gram-positive pathogens. Immunocompromised or neutropenic patients are, of course, at increased risk of infection and are less able to control local infection and therefore should be treated with empiric, broad-spectrum antibiotics at the first clinical signs of infection, including fever.

Several antimicrobials are approved by the FDA for treating SSTIs. It is important to provide anti-MRSA coverage in the empiric regimen of all patients who have severe

---

Box 3
Risk factors for community-associated methicillin-resistant Staphylococcus aureus skin and soft tissue infections

Persons at risk for skin and soft tissue infections caused by community-associated MRSA

Household contacts of a patient who has proven community-associated MRSA infection[29]

Children[30]

Day care center contacts of hospitalized patients who have MRSA infections[31,32]

Men who have sex with men[33]

Soldiers[34,35]

Incarcerated persons[35]

Athletes, particularly those involved in contact sports[36]

Native Americans[37]

Pacific Islanders[38]

Persons with a previous community-associated MRSA infection[39,40]

Intravenous drug users[41]

From Daum RS. Skin and soft tissue infections caused by methicillin-resistant *Staphylococcus aureus*. N Engl J Med 2007;357:380–90; with permission.

SSTIs. A list of anti-MRSA antimicrobials studied in recent cSSTI clinical trials includes:

The most common comparator antimicrobial (vancomycin)
Those currently approved by the FDA (linezolid, daptomycin, tigecycline)
Those in development (dalbavancin, telavancin, ceftobiprole, iclaprim, ceftaroline) **(Table 1**).

A comprehensive review of these studies has recently been published.[42]

When selecting empiric antimicrobials to treat severe cSSTIs, selection of specific antimicrobials that inhibit toxin production may be helpful, particularly in those patients who have evidence of toxic shock syndrome. This is commonly present in patients who have streptococcal and staphylococcal infections. Protein cytotoxins play an important role in the pathogenesis of various staphylococcal infections, and toxin production should be considered when selecting an antimicrobial agent for gram-positive pathogens.[43] The recent identification of a class of secreted staphylococcal peptides [phenol-soluble modulin (PSM) peptides] documents that they have a remarkable ability to recruit, activate, and lyse human neutrophils, thus eliminating the main cellular defense against MRSA infection.[44] The β-lactams actually enhance toxin production. In contrast, both clindamycin and linezolid have the ability to inhibit toxin production by suppressing translation, but not transcription, of toxin genes for *S aureus* and by directly inhibiting synthesis of group A streptococcal toxins. Particularly when patients exhibit signs and symptoms of streptococcal toxic shock syndrome (shock, coagulopathy, organ failure and NSTI), antitoxin antimicrobials should be initiated promptly.[45]

SOURCE CONTROL (IE, EARLY AGGRESSIVE SURGICAL INTERVENTION FOR DRAINAGE OF ABSCESSES AND DEBRIDEMENT OF NECROTIZING SOFT TISSUE INFECTIONS)

Source control includes drainage of infected fluids, debridement of infected soft tissues, removal of infected devices or foreign bodies, and finally, definite measures to correct anatomic derangement resulting in ongoing microbial contamination and restoring optimal function.[46] Source control represents a key component of success in the therapy of sepsis, because it is the best method of prompt reduction of the bacterial inoculum at the site of infection. Source control has been identified best as an important therapeutic strategy in treating complicated abdominal infections,[47] but is of paramount importance for treating cSSTIs also. Appropriate and timely source control is mandatory for treating severe SSTIs, particularly in the case of NSTIs. This is depicted as the main pillar of the treatment triangle of SSTIs in **Fig. 2**.

PATHOGEN IDENTIFICATION AND APPROPRIATE DE-ESCALATION OF ANTIMICROBIAL THERAPY

Given the increasing prevalence of multidrug-resistant pathogens as the etiology of severe SSTIs, pathogen identification is of paramount importance. All patients who have severe SSTIs should have blood cultures obtained on admission, before initiation of empiric antimicrobial therapy if possible. In addition, cultures should be obtained directly from the SSTI site, either abscess fluid when incision and drainage are performed or tissue sample in the case of NSTIs when surgical debridement is performed.

Initial management of cSSTIs should include collection of specimens for culture and antimicrobial susceptibility testing from all patients who have abscesses or purulent lesions. Culture and susceptibility findings are useful for individual patient

Table 1
Clinical trial results for treatment of cSSTIs

Antibiotic	Comparator	Experimental Design	Total Patients	MRSA Patients	Outcome in MRSA Patients Agent Versus Comparator	Outcome in all Patients Agent Versus Comparator
Linezolid[91,a]	Vancomycin	Open-label	1180	285	Clinical cure: 94.0% versus 83.6% Microcure: 88.6% versus 66.9%	Clinically evaluable: 94.4% versus 90.4%
Daptomycin[92,a]	Vancomycin	Double-blind	1092	64	75% versus 69.4%	Clinically evaluable: 83.4% versus 84.2%
Tigecycline[93,a]	Vancomycin	Double-blind	1116	65	78.4% versus 76.5%	Clinically evaluable: 86.5 versus 88.6%
Dalbavancin[94,b]	Linezolid	Double-blind	854	278	91% versus 89%	88.9% versus 91.2%
Televancin[95,b]	Vancomycin	Double-blind	1867	579	Clinical cure: 90.6% versus 86.4% Microcure: 90% versus 85%	Clinically evaluable: 88% versus 87%
Oritavancin[96,b]	Vancomycin/ cephalexin	Double-blind	1769	33	74% versus 80%	Clinically evaluable: 79% versus 76% clinical cure 75% versus 73% microcure
Ceftobiprole[97,b]	Vancomycin	Double-blind	784	121	91.8% versus 90%	Clinical cure ITT: 77.8% versus 77.5% Clinically evaluable: 93.3% versus 93.5%

Agent	Comparator	Design	No. of Patients	Pathogen/MRSA	Microcure MRSA	Efficacy
Ceftobiprole[98,b]	Vancomycin + ceftazidime	Double blind (included Diabetic Foot Infections)	828	123	89.7% versus 86.1%	Clinical cure ITT: 81.9% versus 80.8% Clinically evaluable: 90.5% versus 90.2%
Iclaprim[99,b]	Linezolid	Double-blind	497	70% of pathogens were S aureus, 25% of which were MRSA	—	Clinical cure ITT: 85.5 versus 91.9% Clinically evaluable: 93.8% versus 99.1% Micro cure: 94.7% versus 98.8%
Iclaprim[88,b]	Linezolid	Double-blind	494	60% of pathogens were S aureus, 50% of which were MRSA	Microcure MRSA: 77.0% versus 80.0%	Clinical cure ITT: 84.9% versus 87.2% Clinically evaluable: 89.6% versus 96.4% Microcure: 83.5% versus 84.7% MSSA 77% versus 80% MRSA
Ceftaroline[100,b]	Vancomycin + aztreonam	Double-blind	702	30% with confirmed pathogen were MRSA	Microcure MRSA: 94.9% versus 91.8%	Clinical cure MITT: 86.6% versus 85.6% Clinically evaluable: 91.1% versus 93.3% Microcure: 91.8% versus 92.5%

Abbreviation: MRSA, methicillin-resistant Staphylococcus aureus.

[a] US Food and Drug Administration-approved for treatment of cSSTI caused by MRSA.
[b] Investigational antimicrobial.

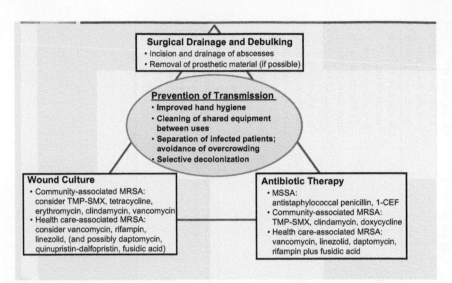

Fig. 2. Treatment triangle for *Staphylococcus aureus* infection. The three components of the treatment of presumed *S aureus* infection include surgical drainage and debridement, obtaining a wound culture, and initiation of appropriate empiric antimicrobial therapy. If methicillin-resistant (MRSA) severe skin and soft tissue infection is confirmed, it is critically important to use all methods to prevent microbial transmission, including hand hygiene. For wound cultures that are positive for community-associated MRSA (usually not a multidrug-resistant phenotype), in vitro susceptibility to trimethoprim–sulfamethoxazole (TMP-SMX), tetracycline, erythromycin, clindamycin, and vancomycin should be assessed. If the isolate is resistant to erythromycin but susceptible to clindamycin, the clindamycin D-zone test should be performed if clindamycin therapy is being considered. For wound cultures that are positive for health care-associated MRSA (usually a multidrug-resistant phenotype), in vitro susceptibility to vancomycin, rifampin, and linezolid should be assessed. Assessment of susceptibility to daptomycin and quinupristin–dalfopristin is not necessary unless therapy with these agents is being considered. Susceptibility to fusidic acid may be assessed in countries where this agent is available. Empiric antibiotic therapy should be reviewed once susceptibility data are known. For methicillin-susceptible *S aureus* (MSSA), antistaphylococcal penicillin or a first-generation cephalosporin (1-CEF) may be suitable. For community-associated MRSA, TMP-SMX, clindamycin, or tetracycline may be suitable. For health care-associated MRSA, vancomycin, linezolid, daptomycin, or rifampin plus fusidic acid may be suitable. (*From* Grayson ML. The treatment triangle for staphylococcal infections [editorial]. N Engl J Med 2006;355:724–7; with permission.)

management and in monitoring local patterns of antimicrobial resistance. It has been documented that physicians and other health care workers cannot predict accurately if an SSTI is caused by MRSA. A prospective observational study conducted in an urban tertiary academic center in ED patients presenting with purulent wounds and abscesses that received wound culture (n=176) documented that physician suspicion of MRSA had a sensitivity of 80% (95% CI 71% to 87%) and a specificity of 23.6% (95% CI 14% to 37%) for the presence of MRSA on wound culture with a positive likelihood ratio (LR) of 1.0 (95% CI 0.9 to 1.3) and a negative LR of 0.8 (95% CI 0.5 to 1.3). Prevalence was 64%. Emergency physicians' suspicion of MRSA infection was a poor predictor of MRSA infection.

Clinicians have a responsibility for appropriate de-escalation of antimicrobial therapy in the treatment of severe SSTIs once culture results return. Pathogen-directed antimicrobial therapy then is initiated, with de-escalation from the initial broad-spectrum empiric antimicrobial regimen, with an attempt to decrease to monotherapy if at all possible.[48] De-escalation of antimicrobial therapy should occur as early as possible, but is only possible if appropriate microbiologic specimens are obtained at the time of SSTI source control. De-escalation is founded on identification of the pathogen and its antibiotic susceptibilities.

In patients who have presumed CA-MRSA SSTIs, it has been recommended that uncomplicated SSTI in healthy individuals may be treated empirically with clindamycin, TMP/SMX, or tetracyclines, although specific data supporting the efficacy of these treatments in large multicenter prospective randomized clinical trials are lacking.[49]

SPECIFIC SEVERE SKIN AND SOFT TISSUE INFECTIONS
Necrotizing Soft Tissue Infections

Necrotizing Soft Tissue Infections (NSTIs) are aggressive soft tissue infections that cause widespread necrosis, and they can include necrotizing cellulitis, fasciitis, and myositis/myonecrosis.[50] Establishing the diagnosis of NSTI can be the main challenge in treating patients who have NSTI, and knowledge of all available tools is key for early and accurate diagnosis.[51] There have been several recent advances in the definition, pathogenesis, diagnostic criteria, and treatment of necrotizing soft tissue infections.[52,53]

Patients who have NSTIs require prompt aggressive surgical debridement, appropriate intravenous antibiotics, and intensive support. Despite aggressive treatment, their mortality and morbidity rates remain high, with some series reporting mortality rates of 25% to 35%.[54] A high index of suspicion should be used in conjunction with laboratory and imaging studies to establish the diagnosis as rapidly as possible. Successful treatment requires early, aggressive surgical debridement of all necrotic tissue, appropriate broad-spectrum systemic antibiotic therapy, and supportive care (fluid resuscitation, organ, and critical care support) to maintain oxygenation and tissue perfusion. Delayed definitive debridement remains the single most important risk factor for death.

A recent single-institution series of 166 patients documented that the overall mortality rate was 16.9%, and limb loss occurred in 26% of patients who had extremity involvement.[55] Independent predictors of mortality included white blood cell count greater than $30,000 \times 10^3/\mu L$, creatinine level greater than 2 mg/dL (176.8 μmol/L), and heart disease at hospital admission. Independent predictors of limb loss included heart disease and shock (systolic blood pressure less than 90 mm Hg) at hospital admission. Clostridial infection was an independent predictor for both limb loss (OR, 3.9 [95% CI, 1.1 to 12.8]) and mortality (OR, 4.1 [95% CI, 1.3 to 12.3]) and was highly associated with intravenous drug use and a high rate of leukocytosis on hospital admission.

Aids to Diagnosis of Necrotizing Soft Tissue Infections

Early operative debridement is a major determinant of outcome in NSTIs. Early recognition of NSTIs, however, is difficult clinically. A novel diagnostic scoring system for distinguishing NSTIs from other severe soft tissue infections based on laboratory tests routinely performed for evaluating severe SSTIs is called the LRINEC score (Table 2).[56]

The LRINEC score initially was developed in a retrospective observational study including 145 patients who had necrotizing fasciitis and 309 patients who had severe cellulitis or abscesses admitted to two tertiary care hospitals. Hematologic and biochemical results done on admission were converted into categorical variables for analysis. Univariate and multivariate logistic regression was used to select significant

Table 2 The laboratory risk indicator for necrotizing fasciitis score	
Variable, Units	Score
C-reactive protein, mg/L	
<150	0
≥150	4
Total white cell count, per mm³	
<15	0
15–25	1
>25	2
Hemoglobin, g/dL	
>13.5	0
11–13.5	1
<11	2
Sodium, mmol/L	
≥135	0
<135	2
Creatinine, μmol/L	
≤141	0
>141	2
Glucose, mmol/L	
≤10	0
>10	1

The maximum score is 13; a score ≥26 should raise the suspicion of necrotizing fasciitis, and a score of ≥8 is strongly predictive of this disease.

predictors. Total white cell count, hemoglobin, sodium, glucose, serum creatinine, and C-reactive protein were selected. The LRINEC score was constructed by converting into integer the regression coefficients of independently predictive factors in the multiple logistic regression model for diagnosing necrotizing fasciitis. The cutoff value for the LRINEC score was 6 points, with a positive predictive value of 92.0% and negative predictive value of 96.0%. Model performance was very good (Hosmer-Lemeshow statistic, $P = .910$); area under the receiver operating characteristic curve was 0.980 and 0.976 in the developmental and validation cohorts, respectively. The LRINEC score is a robust score capable of detecting even clinically early cases of necrotizing fasciitis. The variables used are measured routinely to assess severe soft tissue infections. Patients who have a LRINEC score of greater than or equal to 6 should be evaluated carefully for the presence of necrotizing fasciitis.

Since the initial development of the LRINEC score, several other cohort studies have validated its utility for diagnosing NSTIs.[57] A recent multicenter study in 229 patients who had NSTIs from 2002 to 2005 reported an overall mortality rate of 15.8% and amputation rate of 26.3%. This study also documented that a LRINEC score greater than or equal to 6 was associated with a higher rate of mortality and amputation (receiver operating characteristic curve, area under the curve 0.75).[57]

Diagnostic Imaging in Necrotizing Soft Tissue Infections

A high clinical index of suspicion is required if the diagnosis is to be made sufficiently early for successful treatment. NSTIs necessitate prompt aggressive surgical debridement for satisfactory treatment in addition to antimicrobial therapy. It is critical to remember that because of the rapidly progressive and potentially fatal outcome of this condition, if imaging cannot be performed expeditiously, delaying treatment is not justified.

Plain film findings may reveal extensive soft tissue gas. CT examination can reveal asymmetric thickening of deep fascia in association with gas, and associated abscesses also may be present. MRI additionally can assist in diagnosing NSTIs.[58] MRI has been documented to effectively differentiate between necrotizing and non-necrotizing infection of the lower extremity, but should not delay prompt surgical intervention in NSTI management.[59]

Microbiology of Necrotizing Soft Tissue Infections

Necrotizing fasciitis and myonecrosis typically are caused by infection with group A *Streptococcus, Clostridium perfringens*, or, most commonly, aerobic and anaerobic organisms as part of a polymicrobial infection that may include *S aureus*. In case series, CA-MRSA recently was described as a predominantly monomicrobial cause of necrotizing fasciitis.[60,61] A retrospective review of patients presenting with necrotizing fasciitis between 2000 and 2006 indicated that MRSA was the most common pathogen, accounting for one third of the organisms isolated.[62]

NSTIs are categorized into three specific types based on the microbiologic etiology of the infection.

Type 1, or polymicrobial
Type 2, or group A streptococcal
Type 3, gas gangrene, or clostridial myonecrosis

Increasingly, MRSA has been identified as the causative microbe in NSTIs, but a separate category for this NSTI does not exist.[21,63–66] Given this finding, anti-MRSA empiric antimicrobial therapy should be initiated in all patients who have NSTIs, and pathogen-directed antimicrobial therapy should be considered once tissue culture results are available.

Uncommon microbiologic causes of NSTIs and primary sepsis include *Vibrio* and *Aeromonas* species, virulent gram-negative bacteria and members of the *Vibrionaceae* family that thrive in aquatic environments.[67] These NSTIs are likely to occur in patients who have hepatic disease, diabetes, and immunocompromised conditions.[68] These organisms are found in warm sea waters and are often present in raw oysters, shellfish, and other seafood. The diagnosis of *Vibrio* NSTIs should be suspected when a patient has the appropriate clinical findings and a history of contact with seawater or raw seafood. *Aeromonas hydrophila* is a gram-negative bacillus commonly found in soil, sewage, and fresh or brackish water in many parts of the United States.[69] The contact history of patients who have a rapid onset of SSTIs can alert clinicians to a differential diagnosis of soft tissue infection with *Vibrio vulnificus* (contact with seawater or raw seafood) or *Aeromonas* species (contact with fresh or brackish water, soil, or wood). Early fasciotomy and culture-directed antimicrobial therapy should be performed aggressively in those patients who have hypotensive shock, leukopenia, severe hypoalbuminemia, and underlying chronic illness, especially a combination of hepatic dysfunction and diabetes mellitus. The rate of amputation and mortality is very high in these patients, and early definitive management is of paramount importance.[70–72]

Novel Therapeutic Strategies for Necrotizing Soft Tissue Infections

Several novel therapeutic strategies as adjuncts for treating NSTIs have been described, including vacuum-assisted wound closure (VAC) therapy, intravenous immunoglobulin, and hyperbaric oxygen therapy.

Vacuum-assisted wound closure therapy

Several reports have documented the utility of VAC therapy for managing patients who have acute NSTIs.[73–75] VAC therapy has been associated with reduced time for wound care, improved patient comfort, greater mobility, reduced drainage, and decreased time to wound closure.[76] Although no prospective randomized trials have been conducted comparing VAC therapy with traditional wet dressing techniques, it can be considered, particularly in patients who have large wounds, where conscious sedation or general anesthesia is required for wound dressing changes.

Intravenous immunoglobulin

The use of intravenous immunoglobulin for treating NSTIs remains controversial, but is based upon a potential benefit related to binding of gram-positive organism exotoxins. The clinical studies that have been completed are not randomized blinded trials, but some show evidence of improved outcomes with intravenous immunoglobulin treatment.[77–79] This treatment should be restricted, however, to critically ill patients who have either staphylococcal or streptococcal NSTIs.[80,81]

Hyperbaric oxygen therapy

The benefit of hyperbaric oxygen (HBO) as an adjunctive treatment is controversial, and no prospective randomized clinical trials have been performed. A recent retrospective review investigated the effect of HBO in treating NSTIs.[82] Clinical data were reviewed for 78 patients who had NSTIs. Thirty patients at one center were treated with surgery, antibiotics, and supportive care; 48 patients at a different center received adjunctive HBO treatment. Demographic characteristics and risk factors were similar in the HBO and non-HBO groups. The mean patient age was 49.5 years; 37% of the patients were female, and 49% had diabetes mellitus. Patients underwent a mean of 3.0 excisional debridements. The median hospital length of stay was 16.5 days; the median duration of antibiotic use was 15.0 days. In 36% of patients, cultures were polymicrobial; group A *Streptococcus* was the organism most commonly isolated (28%). No statistically significant differences in outcomes between the two groups were identified. The mortality rate for the HBO group (8.3%) was lower, although not significantly different ($P = .48$) than that observed for the non-HBO group (13.3%). The number of debridements was greater in the HBO group (3.0; $P = .03$). The hospital length of stay and duration of antibiotic use were similar for the two groups. Multivariable analysis showed that hypotension on admission and immunosuppression were significant independent risk factors for death. These authors concluded that the use of HBO to treat NSTIs did not reduce mortality rate, number of debridements, hospital length of stay, or duration of antibiotic use. Immunosuppression and early hypotension were important risk factors associated with higher mortality rates in patients who had NSTIs. Several other published peer-reviewed retrospective studies have identified variable treatment effects with HBO therapy for NSTIs.[83–86] These studies are limited, related to nonrandomized experimental design, retrospective reviews, and poor controls.

Pyomyositis

Myositis is a rare infection that may lead to serious and potentially life-threatening local and systemic complications.[87] The infection can progress rapidly, and early recognition and proper medical and surgical management are therefore the corner-stones of therapy. With the increasing prevalence of community-associated MRSA as a pathogen in severe SSTIs, pyomyositis is more common than in past years. Myositis often occurs in muscle sites that have been compromised by injury, ischemia, malignancy or surgery. The predominant pathogens are *S aureus*, group A strepto-cocci (GAS), gram-negative aerobic and facultative bacilli, and the indigenous aerobic and anaerobic cutaneous and mucous membranes' local microflora.

CT scan imaging is a rapid and sensitive diagnostic test, and it commonly demon-strates diffuse enlargement of the involved muscle. It additionally may demonstrate the presence of fluid or gas collections within the muscle, suggesting the presence of abscesses. MRI is more sensitive in showing early inflammatory changes before development of abscesses in myositis.[88] Emergency surgical exploration is warranted to define the nature of the infective process, which is accomplished by direct exami-nation of the involved muscles. Surgical intervention is required to perform appropriate abscess drainage and debridement and to also evaluate for necrotizing myositis. Fas-ciotomies and extremity amputation are sometimes necessary.

Diabetic Foot Infections as Cause of Severe Skin and Soft Tissue Infections

Diabetic foot infections (DFIs) also can be a cause of severe SSTIs. These patients:

Can present with severe sepsis and septic shock
Frequently require surgical abscess drainage and debridement
May require vascular evaluation for improved arterial inflow
Can require extremity amputation for source control sometimes

Table 3
Risk stratification for patients with diabetic foot infections

Clinical Manifestation of Infection	Infection Severity	PEDIS Grade[a]
Wound lacking purulence or any manifestations of inflammation	Uninfected	1
Presence of ≥2 manifestations of inflammation Any cellulitis/erythema extends ≤2 cm around the ulcer Infection limited to the skin or superficial subcutaneous tissues No other local complications or systemic illness	Mild	2

Patient is systemically well and metabolically stable
≥1 of the following characteristics:
  Cellulitis extending >2 cm
  Lymphangitic streaking
  Spread beneath the superficial fascia
  Deep-tissue abscess
  Gangrene
  Involvement of muscle, tendon, joint, or bone
	Moderate	3

Infection in a patient with systemic toxicity or metabolic instability	Severe	4

Data from Lipsky BA, Berendt AR, Deery HG, et al. Diagnosis and treatment of diabetic foot infec-tions. Clin Infect Dis 2004;39:885–910.
Abbreviation: PEDIS, perfusion, extent/size, depth/tissue loss, infection, and sensation.
Foot ischemia may increase the severity of any infection, and the presence of critical ischemia often makes the infection severe.
[a] International Consensus on the Diabetic Foot.

The Infectious Diseases Society of America Guidelines regarding Diagnosis and Treatment of Diabetic Foot Infections comprehensively review this topic (**Table 3**).[89,90] Aerobic gram-positive cocci (especially *S aureus*) are the predominant pathogens in DFIs. Patients who have chronic wounds or who recently have received antimicrobial therapy also may be infected with gram-negative rods, and those who have foot ischemia or gangrene may have obligate anaerobic pathogens. The fundamental management of patients who have severe cSSTIs related to DFIs is the same as described previously; however, in addition, special attention to a potential diagnosis of concurrent osteomyelitis, potential need for vascular reconstruction for ischemic arterial disease, and assessment of neuropathy and foot offloading must be considered in these patients.

SUMMARY

Severe cSSTIs are associated with significant morbidity and mortality, and it is important to differentiate necrotizing versus non-necrotizing SSTIs early in the course of treatment. Drug-resistant organisms are common causative pathogens in cSSTIs. MRSA is the most common cause of purulent cSSTIs. All patients who present with complicated SSTIs should be treated with broad-spectrum antimicrobial therapy, including mandatory coverage for MRSA. Source control, including abscess drainage and surgical debridement, are the mainstays of therapy in severe cSSTIs. It is of paramount importance to obtain specimens for culture and antimicrobial susceptibilities given the high prevalence of MRSA as a causative pathogen in cSSTIs. Empiric broad-spectrum antimicrobial therapy should be de-escalated to narrower-spectrum agents based on culture pathogen identification and the patient's clinical response.

REFERENCES

1. Napolitano LM. The diagnosis and treatment of skin and soft tissue infections (SSTIs). Surg Infect 2008;9(Suppl 1):s17–27.
2. DiNubile MJ, Lipsky BA. Complicated infections of skin and skin structures: when the infection is more than skin deep. J Antimicrob Chemother 2004; 53(Suppl 2):ii37–50.
3. Vinh DC, Embil JM. Severe skin and soft tissue infections and associated critical illness. Curr Infect Dis Rep 2007;9(5):415–21.
4. May AK. Skin and soft tissue infections. Surg Clin North Am 2009;89(2):403–20.
5. Chan T, Yaghoubian A, Rosing D, et al. Low sensitivity of physical examination findings in necrotizing soft tissue infection is improved with laboratory values: a prospective study. Am J Surg 2008;196(6):926–30 [discussion: 930].
6. Wall DB, deVirgilio C, Black S, et al. Objective criteria may assist in distinguishing necrotizing fasciitis from non-necrotizing soft tissue infection. Am J Surg 2000;179(11):17–21.
7. Wall DB, Klein SR, Black S, et al. A simple model to help distinguish necrotizing fasciitis from non-necrotizing soft tissue infections. J Am Coll Surg 2000;191(3): 227–31.
8. Kollef MH, Sherman G, Ward S, et al. Inadequate antimicrobial treatment of infections: a risk factor for hospital mortality among critically ill patients. Chest 1999;115:462–74.
9. Iregui M, Ward S, Sherman G, et al. Clinical importance of delays in the initiation of appropriate antibiotic treatment for ventilator-associated pneumonia. Chest 2002;122:262–8.

10. Garnacho-Montero J. Impact of adequate empirical antibiotic therapy on the outcome of patients admitted to the intensive care unit with sepsis. Crit Care Med 2003;31:2742–51.
11. Alvarez-Lerma F. Modification of empiric antibiotic treatment in patients with pneumonia acquired in the intensive care unit. ICU-Acquired Pneumonia Study Group. Intensive Care Med 1996;22:387–94.
12. Ruhe JJ, Smith N, Bradsher RW, et al. Community-onset methicillin-resistant *Staphylococcus aureus* skin and soft tissue infections: impact of antimicrobial therapy on outcome. Clin Infect Dis 2007;44:777–84.
13. Schramm GE, Johnson JA, Doherty JA, et al. Methicillin-resistant *Staphylococcus aureus* sterile-site infection: the importance of appropriate initial antimicrobial treatment. Crit Care Med 2006;34(8):2069–74.
14. Chuck EA, Frazee BW, Lambert L, et al. The benefit of empiric treatment for MRSA. J Emerg Med 2008, in press.
15. Gorwitz RJ, Jernigan DB, Powers JH, et al. Strategies for clinical management of MRSA in the community: summary of an experts' meeting convened by the Centers for Disease Control and Prevention. 2006. Available at: http://198.246. 98.21/ncidod/dhqp/pdf/ar/CAMRSA_ExpMtgStrategies.pdf. Accessed April 17, 2009.
16. Kumar A, Roberts D, Wood KE, et al. Duration of hypotension before initiation of effective antimicrobial therapy is the critical determinant of survival in human septic shock. Crit Care Med 2006;34(6):1589–96.
17. Brook I. Microbiology and management of soft tissue and muscle infections. Int J Surg 2008;6(4):328–38.
18. Naimi TS, LeDell KH, Como-Sabetti K, et al. Comparison of community- and health care-associated methicillin-resistant *Staphylococcus aureus* infection. JAMA 2003;290:2976–84.
19. Crum NF, Lee RU, Thornton SA, et al. Fifteen-year study of the changing epidemiology of methicillin-resistant *Staphylococcus aureus*. Am J Med 2006;119:943–51.
20. Moran GJ, Krishnadasan A, Gorwitz RJ, et al. Methicillin-resistant *S aureus* infections among patients in the emergency department. N Engl J Med 2006;355(7):666–74.
21. Miller LG, Perdreau-Remington F, Rieg G, et al. Necrotizing fasciitis caused by community-associated methicillin-resistant *Staphylococcus aureus* in Los Angeles. N Engl J Med 2005;352(14):1445–53.
22. Frazee BW, Lynn J, Charlebois ED, et al. High prevalence of methicillin-resistance in emergency department skin and soft tissue infection. Ann Emerg Med 2005;45:311–20.
23. King MD, Humphrey BJ, Wang YF. Emergence of community acquired methicillin-resistant *Staphylococcus aureus* USA 300 Clone as the predominant cause of skin and soft tissue infections. Ann Intern Med 2006;144:309–17.
24. Awad SS, Elhabash SI, Lee L, et al. Increasing incidence of methicillin-resistant *Staphylococcus aureus* skin and soft tissue infections: reconsideration of empiric antimicrobial therapy. Am J Surg 2007;194:606–10.
25. Hidayat LK, Hsu DI, Quist R, et al. High-dose vancomycin for methicillin-resistant *Staphylococcus aureus* infections. Arch Intern Med 2006;166:2138–44.
26. Howden BP, Ward PB, Charles PGP, et al. Treatment outcomes for serious infections caused by methicillin-resistant *Staphylococcus aureus* with reduced vancomycin susceptibility. Clin Infect Dis 2004;38:521–8.
27. Lipsky BA, Weigelt JA, Gupta V, et al. Skin, soft tissue, bone, and joint infections in hospitalized patients: epidemiology and microbiological, clinical, and economic outcomes. Infect Control Hosp Epidemiol 2007;28(11):1290–8.

28. Stevens DL, Bisno AL, Chambers HF, et al. Infectious Diseases Society of America. Practice guidelines for the diagnosis and management of skin and soft tissue infections. Clin Infect Dis 2005;41(10):1373–406.

29. Dietrich DW, Auld DB, Mermel LA. Community-acquired methicillin-resistant *Staphylococcus aureus* in southern New England children. Pediatrics 2004; 113(4):e347–52.

30. Fridkin SK, Hageman JC, Morrison M, et al. Methicillin-resistant *Staphylococcus aureus* disease in three communities. N Engl J Med 2005;352:1436–44.

31. Adcock PM, Pastor P, Medley F, et al. Methicillin-resistant *Staphylococcus aureus* in two child care centers. J Infect Dis 1998;178:577–80.

32. Shahin R, Johnson IL, Jamieson F, et al. Methicillin-resistant *Staphylococcus aureus* carriage in a child care center following a case of disease. Arch Pediatr Adolesc Med 1999;153:864–8.

33. Lee NE, Taylor MM, Bancroft E, et al. Risk factors for community-associated methicillin-resistant *Staphylococcus aureus* skin infections among HIV-positive men who have sex with men. Clin Infect Dis 2005;40:1529–34 [erratum, Clin Infect Dis 2005;41:135].

34. Ellis MW, Hospenthal DR, Dooley DP, et al. Natural history of community-acquired methicillin-resistant *Staphylococcus aureus* colonization and infection in soldiers. Clin Infect Dis 2004;39:971–9.

35. Aiello AE, Lowy FD, Wright LN, et al. Methicillin-resistant *Staphylococcus aureus* among US prisoners and military personnel: review and recommendations for future studies. Lancet Infect Dis 2006;6:335–41.

36. Kazakova SV, Hageman JC, Matava M, et al. A clone of methicillin-resistant *Staphylococcus aureus* among professional football players. N Engl J Med 2005;352:468–75.

37. Groom AV, Wolsey DH, Naimi TS, et al. Community-acquired methicillin-resistant *Staphylococcus aureus* in a rural American Indian community. JAMA 2001;286: 1201–5.

38. Castrodale LJ, Beller M, Gessner BD. Over-representation of Samoan/Pacific Islanders with methicillin-resistant *Staphylococcus aureus* (MRSA) infections at a large family practice clinic in Anchorage, Alaska, 1996–2000. Ala Med 2004; 46:88–91.

39. Szumowski JD, Cohen DE, Kanaya F, et al. Treatment and outcomes of infections by methicillin-resistant *Staphylococcus aureus* at an ambulatory clinic. Antimicrob Agents Chemother 2007;51:423–8.

40. Skiest DJ, Brown K, Cooper TW, et al. Prospective comparison of methicillin-susceptible and methicillin-resistant community-associated *Staphylococcus aureus* infections in hospitalized patients. J Infect 2007;54:427–34.

41. Young DM, Harris HW, Charlebois ED, et al. An epidemic of methicillin-resistant *Staphylococcus aureus* soft tissue infections among medically underserved patients. Arch Surg 2004;139:947–53.

42. Napolitano LM. Early appropriate parenteral antimicrobial treatment of complicated skin and soft tissue infections caused by methicillin-resistant *Staphylococcus aureus*. Surg Infect (Larchmt) 2008;9(Suppl 1):S15–27.

43. Stevens DL, Ma Y, Salmi DB, et al. Impact of antibiotics on expression of virulence-associated exotoxin genes in methicillin-sensitive and methicillin-resistant *Staphylococcus aureus*. J Infect Dis 2007;195:202–11.

44. Wang R, Braughton KR, Kretschmer D, et al. Identification of novel cytolytic peptides as key virulence determinants for community-associated MRSA. Nat Med 2007;13(12):1510–4.

45. Filbin MR, Ring DC, Wessels MR, et al. Case 2—2009: a 25 year-old man with pain and swelling of the right hand and hypotension. N Engl J Med 2009;360:281–90.
46. Marshall JC, Maier RV, Jimenez M, et al. Source control in the management of severe sepsis and septic shock: an evidence-based review. Crit Care Med 2004;32(Suppl 11):S513–26.
47. Laterre PF. Progress in medical management of intra-abdominal infections. Curr Opin Infect Dis 2008;21(4):393–8.
48. Kuo DC, Chasm RM, Witting MD. Emergency department physician ability to predict methicillin-resistant *Staphylococcus aureus* skin and soft tissue infections. J Emerg Med 2008, in press.
49. Stryjewski ME, Chambers HF. Skin and soft tissue infections caused by community-acquired methicillin-resistant *Staphylococcus aureus*. Clin Infect Dis 2008; 46(Suppl 5):S368–77.
50. Sarani B, Strong M, Pascual J, et al. Necrotizing fasciitis: current concepts and review of the literature. J Am Coll Surg 2009;208(2):279–88.
51. Anaya DA, Dellinger EP. Necrotizing soft tissue infection: diagnosis and management. Clin Infect Dis 2007;44(5):705–10.
52. Cainzos M, Gonzalez-Rodriguez FJ. Necrotizing soft tissue infections. Curr Opin Crit Care 2007;13(4):433–9.
53. Yilmazlar T, Ozturk E, Alsoy A, et al. Necrotizing soft tissue infections: APACHE II score, dissemination, and survival. World J Surg 2007;31(9):1858–62.
54. Cuschieri J. Necrotizing soft tissue infection. Surg Infect (Larchmt) 2008;9(6): 559–62.
55. Anaya DA, McMahon K, Nathens AB, et al. Predictors of mortality and limb loss in necrotizing soft tissue infections. Arch Surg 2005;140:151–7.
56. Wong CH, Khin LW, Heng KS, et al. The LRINEC (Laboratory Risk Indicator for Necrotizing Fasciitis) score: a tool for distinguishing necrotizing fasciitis from other soft tissue infections. Crit Care Med 2004;32(7):1535–41.
57. Su YC, Chen HW, Hong YC, et al. Laboratory risk indicator for necrotizing fasciitis score and the outcomes. ANZ J Surg 2008;78(11):968–72.
58. Struk DW, Munk PL, Lee MJ, et al. Imaging of soft tissue infections. Radiol Clin North Am 2001;39(2):277–303.
59. Brothers TE, Tagge DU, Stutley JE, et al. Magnetic resonance imaging differentiates between necrotizing and non-necrotizing fasciitis of the lower extremity. J Am Coll Surg 1998;187:416–21.
60. Wong CH, Chang HC, Pasupathy S, et al. Necrotizing fasciitis: clinical presentation, microbiology, and determinants of mortality. J Bone Joint Surg Am 2003;85(8):1454–60.
61. McHenry CR, Piotrowski JJ, Petrinic D, et al. Determinants of mortality for necrotizing soft tissue infections. Ann Surg 1995;221(5):558–65.
62. Elhabash S, Lee L, Farrow B, et al. Characteristics and microbiology of patients presenting with necrotizing fasciitis. Presented at the Association of VA Surgeons 31st Annual Meeting. Little Rock, Arkansas, May 10–12, 2007.
63. Lee TC, Carrick MM, Scott BG, et al. Incidence and clinical characteristics of MRSA necrotizing fasciitis in a large urban hospital. Am J Surg 2007;194(6): 809–12.
64. Young LM, Price CS. Community-acquired MRSA emerging as an important cause of necrotizing fasciitis. Surg Infect (Larchmt) 2008;9(4):469–74.
65. Olsen RJ, Burns KM, Chen L, et al. Severe necrotizing fasciitis in a human immunodeficiency virus-positive patient caused by MRSA. J Clin Microbiol 2008; 46(3):1144–7.

66. Dehority W, Wang E, Vernon PS, et al. Community-associated MRSA necrotizing fasciitis in a neonate. Pediatr Infect Dis J 2006;25(11):1080–1.

67. Tsai YH, Hsu RW, Huang TJ, et al. Necrotizing soft tissue infections and sepsis caused by *Vibrio vulnificus* compared with those caused by *Aeromonas* species. J Bone Joint Surg Am 2007;89(3):631–6.

68. Tsai YH, Hsu RW, Huang KC, et al. Systemic *Vibrio* infection presenting as necrotizing fasciitis and sepsis. A series of 13 cases. J Bone Joint Surg Am 2004;86(11):2497–502.

69. Minnaganti VR, Patel PJ, Iancu D, et al. Necrotizing fasciitis caused by *Aeromonas hydrophila*. Heart Lung 2000;29(4):306–8.

70. Bross MH, Soch K, Morales R, et al. *Vibrio vulnificus* infection. diagnosis and treatment. Am Fam Physician 2007;76(4):539–44.

71. Tsai YH, Huang TJ, Hsu RW, et al. Necrotizing soft tissue infections and primary sepsis caused by *Vibrio vulnificus* and *Vibrio cholerae* non-O1. J Trauma 2009; 66(3):899–905.

72. Kuo YL, Shieh SJ, Chiu HY, et al. Necrotizing fasciitis caused by *Vibrio vulnificus*: epidemiology, clinical findings, treatment, and prevention. Eur J Clin Microbiol Infect Dis 2007;26(11):785–92.

73. Huang WS, Hsieh SC, Hsieh CS, et al. Use of vacuum-assisted wound closure to manage limb wounds in patients suffering from acute necrotizing fasciitis. Asian J Surg 2006;29(3):135–9.

74. Steinstraesser L, Sand M, Steinaue HU. Giant VAC in a patient with extensive necrotizing fasciitis. Int J Low Extrem Wounds 2009;8(1):28–30.

75. Silberstein J, Grabowski J, Parsons JK. Use of a vacuum-assisted device for Fournier's gangrene: a new paradigm. Rev Urol 2008;10(1):76–80.

76. Ozturk E, Ozquc H, Yilmazlar T. The use of vacuum-assisted closure therapy in the management of Fournier's gangrene. Am J Surg 2009;197:660–5.

77. Kaul R, McGeer A, Norrby-Teglund A, et al. Intravenous immunoglobulin therapy for streptococcal toxic shock syndrome—a comparative observational study. The Canadian Streptococcal Study Group. Clin Infect Dis 1999;28:800–7.

78. Lamothe F, D'Amico P, Ghosn P, et al. Clinical usefulness of intravenous human immunoglobulins in invasive group A streptococcal infections: case report and review. Clin Infect Dis 1995;21:1469–70.

79. Alejandria MM, Lansang MA, Dans LF, et al. Intravenous immunoglobulin for treating sepsis and septic shock. Cochrane Database Syst Rev 2002;1 CD001090.

80. Darabi K, Abdel-Wahab O, Dzik WH. Current usage of intravenous immune globulin and the rationale behind it: the Massachusetts General Hospital data and a review of the literature. Transfusion 2006;46:741–53.

81. Schrage B, Duan G, Yang LP, et al. Different preparations of intravenous immunoglobulin vary in their efficacy to neutralize streptococcal superantigens: implications for treatment of streptococcal toxic shock syndrome. Clin Infect Dis 2006;43:743–6.

82. George ME, Rueth NM, Skarda DE, et al. Hyperbaric oxygen does not improve outcome in patients with necrotizing soft tissue infection. Surg Infect (Larchmt) 2009;10(1):21–8.

83. Brown DR, Davis NL, Lepawsky M, et al. A multicenter review of the treatment of major truncal necrotizing infections with and without hyperbaric oxygen therapy. Am J Surg 1994;167:485–9.

84. Shupak A, Shoshani O, Golderberg I, et al. Necrotizing fasciitis: an indication for hyperbaric oxygenation therapy? Surgery 1995;118:873–8.

85. Korhonen K. Review Hyperbaric oxygen therapy in acute necrotizing infections. With a special reference to the effects on tissue gas tensions. Ann Chir Gynaecol 2000;89:7–36.
86. Mindrup SR, Kealey GP, Fallon B. Hyperbaric oxygen for the treatment of fournier's gangrene. J Urol 2005;173:1975–7.
87. Brook I. Microbiology and management of myositis. Int Orthop 2004;28(5): 257–60.
88. Garcia J. MRI in inflammatory myopathies. Skeletal Radiol 2000;29:425–38.
89. Lipsky BA, Berendt AR, Deery HG, et al. Infectious Diseases Society of America. Clin Infect Dis 2004;39(7):885–910.
90. Lavery LA, Armstrong DG, Murdoch DP, et al. Validation of the Infectious Diseases Society of America's diabetic foot infection classification system. Clin Infect Dis 2007;44(4):562–5.
91. Weigelt J, Itani K, Stevens D, et al. Linezolid CSSTI Study Group. Linezolid versus vancomycin in treatment of complicated skin and soft tissue infections. Antimicrob Agents Chemother 2005;49:2260–6.
92. Arbeit RD, Maki D, Tally FP, et al. The safety and efficacy of daptomycin for the treatment of complicated skin and skin structure infections. Clin Infect Dis 2004; 38:1673–81.
93. Ellis-Grosse EJ, Babinchak T, Dartois N, et al. The efficacy and safety of tigecycline in the treatment of skin and skin-structure infections: results of 2 double-blind phase 3 comparison studies with vancomycin-aztreonam. Clin Infect Dis 2005;41(Suppl 5):S341–53.
94. Jauregui LE, Babazadeh S, Seltzer E, et al. Randomized, double-blind comparison of once-weekly dalbavancin versus twice-daily linezolid therapy for the treatment of complicated skin and skin structure infections. Clin Infect Dis 2005;41:1407–15.
95. Stryjewski ME, Graham DR, Wilson SE, et al. Telavancin versus vancomycin for the treatment of complicated skin and skin structure infections caused by gram-positive organisms. Clin Infect Dis 2008;46(11):1683–93.
96. Giamarellou H, O'Riordan W, Harris H, et al. Phase 3 trial comparing 3–7 days of oritavancin versus 10–14 days of vancomycin/cephalexin in the treatment of patients with complicated skin and skin structure infections (cSSSI) [abstract L-739]. Presented at the Interscience Conference on Antimicrobial Agents and Chemotherapy. Chicago, 2003.
97. Noel GJ, Strauss RS, Amsler K, et al. Results of a double-blind, randomized trial of ceftobiprole treatment of complicated skin and skin structure infections caused by gram-positive bacteria. Antimicrob Agents Chemother 2008;52: 37–44.
98. Noel GJ, Bush K, Bagchi P, et al. A randomized, double-blind trial comparing ceftobiprole medocaril to vancomycin plus ceftazidime in the treatment of patients with complicated skin and skin structure infection. Clin Infect Dis 2008;46:647–55.
99. ASSIST-1 and ASSIST-2 (Arpida's Skin and Skin Structure Infection Studies). Presented at the 48th Interscience Conference on Antimicrobial Agents and Chemotherapy (ICAAC)/Infectious Diseases Society of America (IDSA) 46th annual meeting. Washington, DC, 2008.
100. Corey R, Wilcox M, Talbot GH, et al. CANVAS-1. Presented at the 48th Interscience Conference on Antimicrobial Agents and Chemotherapy (ICAAC)/Infectious Diseases Society of America (IDSA) 46th annual meeting in Washington, DC, 2008.

Intra-abdominal Sepsis: Newer Interventional and Antimicrobial Therapies

Joseph S. Solomkin, MD[a],*, John Mazuski, MD, PhD[b]

KEYWORDS

- Peritonitis • Abscess • Severity • Source control • Antibiotic
- Percutaneous drainage • Microbiology

Complicated intra-abdominal infections are the second most common cause of septic death in the intensive care unit (ICU).[1] While there have been improvements in the outcome of "sepsis" regardless of etiology, it is apparent that this is even more striking for intra-abdominal infections.[2] From observation, recent advances in interventional techniques, including more aggressive use of percutaneous drainage of abscesses and use of "open abdomen" techniques for peritonitis have significantly affected the morbidity and mortality of physiologically severe complicated intra-abdominal infection.

ALTERED STRATEGIES FOR MANAGING INTRA-ABDOMINAL SEPSIS

The best way of understanding the integration of these advances is as a major change in strategy. During the 1970s and 1980s, an aggressive surgical approach was popular. This provided a definitive operative effort, even in the presence of septic shock, to deal with the process at hand. A more nuanced approach has replaced this previous strategy, much more centered upon temporization. In this case, "damage control" techniques are used for patients with peritonitis, and percutaneous drainage is used in complex settings (such as infected necrotizing pancreatitis) to delay even in the presence of organ failure.[3,4,5] The more aggressive and more

---

The material in this article is derived, in part, from draft guidelines for the management of intra-abdominal infections produced by a joint panel from the Surgical Infections Society and the Infectious Diseases Society of America, co-chaired by the authors.

[a] Department of Surgery, University of Cincinnati College of Medicine, 231 Albert B. Sabin Way, Cincinnati OH 45267-0558, USA
[b] Department of Surgery, Washington University School of Medicine, Saint Louis, MO, USA
* Corresponding author.
E-mail address: joseph.solomkin@uc.edu (J.S. Solomkin).

Infect Dis Clin N Am 23 (2009) 593–608
doi:10.1016/j.idc.2009.04.007
0891-5520/09/$ – see front matter © 2009 Elsevier Inc. All rights reserved.

id.theclinics.com

organized approach to sepsis therapy now undertaken in many emergency departments and critical care units has also benefited patients with severe intra-abdominal infections. Similarly, newer antimicrobial classes and improved understanding of pharmacokinetics and pharmacodynamics have contributed to the evolutionary improvement in outcomes.

At the same time, decisions regarding appropriate empiric antimicrobial therapy have been made more difficult because of increasing rates of antimicrobial resistance in pathogens causing community-acquired infection, an increase in patients at risk of nonhospital health care-associated infection, and an increase in resistance rates in hospital-acquired organisms. These observations mean that antimicrobial therapy must now be routinely considered as part of an antimicrobial stewardship program.

DEFINITIONS USED
Complicated Intra-Abdominal Infections

Complicated intra-abdominal infections extend beyond the hollow viscus of origin into the peritoneal space, and are associated either with abscess formation or peritonitis. This term is not meant to describe the infection's severity or anatomy. Uncomplicated infections involve intramural inflammation of the gastrointestinal (GI) tract, and have a substantial probability of progressing to complicated infection if not adequately treated. Typically, these infections are of lower severity but may present with a picture of severe sepsis syndrome.

Severity of Infection

Severity of infection is defined as a composite of patient age, physiologic derangements, and background medical conditions. These value are captured by anyone of several severity scoring systems, but for the individual patient clinical judgment is at least as accurate as a numerical score.[6,7,8,9]

High Risk

High risk is intended to describe patients with a range of reasons for increased rates of treatment failure, in addition to a higher severity of infection, particularly an anatomically unfavorable infection, or a health care-associated infection (**Box 1**).[10]

Box 1
Clinical factors predicting failure of source control for intra-abdominal infections

Delay in the initial intervention (> 24 hours)

High severity of illness (Acute physiology and chronic health evaluation or APACHE II > 15)

Advanced age

Comorbidity and degree of organ dysfunction

Low albumin

Poor nutritional status

Degree of peritoneal involvement/diffuse peritonitis

Inability to achieve adequate debridement or control of drainage

Presence of malignancy

Health Care-Associated Infection

Healthcare-associated infection is a relatively new term that includes a spectrum of adult patients who have close association with acute care hospitals or reside in chronic care settings.[11] These factors increase their risk for infection caused by multi-drug-resistant bacteria. The definitions for health care-associated infections provided by Klevens and colleagues[11] are used in this guideline. Health care-associated infections include "community-onset" and "hospital-onset." Community-onset health care-associated infections include cases with at least one of the following health care risk factors: history of surgery, hospitalization, dialysis, or residence in a long-term care facility in the previous 12 months preceding the culture date. Hospital-onset includes cases with a positive culture result from a normally sterile site obtained greater than 48 hours after hospital admission.

INITIAL DIAGNOSTIC EFFORTS

Patients with intra-abdominal infections typically present with rapid-onset abdominal pain and symptoms of GI dysfunction (loss of appetite, nausea, vomiting, bloating, obstipation), with or without signs of inflammation (pain, tenderness, fever, tachycardia, tachypnea). The history and physical examination will provide a limited differential diagnosis. This assessment is the basis for decisions regarding the need for and intensity of resuscitation or rehydration, the need for diagnostic imaging, the timing of antibiotic therapy, and the urgency of intervention.

Fluid Resuscitation

Volume depletion is common in febrile patients, and is worsened by poor intake because of nausea or vomiting and in the presence of ileus induced by intra-abdominal inflammation.

For patients with septic shock or organ failure, more aggressive fluid therapy should be provided. The Surviving Sepsis Campaign guidelines for managing septic shock are reasonable, although some recommendations have been found ineffective or harmful.[12] Key recommendations include early goal-directed resuscitation during the first 6 hours after recognition.

It is worth mentioning that resuscitation from hemorrhagic shock in trauma, ultimately a triggering insult for much the same systemic inflammatory response seen in severe sepsis, has moved away from crystalloid therapy.[13,14] The use of whole blood appears to eliminate the problems of expansion of extravascular water volumes seen with crystalloid, and also appears to produce a lower incidence of organ failure. In a randomized prospective study, early transfusion in severe sepsis improved survival.[15]

Initiation of Antimicrobial Therapy

Delaying antimicrobial therapy has been associated with poorer outcomes in patients with septic shock, including those with intra-abdominal infections.[16] The study claiming this finding is, however, a low-quality study as judged by the methodologic quality score system presented by van Nieuwenhoven and colleagues.[17] Other studies have suggested a greater timeframe, and this will likely never been examined in a prospective fashion.[18] The real issue has to do with whether or not those receiving delayed effective therapy were otherwise different than those who received early appropriate therapy, as suggested by more careful studies.[19]

In patients undergoing a source-control procedure, antimicrobial therapy provides, perhaps most importantly, surgical wound prophylaxis and treatment of pathogens potentially disseminated during the procedure, in addition to providing ongoing therapy for the infection. Antimicrobial therapy is, therefore, also considered as wound prophylaxis for all patients undergoing intervention. The rules for prophylaxis in elective surgical procedures include use of agents likely effective against the contaminating organisms, and administration within 1 hour of operation.[20,21] The timing of re-administration of antibiotics to meet these recommendations is dependent on the pharmacokinetics of the agents the patient initially receives. For long-acting agents, sufficient levels may be present during the procedure as to obviate the need for immediate preoperative redosing.

WHAT ARE THE PROPER PROCEDURES FOR OBTAINING ADEQUATE SOURCE CONTROL?

"Source control" is defined as any procedure, or series of procedures, that eliminates infectious foci, controls factors that promote on-going infection, and corrects or controls anatomic derangements to restore normal physiologic function.[5] Source control failure is more likely in patients with delayed (> 24 hours) procedural intervention, higher severity of illness (APACHE II $\geq$ 15), advanced age (> 70 years), pre-existing chronic medical conditions, poor nutritional status, and a higher degree of peritoneal involvement, and is heralded by persistent or recurrent intra-abdominal infection, anastomotic failure, or fistula formation.[22,23,24,25,26]

The timing of the initial intervention is a key decision, particularly in the presence of diffuse peritonitis. Patients with diffuse peritonitis from a perforated viscus cannot be fully resuscitated until on-going soiling has been controlled. In such patients, resuscitation should be continued intra-operatively.

The basis for this has been well studied. In brief, the lymphatic channels of the peritoneum, and particularly the diaphragmatic surface, constitute a high-flow system with relatively large lacunae.[27,28,29,30,31,32,33] These allow rapid efflux of fluid from the peritoneal cavity and, in the presence of infection, rapid efflux of micro-organisms and host defense elements. These enter via the thoracic duct directly into the venous circulation.

For hemodynamically stable patients without peritonitis (eg, abscess), delay of up to 24 hours may be appropriate. This decision is a complex calculation based on a variety of patient-, institution-, and surgeon-specific factors, and greater or lesser delay may be appropriate, with most patients benefiting from a more urgent approach.

USE OF PERCUTANEOUS DRAINAGE FOR ABSCESSES VERSUS OPERATION FOR OTHER PROCESSES

Well-localized fluid collections of appropriate density may be effectively drained percutaneously.[34,35,36,37] Percutaneous drainage of appropriately selected infectious sources may result in significantly less physiologic alterations in patients and may eliminate or reduce the need for open techniques.

Open surgical techniques are typically required for poorly localized, loculated, complex, or diffuse fluid collections, necrotic tissue, high-density fluid, or percutaneously inaccessible collections. The majority of patients respond to a single intervention without significant complication.

Given the range of diseases and the various risk factors for poor outcome, clinical practice has been driven by uncontrolled case series.[38,39,40,41,42,43,44] Percutaneous techniques have continued to evolve and many abscesses are now often approached by interventional radiography.[45]

There are some patients in whom drainage catheter placement is not appropriate, and laparotomy is the procedure of choice. Extraluminal air, and fluid in a "contained" distribution immediately adjacent to underlying diseased bowel (eg, in diverticulitis or appendicitis), can be drained. However, a patient with a similar abscess but with extensive and massive free air or fluid remote from the perforation site should undergo laparotomy.

When laparotomy is undertaken for intra-abdominal infection, a range of factors will determine the extent (if any) of bowel resection, whether an anastamosis or ostomy is created, what tissue is debrided, what type of drainage (if any) is necessary, and what wound-management technique is used. These questions have not been addressed in controlled trials.

OPERATIVE CHOICES IN SEVERE SEPSIS

Two general strategies should be considered for critically ill patients who are either physiologically unstable or at high risk of failed source control. These include laparostomy or the "open abdomen,"[1] and on-demand relaparotomy.[46]

Generally accepted indications for laparostomy, in which neither the fascia nor skin are closed, include severe physiologic derangements intra-operatively that preclude completion of the planned procedure, intra-abdominal hypertension, and loss of abdominal soft tissue preventing immediate fascial closure.

Generally accepted indications for use of an open abdomen technique center upon septic shock, where resuscitation with crystalloid will likely lead to an abdominal compartment syndrome if the fascia is primarily closed.[47,48,49] Another important setting for this procedure is an inability to obtain adequate source control at the index procedure, primarily an inability to achieve control of the site of perforation. Ongoing intestinal ischemia is best managed by a planned re-exploration at 24 hours because of the difficulties in assessing bowel viability.[50]

USE OF THE MICROBIOLOGY LABORATORY IN MANAGING PATIENTS WITH INTRA-ABDOMINAL SEPSIS

There are no data indicating that Gram stain, culture, and susceptibility results alter outcome in patients with a community-acquired complicated intra-abdominal infection. This is in large part a consequence of the fact that most studies primarily include patients with acute appendicitis.

However, there is increasing resistance of community-acquired strains of gram-negative organisms to selected antibiotics in many locales. If resistance for a given antibiotic is greater than 10% to 20% for a common intra-abdominal pathogen in the community, use of that agent should be avoided. Because of widespread resistance of Escherichia coli to ampicillin/sulbactam, that antibiotic is no longer recommended for routine empiric therapy of complicated intra-abdominal infections.[51] There is high penetration of fluoroquinolone-resistant E coli in Latin America and East Asia, and locations with a high prevalence of extended-spectrum beta lactamase-producing strains of Klebsiella sp and E coli.[51] Quinolone-resistant E coli are similarly becoming a problem in some areas and this mandates review of hospital susceptibility data.

In some populations and communities, a relatively high prevalence of more resistant nonenteric gram-negative organisms, such as Pseudomonas aeruginosa, will impact the selection of appropriate empiric antibiotic therapy.[52,53,54]

Routine cultures of patients with community-acquired intra-abdominal infections may facilitate recognition of local changes in resistance, and thereby optimal selection of antimicrobial agents for both definitive treatment and oral step-down therapy. There are marked differences in susceptibility patterns within and between different communities and institutions. These epidemiologic data are of considerable value in defining the most suitable antimicrobial therapy for intra-abdominal infections.

WHY MORE BROAD-SPECTRUM ANTIMICROBIAL THERAPY IS RECOMMENDED FOR SEVERE COMMUNITY-ACQUIRED INFECTION

Several attempts have been made to identify clinical features in patients with complicated intra-abdominal infections that increase the risk of adverse outcomes. These analyses have identified parameters predictive of mortality rather than the risk of recurrent infection. These risk factors include higher APACHE II scores, poor nutritional status, significant cardiovascular disease, and an inability to achieve adequate source control.[55,56,57,58,59,60] Similarly, patients who are immunosuppressed by medical therapy for transplantation, cancer, or inflammatory disease are at higher risk of an adverse outcome. Prolonged prehospital length of stay ($\geq$ 5 days) and prolonged ($\geq$ 2 days) preoperative antimicrobial therapy are significant predictors of failure from recurrent infection, Patients with other acute and chronic diseases may also be immunosuppressed, although this is difficult to define. Intraoperative cultures, including cultures from percutaneous drainage procedures, are therefore central to the prescribing of definitive therapeutic regimens for these patients, and may allow de-escalation to less broad-spectrum therapy.

In patients with such higher severity infections, the consequences of treatment failure may be more significant than in those patients with mild-to-moderate infections. The use of initial empiric antimicrobial regimens that are subsequently identified as lacking in in vitro activity against the organisms actually isolated from the intra-abdominal infection, has been associated with an increased need for additional source-control procedures and more aggressive antimicrobial therapy, increased hospital lengths of stay and costs, and increased mortality.[61] As such, use of broader-spectrum agents providing activity and some gram-negative facultative and aerobic organisms occasionally isolated from such patients have the potential to improve outcome, although this hypothesis has not been rigorously examined in clinical trials.

In these cases, cultures and susceptibility tests are particularly important. The rationale for the widening of coverage to less common organisms is that the risk of treatment failure in such patients is higher and the consequences potentially greater.

Increasing antimicrobial resistance with *Bacteroides fragilis* is similarly of concern, and there are data indicating higher failure rates if these organisms are treated with an inactive agent, particularly cefotetan and cefoxitin.[62,63] No randomized clinical trials have been performed with this agent since resistance was first reported. Similarly, moxifloxacin use for the treatment of patients likely to have *B fragilis* should be avoided if patients have recently received quinolone therapy, as organisms from such patients are likely to have quinolone-resistant isolates.[64,65]

Local microbiology laboratories show great variation in reliably performing in vitro susceptibility tests. Sentinel studies of *B fragilis*, the major pathogen, show uniform susceptibility to metronidazole, carbapenems, and β-lactam/β-lactamase inhibitors.[66,67,68,69,70] Studies of the activity of quinolones against *B fragilis* isolates have yielded conflicting data, in part because of the use of abdominal abscess versus bacteremic isolates.[71,72,73,74] Susceptibility testing of individual anaerobic isolates should be considered when there is persistent isolation of the organism, bacteremia, or when prolonged therapy is needed because of immunosuppression or prosthetic infection. Laboratories can purify and hold isolates for additional testing if requested by the clinician.

THE ROLE OF MICROBIOLOGY FOR PATIENTS WITH HEALTH CARE-ASSOCIATED INFECTIONS

For patients with health care-associated infections, antimicrobial therapy that fails to cover eventual pathogens has been associated with higher rates of treatment failure and mortality. Thus, Gram stains may be of value in detecting gram-positive cocci or yeast that would lead to additional empiric antimicrobial therapy before definitive culture results are available.

Local susceptibility patterns for *Staphylococcus aureus* and for enterococci might warrant addition of a methicillin-resistant *S aureus* (MRSA)-active agent until results of cultures and susceptibility testing are available.[75] For enterococci, local susceptibilities should be monitored for penicillin and vancomycin resistance. If yeast is identified on a Gram stain, additional therapy for *Candida* sp may be considered.

The failure to provide adequate antimicrobial therapy in such patients has been repeatedly associated with an increased incidence of therapeutic failure, and in some cases increased mortality.[61,75]

Numerous prospective, blinded, and randomized trials have compared regimens active against routine isolates of *Enterococcus* for community-acquired infections. In at least six of these studies, the comparator regimen did not have similar coverage.[52,76,77,78,79,80] None of these trials demonstrated an advantage to treatment for enterococci.

There is no evidence that routine use of agents effective against enterococci improves outcome from community-acquired infections, but the presence of this organism appears to increase failure rates in selected patient groups, primarily those with high severity infections.[81]

Isolation of staphylococci and yeast are quite uncommon in patients with community-acquired intra-abdominal infections, and use of agents with effective methicillin-resistant staphylococci and yeast is not indicated in the absence of evidence that such organisms are involved in the infection.

WHAT ANTIMICROBIAL REGIMENS SHOULD BE USED IN PATIENTS WITH HEALTH CARE-ASSOCIATED INTRA-ABDOMINAL INFECTIONS?

Recommended empiric regimens for patients with health care-associated intra-abdominal infections include meropenem, imipenem/cilastatin, doripenem, piperacillin/tazobactam, ciprofloxacin plus metronidazole, ceftazidime or cefepime plus metronidazole, and aztreonam plus metronidazole plus vancomycin. Empiric antibiotic therapy for hospital-acquired intra-abdominal infections should be guided by knowledge of the flora seen at the particular hospital and their antimicrobial susceptibilities. In general, this will necessitate use of multidrug regimens with expanded spectra of activity against gram-negative aerobic and facultative bacilli, which may include aminoglycosides or colistin. Such broad-spectrum antimicrobial therapy should be tailored when culture and susceptibility reports become available to reduce the number and spectra of administered agents.

Health care-associated infections are commonly caused by a more resistant flora, which may include the nonfermenting gram-negatives *P aeruginosa* and *Acinetobacter* sp, extended spectrum β-lactamase-producing *Klebsiella* and *E coli*, *Enterobacter* sp, *Proteus* sp, MRSA, enterococci, and *Candida* sp.[75,82,83,84] For these infections, complex multidrug regimens are recommended because adequate empiric therapy appears important in determining postoperative complications and mortality.[75] Failure to adequately treat resistant organisms has, in similar health care-associated infections, been associated with increased death.[18,19,85] Local resistance patterns of nosocomial isolates seen in the specific hospital should dictate empiric treatment, and treatment should be altered based upon a thorough microbiologic workup of infected fluid.

In infections occurring after elective or emergent operation, a more resistant flora is routinely encountered.[75] The organisms seen are similar to those seen in other nosocomial infections, and anaerobes are not frequently important sources of resistant organisms. The selection of antibiotics would be tailored according to the known nosocomial flora present at the institution where the patient developed the infection.

Fungal infection has been the subject of recent guidelines from the Infectious Diseases Society of America.[86] *Candida albicans* or other fungi are cultured from about 20% of patients with acute perforations of the GI tract. Even when fungi are recovered, antifungal agents are unnecessary in adults unless the patient has recently received immunosuppressive therapy for neoplasm or has a perforation of a gastric ulcer on acid suppression or malignancy, transplantation, or inflammatory disease, or has postoperative or recurrent intra-abdominal infection.[86,87,88] In neonates with necrotizing enterocolitis, *Candida* is not uncommon, and is more likely to represent a true pathogen than in previously healthy adults.

Nonetheless, in the listed settings *Candida* is associated with increased mortality.[82] Patients with health care-associated intra-abdominal infections are at higher risk for *Candida* peritonitis, particularly those with recurrent GI perforations and surgically treated pancreatic infections.[86,87,88] Preemptive antifungal therapy with fluconazole may decrease the incidence of *Candida* peritonitis in such high-risk patients.[89,90]

There has been an evolution of the species of *Candida* seen in candidemia and candida peritonitis.[91] Because of its high susceptibility to fluconazole, *C. albicans* has decreased in frequency and *Candida glabrata* and other species have become somewhat more common. This observation, coupled with the common use of fluconazole prophylaxis in the ICU, suggests empric use of echinocandins (caspofungin, anidulafungin, micafungin).[92,93,94,95,96]

Certain patient groups are at particularly high risk for a poor outcome because of enterococcal infection, and include (*i*) immunocompromised patients, (*ii*) patients with health care-associated postoperative peritonitis, (*iii*) patients with severe sepsis of abdominal origin who have previously received cephalosporins and other broad-spectrum antibiotics selecting for *Enterococcus* spp, and (*iv*) patients with peritonitis and valvular heart disease or prosthetic intravascular material, which place them at high risk of endocarditis.[10,83,84,97]

Isolation of *Enterococcus* is more common in patients with nosocomial intra-abdominal infections, particularly those with postoperative infections, and its isolation is a risk factor for treatment failure and death.[81,98] Thus, in patients with health care-associated intra-abdominal infections, including those with postoperative infections, a reasonable option would be to include coverage of *Enterococcus* in the empiric regimen, until definitive culture results are available. Ampicillin and vancomycin are agents that have activity against this organism, and could be added to a regimen lacking anti-enterococcal activity. Specific risk factors for vancomycin-resistant enterococci have been detailed,[99,100,101,102] which center upon transmission from other colonized or infected patients in an epidemic manner.

MRSA isolates are recovered from patients with postoperative infections, pancreatic infections, and tertiary peritonitis.[103,104] MRSA is not commonly isolated from patients with community-acquired intra-abdominal infections. There are no specific data with regard to antibiotic preferences in treatment of intra-abdominal infections because of MRSA. In general, vancomycin has been used to treat infections caused by this organism. Other antibiotics, including quinupristin/dalfopristin, linezolid, daptomycin, and tigecycline have in vitro activity against methicillin-resistant staphylococci, but there is little published data regarding their efficacy in the treatment of patients with intra-abdominal infections. Thus, vancomycin should probably remain the first-line agent, with use of the others restricted to situations in which vancomycin cannot be used because of severe adverse reactions or when initial therapy with vancomycin is thought to have failed.

PHARMACOKINETIC AND PHARMACODYNAMIC CONSIDERATIONS IN TREATING INTRA-ABDOMINAL SEPSIS

Pharmacokinetic-pharmacodynamic properties of specific antibiotics should be considered in selecting an adequate dosing regimen.[105] Antimicrobial dosing considerations are needed in critically ill patients. Physiologic changes can occur in both of these patient populations, which may alter the apparent volume of distribution or clearance of commonly used antibiotics. In addition, if the estimate of a dosage regimen is dependent on renal function, an accurate estimate of creatinine clearance (CL_{CR}) based on serum creatinine values and body weight may be difficult with commonly used equations and direct measurement of CL_{CR} may be required. For β-lactams and aminoglycosides, the critically ill patient with the early stages of sepsis may have shifts in body fluid and be in hypermetabolic state, resulting in an increase in both volume of distribution and clearance and lower serum antibiotic concentrations.[106,107] These studies suggest that higher doses and more frequent administration of β-lactams may be needed in selected patients who are critically ill, with altered distribution and increased clearance of renally excreted antibiotics. Initial dosing regimens for aminoglycosides and vancomycin should be based on adjusted body weight and total body weight, respectively. Serum drug concentration monitoring is recommended for dosage individualization of aminoglycosides and vancomycin in these patient populations.

There is considerable evidence that less frequent dosing of metronidazole, in particular, is effective. The nitroimidazoles are bactericidal through toxic metabolites, which cause DNA strand breakage. Resistance, both clinical and microbiologic, has been described only rarely. Liver disease leads to a decreased clearance of metronidazole and dosage reduction is recommended.[108,109,110,111]

DURATION OF THERAPY

A duration of therapy no greater than 1 week was appropriate for most patients with intra-abdominal infections, with the exception of those who had inadequate source control.[112,113,114]

Within this window, resolution of clinical signs of infection provide the termination point for antimicrobial therapy. The risk of subsequent treatment failure appears to be quite low in patients who have no clinical evidence of infection at the time of cessation of antimicrobial therapy.[115,116] This usually implies that the patients are afebrile, have normal white blood cell counts, and are tolerating an oral diet.

These conditions are unlikely to occur in a critically ill patient in the ICU who is suffering from a postoperative infection with multisystem organ failure. These patients display persistent or recurrent signs of peritoneal irritation, failure of bowel function to return, or continued fever or leukocytosis, and are at high risk for an intra-abdominal or other infection that may require additional intervention to achieve source control. CT of the abdomen is usually the most accurate method by which to diagnose an ongoing or recurrent intra-abdominal infection. The possibility of an extra-abdominal infection, such as nosocomial pneumonia or urinary tract infection, or a noninfectious cause of fever or leukocytosis, such as venous thrombosis or a pulmonary embolism, should also be considered. For complex patients in the ICU, with multiple organ failures, CT scans may be the only means to determine if conditions for cessation of therapy (no defined collections) are met.

Antimicrobial regimens should be adjusted according to the results of the diagnostic investigations. For patients with a confirmed intra-abdominal infection, this may require broadening the regimen to include agents with activity against health care-associated organisms typically isolated with these infections. Appropriate antimicrobial therapy, based upon cultures of the infected site, should be continued while the investigation proceeds, particularly if the patient manifests signs of sepsis, such as organ dysfunction. The current state of the art would be to terminate antimicrobial therapy and observe for worsening of the overall clinical condition of the patient. If the patient continues to be relatively stable, therapy should not be resumed unless a documented source is identified.

REFERENCES

1. Moss M. Epidemiology of sepsis: race, sex, and chronic alcohol abuse. Clin Infect Dis 2005;41(Suppl 7):S490–7.
2. Martin GS, Mannino DM, Eaton S, et al. The epidemiology of sepsis in the United States from 1979 through 2000. N Engl J Med 2003;348:1546–54.
3. Bohnen JM, Marshall JC, Fry DE, et al. Clinical and scientific importance of source control in abdominal infections: summary of a symposium. Can J Surg 1999;42:122–6.
4. Jimenez MF, Marshall JC. Source control in the management of sepsis. Intensive Care Med 2001;27(Suppl 1):S49–62.
5. Marshall JC, Maier RV, Jimenez M, et al. Source control in the management of severe sepsis and septic shock: an evidence-based review. Crit Care Med 2004;32:S513–26.
6. Knaus WA, Wagner DP, Draper EA, et al. The APACHE III prognostic system. Risk prediction of hospital mortality for critically ill hospitalized adults. [see comments]. Chest 1991;100:1619–36.
7. Le Gall JR, Lemeshow S, Saulnier F. A new Simplified Acute Physiology Score (SAPS II) based on a European/North American multicenter study. [published erratum appears in JAMA 1994 May 4;271(17):1321]. JAMA 1993;270:2957–63.
8. Lemeshow S, Le Gall JR. Modeling the severity of illness of ICU patients. A systems update. JAMA 1994;272:1049–55.
9. Meyer AA, Messick WJ, Young P, et al. Prospective comparison of clinical judgment and APACHE II score in predicting the outcome in critically ill surgical patients. J Trauma 1992;32:747–53.
10. Swenson BR, Metzger R, Hedrick TL, et al. Choosing antibiotics for intra-abdominal infections: what do we mean by "high risk"? Surg Infect (Larchmt) 2009;10: 29–39.
11. Klevens RM, Morrison MA, Nadle J, et al. Invasive methicillin-resistant Staphylococcus aureus infections in the United States. JAMA 2007;298:1763–71.
12. Dellinger RP, Levy MM, Carlet JM, et al. Surviving Sepsis Campaign: international guidelines for management of severe sepsis and septic shock: 2008. Crit Care Med 2008;36:296–327.
13. Hess JR, Holcomb JB. Transfusion practice in military trauma. Transfus Med 2008;18:143–50.
14. Beekley AC. Damage control resuscitation: a sensible approach to the exsanguinating surgical patient. Crit Care Med 2008;36:S267–74.

15. Rivers E, Nguyen B, Havstad S, et al. Early goal-directed therapy in the treatment of severe sepsis and septic shock. N Engl J Med 2001;345:1368–77.

16. Kumar A, Roberts D, Wood KE, et al. Duration of hypotension before initiation of effective antimicrobial therapy is the critical determinant of survival in human septic shock. Crit Care Med 2006;34:1589–96.

17. van Nieuwenhoven CA, Buskens E, van Tiel FH, et al. Relationship between methodological trial quality and the effects of selective digestive decontamination on pneumonia and mortality in critically ill patients. JAMA 2001;286: 335–40.

18. Lodise TP Jr, Patel N, Kwa A, et al. Predictors of 30-day mortality among patients with *Pseudomonas aeruginosa* bloodstream infections: impact of delayed appropriate antibiotic selection. Antimicrob Agents Chemother 2007; 51:3510–5.

19. Kollef MH, Sherman G, Ward S, et al. Inadequate antimicrobial treatment of infections: a risk factor for hospital mortality among critically ill patients. Chest 1999;115:462–74.

20. Bratzler DW, Houck PM. Antimicrobial prophylaxis for surgery: an advisory statement from the National Surgical Infection Prevention Project. Am J Surg 2005; 189:395–404.

21. Bratzler DW, Hunt DR. The surgical infection prevention and surgical care improvement projects: national initiatives to improve outcomes for patients having surgery. Clin Infect Dis 2006;43:322–30.

22. Shlaes DM, Gerding DN, John JF Jr, et al. Society for Healthcare Epidemiology of America and Infectious Diseases Society of America Joint Committee on the Prevention of Antimicrobial Resistance: guidelines for the prevention of antimicrobial resistance in hospitals. Clin Infect Dis 1997;25:584–99.

23. Koperna T, Schulz F. Prognosis and treatment of peritonitis. Do we need new scoring systems? Arch Surg 1996;131:180–6.

24. Koperna T, Schulz F. Relaparotomy in peritonitis: prognosis and treatment of patients with persisting intraabdominal infection. World J Surg 2000;24:32–7.

25. Mulier S, Penninckx F, Verwaest C, et al. Factors affecting mortality in generalized postoperative peritonitis: multivariate analysis in 96 patients. World J Surg 2003;27:379–84.

26. Grunau G, Heemken R, Hau T. Predictors of outcome in patients with postoperative intra-abdominal infection. Eur J Surg 1996;162:619–25.

27. Hall JC, Heel KA, Papadimitriou JM, et al. The pathobiology of peritonitis. Gastroenterology 1998;114:185–96.

28. Li JC, Yu SM. Study on the ultrastructure of the peritoneal stomata in humans. Acta Anat (Basel) 1991;141:26–30.

29. Michailova KN. Ultrastructural observations on the human visceral pleura. Eur J Morphol 1997;35:125–35.

30. Michailova KN. Postinflammatory changes of the diaphragmatic stomata. Ann Anat 2001;183:309–17.

31. Shao XJ, Ohtani O, Saitoh M, et al. Development of diaphragmatic lymphatics: the process of their direct connection to the peritoneal cavity. Arch Histol Cytol 1998;61:137–49.

32. Li J, Zhao Z, Zhou J, et al. A study of the three-dimensional organization of the human diaphragmatic lymphatic lacunae and lymphatic drainage units. Ann Anat 1996;178:537–44.

33. bu-Hijleh MF, Habbal OA, Moqattash ST. The role of the diaphragm in lymphatic absorption from the peritoneal cavity. J Anat 1995;186(Pt 3):453–67.

34. Akinci D, Akhan O, Ozmen MN, et al. Percutaneous drainage of 300 intraperitoneal abscesses with long-term follow-up. Cardiovasc Intervent Radiol 2005;28: 744–50.

35. Betsch A, Wiskirchen J, Trubenbach J, et al. CT-guided percutaneous drainage of intra-abdominal abscesses: APACHE III score stratification of 1-year results. Acute physiology, age, chronic health evaluation. Eur Radiol 2002;12:2883–9.

36. Bufalari A, Giustozzi G, Moggi L. Postoperative intraabdominal abscesses: percutaneous versus surgical treatment. Acta Chir Belg 1996;96:197–200.

37. Theisen J, Bartels H, Weiss W, et al. Current concepts of percutaneous abscess drainage in postoperative retention. J Gastrointest Surg 2005;9:280–3.

38. Pruett TL, Simmons RL. Status of percutaneous catheter drainage of absceses. Surg Clin North Am 1988;68:89–105.

39. Gerzof SG, Robbins AH, Birkett DH. Computed tomography in the diagnosis and management of abdominal abscesses. Gastrointest Radiol 1978;3:287–94.

40. Gerzof SG, Johnson WC, Robbins AH, et al. Expanded criteria for percutaneous abscess drainage. Arch Surg 1985;120:227–32.

41. Gerzof SG, Robbins AH, Johnson WC, et al. Percutaneous catheter drainage of abdominal abscesses: a five-year experience. N Engl J Med 1981;305:653–7.

42. vanSonnenberg E, Mueller PR, Ferrucci JT Jr. Percutaneous drainage of 250 abdominal abscesses and fluid collections. Part I: results, failures, and complications. Radiology 1984;151:337–41.

43. Levison MA. Percutaneous versus open operative drainage of intra-abdominal abscesses. Infect Dis Clin North Am 1992;6:525–44.

44. Sones PJ. Percutaneous drainage of abdominal abscesses. Am J Roentgenol 1984;142:35–9.

45. Maher MM, Gervais DA, Kalra MK, et al. The inaccessible or undrainable abscess: how to drain it. Radiographics 2004;24:717–35.

46. van RO, Mahler CW, Boer KR, et al. Comparison of on-demand vs planned relaparotomy strategy in patients with severe peritonitis: a randomized trial. JAMA 2007;298:865–72.

47. Schein M, Wittmann DH, Aprahamian CC, et al. The abdominal compartment syndrome: the physiological and clinical consequences of elevated intra-abdominal pressure. J Am Coll Surg 1995;180:745–53.

48. Miller PR, Meredith JW, Johnson JC, et al. Prospective evaluation of vacuum-assisted fascial closure after open abdomen: planned ventral hernia rate is substantially reduced. Ann Surg 2004;239:608–14.

49. Fabian TC. Damage control in trauma: laparotomy wound management acute to chronic. Surg Clin North Am 2007;87:73–93, vi.

50. Schein M. Planned relaparotomies and laparostomy. In: Schein M, Marshall JC, editors. A guide to the management of surgical infections. Heidelberg: Springer; 2003. p. 412–23.

51. Paterson DL, Rossi F, Baquero F, et al. In vitro susceptibilities of aerobic and facultative gram-negative bacilli isolated from patients with intra-abdominal infections worldwide: the 2003 Study for Monitoring Antimicrobial Resistance Trends (SMART). J Antimicrob Chemother 2005;55:965–73.

52. Yellin AE, Heseltine PN, Berne TV, et al. The role of *Pseudomonas* species in patients treated with ampicillin and Sulbactam for gangrenous and perforated appendicitis. Surg Gynecol Obstet 1985;161:303–7.

53. Bradley JS, Behrendt CE, Arrieta AC, et al. Convalescent phase outpatient parenteral antiinfective therapy for children with complicated appendicitis. Pediatr Infect Dis J 2001;20:19–24.

54. Lin WJ, Lo WT, Chu CC, et al. Bacteriology and antibiotic susceptibility of community-acquired intra-abdominal infection in children. J Microbiol Immunol Infect 2006;39:249–54.
55. Christou NV, Barie PS, Dellinger EP, et al. Surgical Infection Society intra-abdominal infection study. Prospective evaluation of management techniques and outcome. Arch Surg 1993;128:193–8 [discussion: 198–9].
56. Dellinger EP, Wertz MJ, Meakins JL, et al. Surgical infection stratification system for intra-abdominal infection. Multicenter trial. Arch Surg 1985;120:21–9.
57. Nystrom PO, Bax R, Dellinger EP, et al. Proposed definitions for diagnosis, severity scoring, stratification, and outcome for trials on intraabdominal infection. Joint Working Party of SIS North America and Europe. [Review]. World J Surg 1990;14:148–58.
58. Ohmann C. Prognostic scores and design of clinical studies. Infection 1998;26: 342–4.
59. Ohmann C, Wittmann DH, Wacha H. Prospective evaluation of prognostic scoring systems in peritonitis. Peritonitis Study Group. Eur J Surg 1993;159: 267–74.
60. Wacha H, Hau T, Dittmer R, et al. Risk factors associated with intraabdominal infections: a prospective multicenter study. Peritonitis Study Group. Langenbecks Arch Surg 1999;384:24–32.
61. Mosdell DM, Morris DM, Voltura A, et al. Antibiotic treatment for surgical peritonitis. Ann Surg 1991;214:543–9.
62. Bieluch VM, Cuchural GJ, Snydman DR, et al. Clinical importance of cefoxitin-resistant Bacteroides fragilis isolates. Diagn Microbiol Infect Dis 1987;7:119–26.
63. Snydman DR, Cuchural GJ Jr, McDermott L, et al. Correlation of various in vitro testing methods with clinical outcomes in patients with Bacteroides fragilis group infections treated with cefoxitin: a retrospective analysis. Antimicrob Agents Chemother 1992;36:540–4.
64. Oh H, Nord CE, Barkholt L, et al. Ecological disturbances in intestinal microflora caused by clinafloxacin, an extended-spectrum quinolone. Infection 2000;28: 272–7.
65. Sullivan A, Edlund C, Nord CE. Effect of antimicrobial agents on the ecological balance of human microflora. Lancet Infect Dis 2001;1:101–14.
66. Aldridge KE, O'Brien M. In vitro susceptibilities of the Bacteroides fragilis group species: change in isolation rates significantly affects overall susceptibility data. J Clin Microbiol 2002;40:4349–52.
67. Cuchural GJ Jr, Tally FP, Jacobus NV, et al. Susceptibility of the Bacteroides fragilis group in the United States: analysis by site of isolation. Antimicrob Agents Chemother 1988;32:717–22.
68. Snydman DR, McDermott L, Cuchural GJ Jr, et al. Analysis of trends in antimicrobial resistance patterns among clinical isolates of Bacteroides fragilis group species from 1990 to 1994. Clin Infect Dis 1996;23(Suppl 1):S54–65.
69. Snydman DR, Jacobus NV, McDermott LA, et al. Multicenter study of in vitro susceptibility of the Bacteroides fragilis group, 1995 to 1996, with comparison of resistance trends from 1990 to 1996. Antimicrob Agents Chemother 1999; 43:2417–22.
70. Snydman DR, Jacobus NV, McDermott LA, et al. National survey on the susceptibility of Bacteroides Fragilis Group: report and analysis of trends for 1997–2000. Clin Infect Dis 2002;35:S126–34.
71. Golan Y, McDermott LA, Jacobus NV, et al. Emergence of fluoroquinolone resistance among Bacteroides species. J Antimicrob Chemother 2003;52:208–13.

72. Goldstein EJ, Citron DM, Warren YA, et al. In vitro activity of moxifloxacin against 923 anaerobes isolated from human intra-abdominal infections. Antimicrob Agents Chemother 2006;50:148–55.

73. Snydman DR, Jacobus NV, McDermott LA, et al. In vitro activities of newer quinolones against Bacteroides group organisms. Antimicrob Agents Chemother 2002;46:3276–9.

74. Snydman DR, Jacobus NV, McDermott LA, et al. National survey on the susceptibility of Bacteroides fragilis group: report and analysis of trends in the United States from 1997 to 2004. Antimicrob Agents Chemother 2007;51:1649–55.

75. Montravers P, Gauzit R, Muller C, et al. Emergence of antibiotic-resistant bacteria in cases of peritonitis after intraabdominal surgery affects the efficacy of empirical antimicrobial therapy. Clin Infect Dis 1996;23:486–94.

76. Cohn SM, Lipsett PA, Buchman TG, et al. Comparison of intravenous/oral ciprofloxacin plus metronidazole versus piperacillin/tazobactam in the treatment of complicated intraabdominal infections. Ann Surg 2000;232:254–62.

77. Ohlin B, Cederberg A, Forssell H, et al. Piperacillin/tazobactam compared with cefuroxime/ metronidazole in the treatment of intra-abdominal infections. Eur J Surg 1999;165:875–84.

78. Polk HC Jr, Fink MP, Laverdiere M, et al. Prospective randomized study of piperacillin/tazobactam therapy of surgically treated intra-abdominal infection. The Piperacillin/Tazobactam Intra-Abdominal Infection Study Group. Am Surg 1993;59:598–605.

79. Sirinek KR, Levine BA. A randomized trial of ticarcillin and clavulanate versus gentamicin and clindamycin in patients with complicated appendicitis. Surg Gynecol Obstet 1991;172(Suppl):30–5.

80. Walker AP, Nichols RL, Wilson RF, et al. Efficacy of a beta-lactamase inhibitor combination for serious intraabdominal infections. Ann Surg 1993;217:115–21.

81. Burnett RJ, Haverstock DC, Dellinger EP, et al. Definition of the role of enterococcus in intraabdominal infection: analysis of a prospective randomized trial. Surgery 1995;118:716–21.

82. Montravers P, Dupont H, Gauzit R, et al. Candida as a risk factor for mortality in peritonitis. Crit Care Med 2006;34:646–52.

83. Montravers P, Lepape A, Dubreuil L, et al. Clinical and microbiological profiles of community-acquired and nosocomial intra-abdominal infections: results of the French prospective, observational EBIIA study. J Antimicrob Chemother 2009; 63:785–94.

84. Montravers P, Chalfine A, Gauzit R, et al. Clinical and therapeutic features of nonpostoperative nosocomial intra-abdominal infections. Ann Surg 2004;239: 409–16.

85. Ibrahim EH, Sherman G, Ward S, et al. The influence of inadequate antimicrobial treatment of bloodstream infections on patient outcomes in the ICU setting. Chest 2000;118:146–55.

86. Pappas PG, Rex JH, Sobel JD, et al. Guidelines for treatment of candidiasis. Clin Infect Dis 2004;38:161–89.

87. Calandra T, Bille J, Schneider R, et al. Clinical significance of Candida isolated from peritoneum in surgical patients. Lancet 1989;2:1437–40.

88. Solomkin JS, Flohr AB, Quie PG, et al. The role of Candida in intraperitoneal infections. Surgery 1980;88:524–30.

89. Eggimann P, Francioli P, Bille J, et al. Fluconazole prophylaxis prevents intra-abdominal candidiasis in high-risk surgical patients. Crit Care Med 1999;27: 1066–72.

90. Mean M, Marchetti O, Calandra T. Bench-to-bedside review: *Candida* infections in the intensive care unit. Crit Care 2008;12:204.
91. Hof H. Developments in the epidemiolgy of invasive fungal infections—implications for the empiric and targeted antifungal therapy. Mycoses 2008;51(Suppl 1):1–6.
92. Pfaller MA, Boyken L, Hollis RJ, et al. In vitro susceptibility of invasive isolates of *Candida* spp. to anidulafungin, caspofungin, and micafungin: six years of global surveillance. J Clin Microbiol 2008;46:150–6.
93. Pfaller MA, Messer SA, Boyken L, et al. Use of fluconazole as a surrogate marker to predict susceptibility and resistance to voriconazole among 13,338 clinical isolates of *Candida* spp. Tested by clinical and laboratory standards institute-recommended broth microdilution methods. J Clin Microbiol 2007;45:70–5.
94. Mora-Duarte J, Betts R, Rotstein C, et al. Comparison of caspofungin and amphotericin B for invasive candidiasis. N Engl J Med 2002;347:2020–9.
95. Reboli AC, Rotstein C, Pappas PG, et al. Anidulafungin versus fluconazole for invasive candidiasis. N Engl J Med 2007;356:2472–82.
96. Pappas PG, Rotstein CM, Betts RF, et al. Micafungin versus caspofungin for treatment of candidemia and other forms of invasive candidiasis. Clin Infect Dis 2007;45:883–93.
97. Blot S, De Waele JJ. Critical issues in the clinical management of complicated intra-abdominal infections. Drugs 2005;65:1611–20.
98. Sitges-Serra A, Lopez MJ, Girvent M, et al. Postoperative enterococcal infection after treatment of complicated intra-abdominal sepsis. Br J Surg 2002;89:361–7.
99. Mascini EM, Bonten MJ. Vancomycin-resistant enterococci: consequences for therapy and infection control. Clin Microbiol Infect 2005;11(Suppl 4):43–56.
100. Leavis HL, Willems RJ, Top J, et al. Epidemic and nonepidemic multidrug-resistant *Enterococcus faecium*. Emerg Infect Dis 2003;9:1108–15.
101. Bonten MJ, Willems R, Weinstein RA. Vancomycin-resistant enterococci: why are they here, and where do they come from? Lancet Infect Dis 2001;1:314–25.
102. Mazuski JE. Vancomycin-resistant enterococcus: risk factors, surveillance, infections, and treatment. Surg Infect (Larchmt) 2008;9:567–71.
103. Fierobe L, Decre D, Muller C, et al. Methicillin-resistant *Staphylococcus aureus* as a causative agent of postoperative intra-abdominal infection: relation to nasal colonization. Clin Infect Dis 1999;29:1231–8.
104. Patel M, Kumar RA, Stamm AM, et al. USA300 genotype community-associated methicillin-resistant *Staphylococcus aureus* as a cause of surgical site infections. J Clin Microbiol 2007;45:3431–3.
105. Drusano GL. Antimicrobial pharmacodynamics: critical interactions of 'bug and drug'. Nat Rev Microbiol 2004;2:289–300.
106. Edmiston CE, Krepel C, Kelly H, et al. Perioperative antibiotic prophylaxis in the gastric bypass patient: do we achieve therapeutic levels? Surgery 2004;136:738–47.
107. Pai MP, Bearden DT. Antimicrobial dosing considerations in obese adult patients. Pharmacotherapy 2007;27:1081–91.
108. Lamp KC, Freeman CD, Klutman NE, et al. Pharmacokinetics and pharmacodynamics of the nitroimidazole antimicrobials. Clin Pharmacokinet 1999;36:353–73.
109. Sprandel KA, Drusano GL, Hecht DW, et al. Population pharmacokinetic modeling and Monte Carlo simulation of varying doses of intravenous metronidazole. Diagn Microbiol Infect Dis 2006;55:303–9.

110. Lau AH, Emmons K, Seligsohn R. Pharmacokinetics of intravenous metronidazole at different dosages in healthy subjects. Int J Clin Pharmacol Ther Toxicol 1991;29:386–90.

111. Ljungberg B, Nilsson-Ehle I, Ursing B. Metronidazole: pharmacokinetic observations in severely ill patients. J Antimicrob Chemother 1984;14:275–83.

112. Solomkin JS, Mazuski JE, Baron EJ, et al. Guidelines for the selection of anti-infective agents for complicated intra-abdominal infections. Clin Infect Dis 2003;37:997–1005.

113. Mazuski JE, Sawyer RG, Nathens AB, et al. The Surgical Infection Society guidelines on antimicrobial therapy for intra-abdominal infections: an executive summary. Surgical Infections 2002;3:161–74.

114. Mazuski JE, Sawyer RG, Nathens AB, et al. The Surgical Infection Society guidelines on antimicrobial therapy for intra-abdominal infections: evidence for the recommendations. Surgical Infections 2002;3:175–234.

115. Hedrick TL, Evans HL, Smith RL, et al. Can we define the ideal duration of antibiotic therapy? Surg Infect (Larchmt) 2006;7:419–32.

116. Lennard ES, Dellinger EP, Wertz MJ, et al. Implications of leukocytosis and fever at conclusion of antibiotic therapy for intra-abdominal sepsis. Ann Surg 1982; 195:19–24.

Central Nervous System Infections: Meningitis and Brain Abscess

Hitoshi Honda, MD, David K. Warren, MD, MPH*

KEYWORDS

- Meningitis • Brain abscess • Subdural empyema
- Diagnosis • Treatment

Despite advances in antimicrobial and antiviral therapy, meningitis and brain abscess are infections that result in significant morbidity and mortality. A multidisciplinary approach, including intensive care, is often required in the treatment of these infections. Meningitis is defined by the presence of the inflammation of the meninges, with characteristic changes of cerebrospinal fluid. Brain abscess is a focal infection of the brain parenchyma, commonly caused by bacterial, fungal, and parasitic pathogens. This article reviews the common infectious etiologies of central nervous system infections, especially bacterial meningitis and brain abscess, and their subsequent management in the intensive care unit (ICU).

MENINGITIS
Epidemiology and Etiology

Bacterial meningitis

Bacterial meningitis can be divided into community-onset and nosocomial infections. The development of effective vaccines against *Hemophilus influenzae* type-b and *Streptococcus pneumoniae* resulted in a profound decline in the incidence of community-acquired bacterial mening itis among children in the United States since the 1980s.[1,2] However, among adults, the annual incidence of community-onset bacterial meningitis (three to six cases per 100,000 persons) has not changed over the past decade.[3–5] Common causes of community-onset bacterial meningitis in the United States and Northern Europe include *Streptococcus pneumoniae* (47%–51% of cases), *Neiserria meningitidis* (25%–37%), and *Listeria monocytogenes* (4%–8%).[6,7]

Meningitis caused by *S. pneumoniae* results in a 20% to 30% in-hospital mortality and up to a 40% rate of intracranial complications (eg, brain edema, hydrocephalus,

Division of Infectious Diseases, Washington University of School of Medicine, 660 South Euclid Avenue, Campus Box, 8051 Saint Louis, MO 63110, USA
* Corresponding author.
E-mail address: dwarren@im.wustl.edu (D.K. Warren).

Infect Dis Clin N Am 23 (2009) 609–623
doi:10.1016/j.idc.2009.04.009
0891-5520/09/$ – see front matter © 2009 Elsevier Inc. All rights reserved.

id.theclinics.com

and intracranial hemorrhage).[7,8] Immunodeficient states (eg, asplenia or agamma-globulinemia) are risk factors for pneumococcal meningitis.[9]

Outside of the United States and Europe, N meningitidis is the leading cause of meningitis in healthy individuals.[10] The annual incidence of meningococcal meningitis in the United States has been stable since the 1960s, at approximately 0.9 to 1.5 cases per 100,000 population.[11] Serogroups B, C, and Y account for the majority of endemic cases in the United States.[10,12] Individuals with asplenia or terminal complement deficiency are predisposed to meningococcal meningitis.[9]

L monocytogenes is a Gram-positive bacillus, commonly found in soil and fecal flora of human beings.[13] While ingestion of a large inoculum may cause gastroenteritis in healthy individuals, bacteremia and meningitis can occur in individuals over 50 years of age or among persons with deficiencies in cell-mediated immunity.[14] L monocytogenes rarely causes meningitis in younger, healthy individuals; screening for HIV infection is warranted if L monocytogenes meningitis occurs in this patient group.[9,15]

Other pathogens infrequently cause bacterial meningitis. H influenzae meningitis in adults is associated with asplenia or other immunocompromised states.[9] Streptococcus pyogenes meningitis, often secondary to otitis media, is a rare cause of community onset meningitis, with an incidence of 0.5% to 1.5% of bacterial meningitis cases.[7,16] Streptococcus agalactiae may cause bacterial meningitis in patients over 65 years of age or with diabetes mellitus.[17] Zoonotic pathogens, such as Capnocytophaga canimorsus acquired from an animal bite, may rarely result in meningitis following bacteremia in patients with predisposing factors (eg, immunosuppressive states or alcoholism).[18] Rickettsial diseases, ehrlichiosis, or leptospirosis may clinically manifest as meningitis; however, cerebrospinal fluid analysis findings are consistent with aseptic rather than bacterial meningitis.

Nosocomial bacterial meningitis has been a growing concern in critical care medicine.[19,20] Neurosurgical procedures (eg, cerebrospinal fluid shunt placement) or cerebrospinal fluid leakage (eg, recent head injury) predisposes to nosocomial meningitis. The incidence of nosocomial meningitis ranges from 1% to 6% among neurosurgical patients.[21–23] Although S pneumoniae is the most common cause of nosocomial meningitis, Staphylococcus spp is frequently isolated in meningitis after neurosurgery (37%).[23] Aerobic, Gram-negative bacilli (especially Enterobacteriaceae) cause up to 33% of nosocomial meningitis.[24]

Viral meningitis

Enteroviruses, such as coxsackieviruses and echoviruses, are the leading cause of viral meningitis in adults.[25] Enteroviruses are transmitted via a fecal-oral route, with peak disease incidence in the late summer and fall. Many of the herpes viruses cause a meningitis or encephalitis syndrome. Herpes simplex virus (HSV) encephalitis is usually caused by HSV-1 and has an annual incidence of one case per 250,000 population in the United States.[26] HSV encephalitis has a bimodal age distribution, commonly occurring in patients younger than 20 and older than 50 years of age. HSV-2 is an important cause of viral meningitis, accounting for 17% of cases of aseptic meningitis.[27] HSV-2 meningitis can occur independently of HSV-2 genital lesions.[28] Varicella zoster virus (VZV) accounted for 8% case of viral meningitis among adults and was under-recognized as a cause of meningitis until polymerase chain reaction (PCR) was widely available.[27]

Arboviruses (eg, California encephalitis virus group, St. Louis encephalitis virus, and West Nile virus) can also cause meningoencephalitis. In the past 10 years, West Nile virus (WNV) has emerged as a notable cause of meningoencephalitis in the United States. An epidemic investigation in 1999 identified 59 cases in New York City. Within

2 to 3 years, WNV had spread throughout the East Coast.[29–31] This epidemic has since shifted to the Midwest and western United States.[30] About 34% of the domestic reported cases in 2007 were West Nile neuroinvasive disease, characterized by fever, headache, seizure, and flaccid paralysis (polio-like syndrome).[31,32] In the United States, WNV is primarily transmitted by the *Culex* species mosquito.[33]

Other less common viral pathogens can causes aseptic meningitis. The incidence of mumps meningitis has decreased because of widespread of vaccination. Eleven cases of mumps meningoencephalitis were reported in a 2005 to 2006 outbreak affecting over 2,500 patients in 11 states.[34] Lymphocytic choriomeningitis virus, a rare cause of viral meningitis, is transmitted by contact with infected rodents, their excretion, or through transplanted organs.[35] Acute HIV infection may manifests as aseptic meningoencephalitis.[36]

Fungal and parasitic meningitis

Although many other pathogens have been reported to cause meningitis, several important pathogens should be considered in certain circumstances. Cryptococcal meningitis is common among immunosuppressed individuals, particularly AIDS patients, but it can also occur in immunocompetent hosts.[37] The incidence of crypotococcal meningitis has significantly declined in the era of highly active antiretroviral therapy with the recent annual incidence being approximately two to seven cases per 1,000 persons with AIDS.[38] *Mycobacterium tuberculosis* meningitis is often a difficult diagnoses. A total of 186 cases of tuberculous meningitis (1.3% of all cases of tuberculosis) were reported in 2005 in the United States.[39] Despite the decline of incidence of tuberculosis in the United States, the incidence of tuberculous meningitis has changed little.[40]

Primary amebic meningoencephalitis is caused by *Naegleria fowleri,* a thermophilic, free-living, fresh-water amoeba. Primary amebic meningoencephalitis is very rare—only six cases were reported in the United States in 2007—but nearly always fatal.[41] A history of fresh water exposure and a high index of clinical suspicion are a key to make the diagnosis.

Clinical Manifestation and Physical Examination

Diagnosing meningitis, especially in elderly and neonatal patients, can be challenging because of considerable variability in clinical manifestations (**Table 1**). The sensitivity

Table 1 Presenting symptoms and signs of in patients with bacterial meningitis	
Symptom or Sign	**Relative Frequency (%)**
Headache	≥90
Fever	≥90
Meningismus	≥85
Altered sensorium	>80
Vomiting	~35
Seizures	~30
Focal neurologic findings	10~20
Papilledema	<5

From Tunkel AR, Scheld WM. Acute meningitis. In: Mandel GL, Bennett JE, Dolin R, editors. Principles and Practice of Infectious Disease 6th edition. Philadelphia. Elsevier Churchill Livingstone; 2005. p.1099; with permission.

of the classic triad of bacterial meningitis (ie, fever, neck stiffness, and altered mental status) is approximately 40%.[7,42] In severe cases, bacterial meningitis may present with coma, seizure, and focal neurologic deficits, which are associated with an unfavorable prognosis.[7,43,44] Severity of symptoms may be influenced by host factors, such as age, anatomic abnormalities, concurrent illness, immune function, and causative pathogens. Evaluation of a suspected meningitis patient should include a complete neurologic examination, in addition to general examination with emphasis on the head, ear, nose, and oropharynx. Additional maneuvers specifically for meningitis, such as Kernig's sign, Brudzinski's sign, and jolt accentuation of headache may indicate the presence of meningeal irritation.[42]

Laboratory Diagnosis

Opening pressure, cell count, and chemistries

Given the lack of specific symptoms or physical findings, the diagnosis of meningitis is based on the analysis of cerebrospinal fluid. Careful interpretation of cerebrospinal fluid is required to avoid misdiagnosis. Opening pressure is typically elevated in bacterial meningitis; however, the range can be variable. Measurement of opening pressure is particularly important for cryptococcal meningitis because high opening pressure (>250 mm Hg) is a poor prognostic indicator.[45] A pleocytosis (100 cells/mm^3–10,000 cells/mm^3) is usually seen in patients with bacterial meningitis with 80% to 95% of cases having a neutrophil-predominant pleocytosis.[7,46] A normal, or mildly elevated, cerebrospinal fluid leukocyte count can occur in up to 10% of patients with bacterial meningitis and suggests poor prognosis.[7] A lymphocyte-predominant pleocytosis is generally seen in viral, fungal, or tuberculous meningitis; however, predominance of lymphocyte in cerebrospinal fluid does not exclude the possibility of bacterial meningitis.[7,24] An increase in cerebrospinal fluid protein is seen in virtually all patients with bacterial meningitis.[47] A decreased cerebrospinal fluid glucose level ($\leq$ 40 mg/dL) supports a diagnosis of bacterial meningitis.[47] Other biochemical markers, such as elevated cerebrospinal fluid lactate level or elevated serum procalcitonin level, may be beneficial in distinguishing bacterial meningitis from other etiologies of meningeal irritation.[48,49]

Gram stain and cultures

A rapidly performed Gram stain of cerebrospinal fluid can provide timely identification of the causative pathogen because the sterilization of cerebrospinal fluid can occur as quickly as 15 minutes after parenteral antimicrobial therapy.[50] Even if the cerebrospinal fluid culture is subsequently negative, a Gram stain of the cerebrospinal fluid may show the causative organism. Sensitivity of Gram stain in bacterial meningitis ranges from 60% to 90%, depending on the concentration of bacteria in the cerebrospinal fluid.[7,51] A positive Gram stain is highly specific for bacterial meningitis. Centrifugation of specimen may increase the yield of Gram stain. Cerebrospinal fluid culture is essential in the diagnostic workup of bacterial meningitis. Communication with the microbiology laboratory is crucial, as certain pathogens require prolonged incubation or special techniques.

PCR, latex agglutination, and serology

PCR assays have been particularly useful in the diagnosis of viral meningitis.[27] The sensitivity and specificity of PCR for both bacterial (N meningitidis, S pneumoniae, and H influenzae) and viral (HSV, VZV, and enteroviruses) meningitis exceed 90%.[52,53] Although PCR assays have become the gold standard for diagnosing viral meningitis, clinical correlation is always warranted, given the possibility of false-negative and false-positive results. Cryptococcal antigen latex agglutination of testing of cerebrospinal fluid has both excellent sensitivity and specificity in the diagnosis of cryptococcal meningitis (sensitivity: 93%–100%; specificity: 93%–98%).[54] Serologic testing to cerebrospinal fluid (ie, anti-WNV IgM) is crucial to confirm the diagnosis of WNV neuroinvasive disease.[31]

The Dilemma Between Diagnosis and Early Treatment

Lumbar puncture should not delay initiation of antimicrobial therapy in cases in which bacterial meningitis is suspected. A delay in treatment is strongly associated with adverse outcome.[55–58] The most common factors associated with delay of antimicrobial therapy are cranial imaging before lumbar puncture and transfer of the patient to another hospital.[46] The mean time to administration of antimicrobial agents from presentation in United States hospitals is between 1 and 4.9 hours.[44,56–58] Delayed administration of antimicrobial agents greater than 6 hours after presentation is associated with increased mortality and neurologic sequelae.[58] CT scan of the brain is routinely performed before lumbar puncture, despite the low prevalence (2%) of pre-existing mass effect or space-occupying lesions in the general patient population.[59] Established clinical criteria can reduce the need for unnecessary cranial imaging before lumbar puncture. Guidelines from the Infectious Disease Society of America (IDSA) recommend cranial imaging before lumbar puncture be restricted to certain high-risk patients (eg, immunocompromised patients, history of central nervous system disease, new onset seizure, papilledema, abnormal level of consciousness, and focal neurologic deficits).[47] Whenever a CT scan of the brain is indicated, the administration of the first dose of antimicrobials is recommended before cranial imaging.[47]

Treatment

Antimicrobial therapy

Although the basic approach to patients with meningitis is similar to other infectious diseases, empiric antibiotic treatment should be instituted without delay. The choice of empiric antimicrobials should be based on those agents with activity against most likely pathogens, epidemiologic data, age, patient immune status, or other predisposing factors (eg, history of basal skull fracture or penetrating trauma). Another important factor is antimicrobial penetration into the central nervous system. While meningitis disrupts the blood-brain barrier and facilitates drug penetration, the cerebrospinal fluid concentration of antimicrobials is often limited.[60] Once a causative pathogen is identified, antimicrobial therapy should be modified. The choice of pathogen-targeted therapy depends on in vitro antimicrobial susceptibility and the penetration of the antimicrobial agent into cerebrospinal fluid. An antibiotic with bactericidal activity is strongly preferred to one with bacteriostatic activity, as the concentration of antimicrobial agents in cerebrospinal fluid is variable. Third-generation cephalosporins (eg, ceftriaxone and cefotaxime) have been used as first-line agents, because approximately 80% of community-onset meningitis is caused by S pneumoniae and N meningitidis.[6,7] However, analysis of over 27,000 strains of S pneumoniae isolates from the United States between 1998 and 2002 revealed that the prevalence of penicillin resistance (minimal inhibitory concentration ≥ 2 µg/ml) was 18.4%, and isolates with resistance to both penicillin and third-generation cephalosporins was 9.1%.[61] Meningitis caused by penicillin-resistant S pneumoniae is associated with higher mortality.[62] Given increased cephalosporin resistance, empiric therapy for community-onset bacterial meningitis in the United States is both vancomycin and a third-generation cephalosporin.[47]

Ampicillin should be used if listerial meningitis is suspected; *L monocytogenes* is intrinsically resistant to cephalosporins.[13] Concomitant use of gentamicin should be considered, as it gives synergistic bactericidal activity in vitro. However, there is no clinical trial data to prove the efficacy of adding gentamicin for listerial meningitis. Patients presenting with encephalitis should receive acyclovir until HSV infection is ruled out.[63]

Broader spectrum antimicrobial agents are required to treat nosocomial meningitis, as the causative organisms differ from those seen in community-onset meningitis. Vancomycin, combined with either third- or fourth-generation cephalosporins or a carbapenem, are appropriate empiric antimicrobial regimens. Successful treatment of staphylococcal meningitis using newer antistaphylococcal agents (ie, linezolid or daptomycin) has been reported; however, no clinical trials have been conducted to compare these agents with vancomycin.[64–66] Removal of retained foreign bodies (eg, intraventricular catheter) is recommended in cases of nosocomial meningitis.

Supportive care
Comprehensive supportive care is required in the management of meningitis. Appropriate circulatory resuscitation is essential. Many experts recommend that euvolemic states are preferred to restricted volume states to reduce adverse neurologic outcome by under-hydration.[67] Periodic mental status assessment is useful for evaluation of recovery, as well as prompt recognition of new-onset focal neurologic changes or seizures. Alteration of mental status in patients with meningitis may be caused by multiple factors: exacerbation of meningeal inflammation, abscess with surrounding cerebral edema, fever, hyponatremia because of the syndrome of inappropriate antidiuretic hormone (SIADH), or toxicity because of high doses of antimicrobials, especially beta-lactams or carbapenems.

Adjuvant therapy
In randomized trials, corticosteroid therapy for tuberculous meningitis reduced mortality.[68–70] Corticosteroids also have been used for bacterial meningitis among pediatric patients, based on a randomized, controlled trial in the late 1980s.[71] Dexamethasone therapy in the pediatric population with bacterial meningitis is associated with a lower mortality and decreased incidence of neurologic or audiologic sequelae because of the reduction of the host inflammatory response in the subarachnoid space.[72,73] One clinical trial conducted in Europe found a benefit for dexamethasone use in pneumococcal meningitis among adults, but did not find the same benefit in meningococcal or listerial meningitis.[74] Corticosteroids should be administered simultaneously with antimicrobial agents because the lysis of bacteria by antimicrobial agents triggers the release of inflammatory cytokine, which is felt to worsen local tissue damage.[74,75] Corticosteroids do not reduce the concentration of ceftriaxone or vancomycin level in cerebrospinal fluid, provided these antimicrobial agents are appropriately dosed.[76,77] Current guidelines from the IDSA and a meta analysis support the use of corticosteroid in patients with bacterial meningitis.[47,78] However, two recent clinical trials revealed conflicting results regarding the clinical efficacy of empiric dexamethasone for suspected bacterial meningitis among Asians and a high-prevalence of the HIV population.[79,80] The overall benefit of corticosteroid therapy in the treatment of bacterial meningitis is still not clearly understood.

Management of complications
Lack of clinical response after 24 to 48 hours of antimicrobial therapy should be considered treatment failure.[47,63] A repeat lumbar puncture is the most effective way assess for inadequate response to antimicrobial therapy. Resolution of

hypoglycorrhachia and reduction of the cerebrospinal fluid lactate level are the earliest indicators of improvement.[63]

Hyponateremia and seizure are the most common complications of meningitis. Approximately 25% of patients with bacterial meningitis develop hyponatremia.[48] Etiologies of hyponateremia can be multifactorial, such as salt wasting, SIADH, aggressive hydration, or adrenal insufficiency. Serum electrolytes should be appropriately corrected with serial monitoring of serum electrolytes. Seizures occur in 13% to 15% of patients with bacterial meningitis.[7,43] Electroencephalographic monitoring, especially in patients with history of seizure or fluctuating mental status, should be considered.[46] Although the need for an anticonvulsant as seizure prophylaxis for all patients with bacterial meningitis is not clear, use of anticonvulsants is warranted once clinical evidence of seizure is noted or if a mass lesion is identified.

Acute hydrocephalus occurs in 3% to 8% of cases of bacterial meningitis.[46] Hydrocephalus caused by meningitis usually results from interference with cerebrospinal fluid flow through the ventricular system. Elevated opening pressure may suggest the presence of hydrocephalus and the diagnosis is confirmed by cranial imaging. Elevated intracranial pressure is commonly seen in more than 50% of patients with cryptococcal meningitis.[45] A repeat lumbar puncture, ventriculostomy, or ventricular shunt placement should be considered to treat acute hydrocephalus or elevated intracranial pressure.[45–47]

BRAIN ABSCESS
Epidemiology and Etiology

Because of improvements in the treatment of ear, sinus, and orofacial infections over the last half century, brain abscesses are rare, with only 1,500 to 2,500 infections each year in the United States.[81] Delays in hospitalization, focal neurologic deficits at admission, impaired host immunity, uncontrolled diabetes, and Glasgow Coma Scale less than 12 are associated with death and permanent neurologic deficits because of brain abscesses.[82–85] Understanding the pathogenesis of brain abscesses is important in determining the most likely causative microorganisms and subsequent treatment.

Bacterial brain abscesses most commonly are the result of contiguous spread of infection from the oropharynx, middle ear, and paranasal sinuses.[86] How microorganisms seed the brain from these sources is not fully understood; valveless emissary veins may allow microorganism to flow into the venous system of the brain from these sites.[86] Cranial trauma is another source of brain abscess by contiguous means. The prevalence of brain abscesses after penetrating trauma or neurosurgical procedures ranges from 2% to 14%.[83–85,87]

Hematogenous spread from distant focus of infection is also other important cause of brain abscess, and can occur in the setting of chronic pyogenic lung disease, endocarditis, intra-abdominal abscess, and urinary tract infections.[88]

Streptococci (eg, *Streptococcus milleri* group and viridian group streptococci) are the most common cause of pyogenic brain abscesses because of extension from the nasopharynx and oropharynx. Anaerobic bacteria (eg, *Bacteroides* spp, *Prevotella* spp, *Peptostreptococcus*, *Fusobacterium* spp, or *Actinomyces* spp) are another major cause of brain abscesses, often as a part of polymicrobial infection.

The microbiology of brain abscesses depends on the initial site of infection. *Streptococcus* spp and anaerobic organisms are often isolated in patients with lung abscesses. *Staphylococcus aureus* or viridians group streptococci are often seen among patients with brain abscesses resulting from endocarditis.

Enteric Gram-negative bacilli are often recovered in association with an intra-abdominal or genitourinary source. *Pseudomonas* spp can be seen in brain abscesses arising from otitis media or otitis extrena.[86] *Staphylococcus* spp and aerobic, Gram-negative bacilli are also frequently isolated from brain abscesses related to head trauma or neurosurgical procedures.[89]

Opportunistic pathogens can be a cause of brain abscesses in the immunocompromised or elderly population. Brain abscesses due to *Nocardia* spp often result from dissemination of cutaneous or pulmonary infection. Brain abscesses caused by *M tuberculosis* and nontuberculous mycobacteria have been reported in patients with HIV infection.[90] *L monocytogenes* may cause brain abscesses in immunosuppressed individuals.[91]

Fungal brain abscesses caused by yeast (eg, *Candida* spp, *Cryptococcus* spp), dimorphic fungi (eg, *Histoplasma* spp, *Coccidioides* spp, *Blastomyces* spp), and molds (eg, *Aspergillus* spp, *Rhizopus*) are associated with immunocompromised states, and in the case of zygomycosis, poorly controlled diabetes.

Protozoa and helminths can cause parasitic brain abscesses. Central nervous system toxoplasmosis, because of *Toxoplasma gondii*, and neurocystcercosis, caused by the larval form of *Taenia solium*, are notable examples of parasitic infections and can be suggested by obtaining a relevant social history (eg, cat exposure, exposure to livestock in high prevalence areas).

Clinical Manifestation

Headache, mental status changes, focal neurologic deficit, and fever are hallmark of symptoms of brain abscess (**Table 2**). New-onset seizures can also be an initial symptom of brain abscess. One study reported the sensitivity of the classic clinical triad of fever, headache, and focal neurologic deficits to be only 17%.[84] Clinical manifestations are dependent on the location and size of the brain abscess, host immune status, and the virulence of the causative microorganism.

Diagnosis

The wide availability of imaging studies has improved the diagnosis of brain abscess. CT with intravenous contrast may reveal single- or multiple-ring enhancing lesions, particularly in well-established or chronic brain abscess. MRI with gadolinium contrast

Table 2
Common symptoms and signs of in brain abscess

Symptom or Sign	Frequency (%)
Headache	~70
Mental status changes	70
Focal neurologic deficits	>60
Fever	45–50
Seizures	25~35
Nausea and vomiting	25~50
Nucheal rigidity	~25
Papilledema	~25

From Tunkel AR. Brain abscess. In: Mandel GL, Bennett JE, Dolin R, editors. Principles and Practice of Infectious Disease 6th edition. Philadelphia. Elsevier Churchill Livingstone; 2005. p. 1154; with permission.

is more sensitive and specific than CT scan with contrast study to diagnose brain abscess.[88] Once a diagnosis of brain abscess is considered by radiographic imaging, microbiologic investigation should be performed. A CT-guided stereotactic biopsy with aspiration of abscesses lessens the necessity of open craniotomy and can be both diagnostic and therapeutic.[92] Comprehensive microbiologic investigations should be performed, as repeated sampling is usually not feasible.

Treatment

Antimicrobial therapy

The treatment of brain abscess requires a multidisciplinary approach involving intensivists, neurosurgeons, radiologists, and infectious disease specialists. While empiric antimicrobial therapy should be started, particularly in patients with sepsis or impending herniation, every effort should be made to quickly obtain microbiologic or tissue diagnosis before initiating antimicrobial therapy.[63] As brain abscesses are frequently polymicrobial, empiric antimicrobial therapy should cover Gram-positive, Gram-negative, and anaerobic microorganisms. An example regimen would include a third- or fourth-generation cephalosporin, metronidazole, and vancomycin, based on predisposing factors. Carbapenems can be used in place of the combination of cephalosporins and metronidazole. Once a causative microorganism is identified, antimicrobial therapy can be tailored. Similar to meningitis, the choice of optimal therapy is determined by antimicrobial penetration to the brain parenchyma and in vitro susceptibilities of the pathogens.

Duration of therapy is influenced by causative microorganisms and reduction in the size of the abscess. Cerebral nocardiosis or actinomycosis may require a prolonged course (eg, ≥ 12 months) of therapy. While at least 6 to 8 weeks of parenteral therapy has been traditionally given for bacterial brain abscesses, there is no convincing data supporting the optimal duration of therapy. Duration of antimicrobial therapy should be determined individually, based on the size of abscess, combination of surgical treatment, causative organism and response to treatment.[86]

Surgical therapy

Indications for closed drainage and aspiration of brain abscess versus open craniotomy are controversial. However, most experts feel that brain abscesses greater than 2.5 cm in diameter should be surgically treated (ie, open craniotomy or stereotactic aspiration), because of poor response with antimicrobial therapy alone.[81] Although open craniotomy is often not necessary, it should be considered in special clinical situations. A traumatic brain abscess may require craniotomy to remove foreign material or bone chips. Cerebellar or brain stem abscesses are often indication for posterior fossa craniotomy because of the potential for brain herniation due to the small volume of posterior fossa.[86] Periventricular brain abscesses often require craniotomy given the risk of intraventricular rupture.[93] A ventriculostomy placement is indicated for significantly elevated intracranial pressure. The etiology of high intracranial pressure (eg, obstructive hydrocephalus, ventricular rupture, or mass effect because of brain abscesses) also should be investigated at the same time.

Adjuvant therapy

Dexamethasone has been used for reducing intracranial pressure, especially in patients with impending brain herniation. The benefit of dexamethasone in treatment of brain abscess remains unclear.[82,85,87,94] Unnecessary or prolonged use of corticosteroids should be avoided because of its numerous adverse effects.

Seizure is a common complication in patients with brain abscesses, occurring in 13% to 25% of cases.[84,88] Although seizures may not affect the overall mortality rate, an anticonvulsant should be prescribed to prevent seizure in early course of therapy.[83,84,94]

SUBDURAL EMPYEMA

Subdural empyema, which is defined as a purulent infection of the space between the cranial dura and arachnoid membrane, is a neurosurgical emergency, with approximately 10% to 13% mortality, despite aggressive neurosurgical management.[95,96] The pathogenesis of subdural empyema is similar to those of brain abscess: direct extension from a contiguous foci (eg, paranasal sinus diseases, cranial osteomyelitis, or cranial trauma), or hematogenous spread from distant foci. The microbiology of subdural empyema is also similar to brain abscesses. Once bacteria invade into the subdural space, it may spread across the cerebral hemisphere because of lack of an anatomic barrier. Major symptoms include headache, altered mental status, and focal signs, depending on the extent of empyema.[97] Clinical course can be rapidly deteriorated because of rapid accumulation of pus in the subdural space. Cranial imaging is essential to diagnose subdural empyema. CT scan of the brain usually shows a hypodense subdural lesion with medial membrane enhancement.[98] MRI may be more sensitive to visualize subdural lesions. Combination of antimicrobial therapy and adequate surgical irrigation of subdural space via burr hole or craniotomy is a mainstay of therapy.[97]

SUMMARY

Meningitis and brain abscess are life-threatening infectious diseases requiring the highest medical attention. A multidisciplinary approach, including emergency medicine, infectious diseases, neurology, and neurosurgery facilitates prompt diagnosis and treatment. Acknowledgment of treatment strategy will lead to improving the outcome of central nervous system infection.

REFERENCES

1. Adams WG, Adams WG, Deaver KA, et al. Decline of childhood *Haemophilus influenzae* type b (Hib) disease in the Hib vaccine era. JAMA 1993;269(2):221–6.
2. Centers for Disease Control and Prevention. Direct and indirect effects of routine vaccination of children with 7-valent pneumococcal conjugate vaccine on incidence of invasive pneumococcal disease–United States, 1998–2003. Morb Mortal Wkly Rep 2005;54(36):893–7.
3. Choi C. Bacterial meningitis in aging adults. Clin Infect Dis 2001;33(8):1380–5.
4. Short WR, Tunkel AR. Changing epidemiology of bacterial meningitis in the United States. Curr Infect Dis Rep 2000;2(4):327–31.
5. Weisfelt M, van de Beek D, Spanjaard L, et al. Community-acquired bacterial meningitis in older people. J Am Geriatr Soc 2006;54(10):1500–7.
6. Schuchat A, Robinson K, Wenger JD, et al. Bacterial meningitis in the United States in 1995. Active Surveillance Team. N Engl J Med 1997;337(14):970–6.
7. van de Beek D, de Gans J, Spanjaard L, et al. Clinical features and prognostic factors in adults with bacterial meningitis. N Engl J Med 2004;351(18):1849–59.
8. Weisfelt M, van de Beek D, Spanjaard L, et al. Clinical features, complications, and outcome in adults with pneumococcal meningitis: a prospective case series. Lancet Neurol 2006;5(2):123–9.
9. Overturf GD. Indications for the immunological evaluation of patients with meningitis. Clin Infect Dis 2003;36(2):189–94.

10. Tzeng YL, Stephens DS. Epidemiology and pathogenesis of *Neisseria meningitidis*. Microbes Infect 2000;2(6):687–700.
11. Rosenstein NE, Perkins BA, Stephens DS, et al. Meningococcal disease. N Engl J Med 2001;344(18):1378–88.
12. Stephens DS. Uncloaking the meningococcus: dynamics of carriage and disease. Lancet 1999;353(9157):941–2.
13. Southwick FS, Purich DL. Intracellular pathogenesis of listeriosis. N Engl J Med 1996;334(12):770–6.
14. Brouwer MC, van de Beek D, Heckenberg SG, et al. Community-acquired *Listeria monocytogenes* meningitis in adults. Clin Infect Dis 2006;43(10):1233–8.
15. Zuniga M, Aguado JM, Vada J. *Listeria monocytogenes* meningitis in previously healthy adults: long-term follow-up. QJM 1992;85(307–308):911–5.
16. Samuels MA, Gonzalez RG, Kim AY, et al. Case records of the Massachusetts General Hospital. Case 34–2007. A 77-year-old man with ear pain, difficulty speaking, and altered mental status. N Engl J Med 2007;357(19):1957–65.
17. Jackson LA, Hilsdon R, Farley MM, et al. Risk factors for group B streptococcal disease in adults. Ann Intern Med 1995;123(6):415–20.
18. Le Moal G, Landron C, Grollier G, et al. Meningitis due to *Capnocytophaga canimorsus* after receipt of a dog bite: case report and review of the literature. Clin Infect Dis 2003;36(3):e42–6.
19. Weisfelt M, van de Beek D, Spanjaard L, et al. Nosocomial bacterial meningitis in adults: a prospective series of 50 cases. J Hosp Infect 2007;66(1):71–8.
20. Palabiyikoglu I, Tekeli E, k Cokca F, et al. Nosocomial meningitis in a university hospital between 1993 and 2002. J Hosp Infect 2006;62(1):94–7.
21. Lyke KE, Obasanjo OO, Williams MA, et al. Ventriculitis complicating use of intraventricular catheters in adult neurosurgical patients. Clin Infect Dis 2001;33(12):2028–33.
22. Korinek AM, Baugnon T, Golmard JL, et al. Risk factors for adult nosocomial meningitis after craniotomy: role of antibiotic prophylaxis. Neurosurgery 2006;59(1):126–33.
23. Kourbeti IS, Jacobs AV, Koslow M, et al. Risk factors associated with postcraniotomy meningitis. Neurosurgery 2007;60(2):317–25.
24. Durand ML, Calderwood SB, Weber DJ, et al. Acute bacterial meningitis in adults. A review of 493 episodes. N Engl J Med 1993;328(1):21–8.
25. Connolly KJ, Hammer SM. The acute aseptic meningitis syndrome. Infect Dis Clin North Am 1990;4(4):599–622.
26. Tyler KL. Herpes simplex virus infections of the central nervous system: encephalitis and meningitis, including Mollaret's. Herpes 2004;11(Suppl 2):57A–64A.
27. Kupila L, Vuorinen T, Vainionpaa R, et al. Etiology of aseptic meningitis and encephalitis in an adult population. Neurology 2006;66(1):75–80.
28. Schlesinger Y, Tebas P, Gaudreault-Keener M, et al. Herpes simplex virus type 2 meningitis in the absence of genital lesions: improved recognition with use of the polymerase chain reaction. Clin Infect Dis 1995;20(4):842–8.
29. Nash D, Mostashari F, Fine A, et al. The outbreak of West Nile virus infection in the New York City area in 1999. N Engl J Med 2001;344(24):1807–14.
30. Gubler DJ. The continuing spread of West Nile virus in the Western hemisphere. Clin Infect Dis 2007;45(8):1039–46.
31. Solomon T. Flavivirus encephalitis. N Engl J Med 2004;351(4):370–8.
32. Center for Disease Control and Prevention. West Nile virus activity–United States, 2007. Morb Mortal Wkly Rep 2008;57(26):720–3.

33. Center for Disease Control and Prevention. West Nile virus. Statistics, surveillance and control. Available at: http://www.cdc.gov/ncidod/dvbid/westnile/surv&controlCaseCount02_detailed.htm. Accessed January 29, 2009.

34. Center for Disease Control and Prevention. Update: multistate outbreak of mumps–United States, January 1–May 2, 2006. Morb Mortal Wkly Rep 2006; 55(20):559–63.

35. Fischer SA, Graham MB, Kuehnert MJ, et al. Transmission of lymphocytic choriomeningitis virus by organ transplantation. N Engl J Med 2006;354:2235–49.

36. Newton PJ, Newsholme W, Brink NS, et al. Acute meningoencephalitis and meningitis due to primary HIV infection. BMJ 2002;325(7374):1225–7.

37. Ecevit IZ, Clancy CJ, Schmalfuss IM, et al. The poor prognosis of central nervous system cryptococcosis among nonimmunosuppressed patients: a call for better disease recognition and evaluation of adjuncts to antifungal therapy. Clin Infect Dis 2006;42(10):1443–7.

38. Mirza SA, Phelan M, Rimland D, et al. The changing epidemiology of cryptococcosis: an update from population-based active surveillance in 2 large metropolitan areas, 1992-2000. Clin Infect Dis 2003;36(6):789–94.

39. Center for Disease Control and Prevention. Reported tuberculosis in the United States 2005. Available at: http://www.cdc.gov/tb/surv/surv2005/PDF/TBSurvFULLReport.pd. Accessed May 27, 2009.

40. Center for Disease Control and Prevention. Trends in tuberculosis incidence–United States, 2006. Morb Mortal Wkly Rep 2007;56(11):245–50.

41. Center for Disease Control and Prevention. Primary amebic meningoencephalitis–Arizona, Florida, and Texas, 2007. Morb Mortal Wkly Rep 2008;57(21):573–7.

42. Attia J, Hatala R, Cook DJ, et al. The rational clinical examination. Does this adult patient have acute meningitis? JAMA 1999;282(2):175–81.

43. Aronin SI, Peduzzi P, Quagliarello VJ. Community-acquired bacterial meningitis: risk stratification for adverse clinical outcome and effect of antibiotic timing. Ann Intern Med 1998;129(11):862–9.

44. Flores-Cordero JM, Amaya-Villar R, Rincon-Ferrari MD, et al. Acute community-acquired bacterial meningitis in adults admitted to the intensive care unit: clinical manifestations, management and prognostic factors. Intensive Care Med 2003; 29(11):1967–73.

45. Saag MS, Graybill RJ, Larsen RA, et al. Practice guidelines for the management of cryptococcal disease. Infectious Diseases Society of America. Clin Infect Dis 2000;30(4):710–8.

46. van de Beek D, de Gans J, Tunkel AR, et al. Community-acquired bacterial meningitis in adults. N Engl J Med 2006;354(1):44–53.

47. Tunkel AR, Hartman BJ, Kaplan SL, et al. Practice guidelines for the management of bacterial meningitis. Clin Infect Dis 2004;39(9):1267–84.

48. Genton B, Berger JP. Cerebrospinal fluid lactate in 78 cases of adult meningitis. Intensive Care Med 1990;16(3):196–200.

49. Viallon A, Zeni F, Lambert C, et al. High sensitivity and specificity of serum procalcitonin levels in adults with bacterial meningitis. Clin Infect Dis 1999;28(6):1313–6.

50. Kanegaye JT, Soliemanzadeh P, Bradley JS. Lumbar puncture in pediatric bacterial meningitis: defining the time interval for recovery of cerebrospinal fluid pathogens after parenteral antibiotic pretreatment. Pediatrics 2001;108(5):1169–74.

51. La Scolea LJ Jr, Dryja D. Quantitation of bacteria in cerebrospinal fluid and blood of children with meningitis and its diagnostic significance. J Clin Microbiol 1984; 19(2):187–90.

52. Radstrom P, Backman A, Qian N, et al. Detection of bacterial DNA in cerebrospinal fluid by an assay for simultaneous detection of *Neisseria meningitidis*, *Haemophilus influenzae*, and streptococci using a seminested PCR strategy. J Clin Microbiol 1994;32(11):2738–44.

53. DeBiasi RL, Tyler KL. Polymerase chain reaction in the diagnosis and management of central nervous system infections. Arch Neurol 1999;56(10): 1215–9.

54. Tanner DC, Weinstein MP, Fedorciw B, et al. Comparison of commercial kits for detection of cryptococcal antigen. J Clin Microbiol 1994;32(7):1680–4.

55. Bryan CS, Reynolds KL, Crout L. Promptness of antibiotic therapy in acute bacterial meningitis. Ann Emerg Med 1986;15(5):544–7.

56. Talan DA, Guterman JJ, Overturf GD, et al. Analysis of emergency department management of suspected bacterial meningitis. Ann Emerg Med 1989;18(8): 856–62.

57. Miner JR, Heegaard W, Mapes A, et al. Presentation, time to antibiotics, and mortality of patients with bacterial meningitis at an urban county medical center. J Emerg Med 2001;21(4):387–92.

58. Proulx N, Frechette D, Toye B, et al. Delays in the administration of antibiotics are associated with mortality from adult acute bacterial meningitis. QJM 2005;98(4): 291–8.

59. Hasbun R, Abrahams J, Jekel J, et al. Computed tomography of the head before lumbar puncture in adults with suspected meningitis. N Engl J Med 2001;345(24): 1727–33.

60. Lutsar I, McCracken GH Jr, Friedland IR. Antibiotic pharmacodynamics in cerebrospinal fluid. Clin Infect Dis 1998;27(5):1117–27.

61. Karlowsky JA, Thornsberry C, Jones ME, et al. Factors associated with relative rates of antimicrobial resistance among *Streptococcus pneumoniae* in the United States: results from the TRUST Surveillance Program (1998–2002). Clin Infect Dis 2003;36(8):963–70.

62. Auburtin M, Wolff M, Charpentier J, et al. Detrimental role of delayed antibiotic administration and penicillin-nonsusceptible strains in adult intensive care unit patients with pneumococcal meningitis: the PNEUMOREA prospective multicenter study. Crit Care Med 2006;34(11):2758–65.

63. Cunha BA. Central nervous system infections in the compromised host: a diagnostic approach. Infect Dis Clin North Am 2001;15(2):567–90.

64. Ntziora F, Falagas ME. Linezolid for the treatment of patients with central nervous system infection. Ann Pharmacother 2007;41(2):296–308.

65. Kallweit U, Harzheim M, Marklein G, et al. Successful treatment of methicillin-resistant *Staphylococcus aureus* meningitis using linezolid without removal of intrathecal infusion pump. Case report. J Neurosurg 2007;107(3):651–3.

66. Lee DH, Palermo B, Chowdhury M. Successful treatment of methicillin-resistant *Staphylococcus aureus* meningitis with daptomycin. Clin Infect Dis 2008;47(4): 588–90.

67. Maconochie I, Baumer H, Stewart ME. Fluid therapy for acute bacterial meningitis. Cochrane Database Syst Rev 2008;(1):CD004786.

68. Kumarvelu S, Prasad K, Khosla A, et al. Randomized controlled trial of dexamethasone in tuberculous meningitis. Tuber Lung Dis 1994;75(3):203–7.

69. Schoeman JF, Van Zyl LE, Laubscher JA, et al. Effect of corticosteroids on intracranial pressure, computed tomographic findings, and clinical outcome in young children with tuberculous meningitis. Pediatrics 1997;99(2):226–31.

70. Thwaites GE, Nguyen DB, Nguyen HD, et al. Dexamethasone for the treatment of tuberculous meningitis in adolescents and adults. N Engl J Med 2004;351(17): 1741–51.
71. Lebel MH, Freij BJ, Syrogiannopoulos GA, et al. Dexamethasone therapy for bacterial meningitis. Results of two double-blind, placebo-controlled trials. N Engl J Med 1988;319(15):964–71.
72. Odio CM, Faingezicht I, Paris M, et al. The beneficial effects of early dexamethasone administration in infants and children with bacterial meningitis. N Engl J Med 1991;324(22):1525–31.
73. Schaad UB, Lips U, Gnehm HE, et al. Dexamethasone therapy for bacterial meningitis in children. Swiss Meningitis Study Group. Lancet 1993;342(8869):457–61.
74. de Gans J, van de Beek D. Dexamethasone in adults with bacterial meningitis. N Engl J Med 2002;347(20):1549–56.
75. van de Beek D, de Gans J, McIntyre P, et al. Steroids in adults with acute bacterial meningitis: a systematic review. Lancet Infect Dis 2004;4(3):139–43.
76. Gaillard JL, Abadie V, Cheron G, et al. Concentrations of ceftriaxone in cerebrospinal fluid of children with meningitis receiving dexamethasone therapy. Antimicrobial Agents Chemother 1994;38(5):1209–10.
77. Ricard JD, Wolff M, Lacherade JC, et al. Levels of vancomycin in cerebrospinal fluid of adult patients receiving adjunctive corticosteroids to treat pneumococcal meningitis: a prospective multicenter observational study. Clin Infect Dis 2007; 44(2):250–5.
78. van de Beek D, de Gans J, McIntyre P, et al. Corticosteroids for acute bacterial meningitis. Cochrane Database Syst Rev 2007;(1):CD004405.
79. Nguyen TH, Tran TH, Thwaites G, et al. Dexamethasone in Vietnamese adolescents and adults with bacterial meningitis. N Engl J Med 2007;357(24):2431–40.
80. Scarborough M, Gordon SB, Whitty CJ, et al. Corticosteroids for bacterial meningitis in adults in sub-Saharan Africa. N Engl J Med 2007;357(24):2441–50.
81. Mamelak AN, Mampalam TJ, Obana WG, et al. Improved management of multiple brain abscesses: a combined surgical and medical approach. Neurosurgery 1995;36(1):76–85.
82. Seydoux C, Francioli P. Bacterial brain abscesses: factors influencing mortality and sequelae. Clin Infect Dis 1992;15(3):394–401.
83. Xiao F, Tseng MY, Teng LJ, et al. Brain abscess: clinical experience and analysis of prognostic factors. Surg Neurol 2005;63(5):442–9.
84. Tseng JH, Tseng MY. Brain abscess in 142 patients: factors influencing outcome and mortality. Surg Neurol 2006;65(6):557–62.
85. Tonon E, Scotton PG, Gallucci M, et al. Brain abscess: clinical aspects of 100 patients. Int J Infect Dis 2006;10(2):103–9.
86. Mathisen GE, Johnson JP. Brain abscess. Clin Infect Dis 1997;25(4):763–79.
87. Kao PT, Tseng HK, Liu CP, et al. Brain abscess: clinical analysis of 53 cases. J Microbiol Immunol Infect 2003;36(2):129–36.
88. Heilpern KL, Lorber B. Focal intracranial infections. Infect Dis Clin North Am 1996;10(4):879–98.
89. Yang KY, Chang WN, Ho JT, et al. Postneurosurgical nosocomial bacterial brain abscess in adults. Infection 2006;34(5):247–51.
90. Farrar DJ, Flanigan TP, Gordon NM, et al. Tuberculous brain abscess in a patient with HIV infection: case report and review. Am J Med 1997;102(3):297–301.
91. Mylonakis E, Hohmann EL, Calderwood SB. Central nervous system infection with *Listeria monocytogenes*. 33 years' experience at a general hospital and review of 776 episodes from the literature. Medicine (Baltimore) 1998;77(5):313–36.

92. Mampalam TJ, Rosenblum ML. Trends in the management of bacterial brain abscesses: a review of 102 cases over 17 years. Neurosurgery 1988;23(4): 451–8.
93. Zeidman SM, Geisler FH, Olivi A. Intraventricular rupture of a purulent brain abscess: case report. Neurosurgery 1995;36(1):189–93.
94. Hakan T, Ceran N, Erdem I, et al. Bacterial brain abscesses: an evaluation of 96 cases. J Infect 2006;52(5):359–66.
95. Dill SR, Cobbs CG, McDonald CK. Subdural empyema: analysis of 32 cases and review. Clin Infect Dis 1995;20(2):372–86.
96. Nathoo N, Nadvi SS, van Dellen JR, et al. Intracranial subdural empyemas in the era of computed tomography: a review of 699 cases. Neurosurgery 1999;44: 529–35.
97. Osborn MK, Steinberg JP. Subdural empyema and other suppurative complications of paranasal sinusitis. Lancet Infect Dis Jan 2007;7(1):62–7.
98. Weisberg L. Subdural empyema. Clinical and computed tomographic correlations. Arch Neurol 1986;43(5):497–500.

Fungal Infections in the ICU

Marya D. Zilberberg, MD, MPH[a,b,]*, Andrew F. Shorr, MD, MPH[c,d]

KEYWORDS

- Critical illness • ICU • Fungal infection • *Candida*
- *Aspergillus* • Invasive

Pulmonologists and intensivists often care for patients at risk for infections caused by both *Aspergillus* and *Candida*. Infection with either can lead to severe life- threatening disease. Mortality rates for invasive fungal disease often exceed 30%. Furthermore, immunosuppressed patients are at increased risk for disease caused by both pathogens. despite these similarities, however, important differences exist between infections caused by mold as compared with those related to yeast. For mold, the lungs (in addition to the central nervous system) remain the key affected organ system, while yeast rarely are implicated as a cause of pneumonia. Conversely, colonization by *Aspergillus* has clearly different implications for the patient than does colonization with *Candida*. For both organisms, however, multiple diagnostic challenges remain. Fortunately, therapeutic paradigms are shifting, and clinicians have many new agents in their armamentarium for combating fungal infection. Given the rapidly changing literature in this broad area, it is imperative that physicians caring for the immunosuppressed patient and for the critically ill remain abreast of this evolving field.

INVASIVE PULMONARY ASPERGILLOSIS

Invasive pulmonary aspergillosis (IPA) represents a dreaded complication in critically ill patients. Several species of *Aspergillus* remain major causes of IPA. In particular, *A fumigatus*, *A flavus* and *A niger* account for nearly all human disease. Although *Aspergillus* can lead to disease in both immunocompetent and immunocompromised hosts, the intensivist often is addressing disease in the systemically immunosuppressed patient. The pulmonologist, alternatively, may face several types of noninvasive disease such as allergic bronchopulmonary aspergillosis (ABPA), mycetomoa

[a] Department of Health Policy and Management, School of Public Health and Health Sciences, University of Massachusetts, Amherst, MA 01003, USA
[b] EviMed Research Group, LLC, Post Office Box 303, Goshen, MA 01032, USA
[c] Division of Pulmonary and Critical Care Medicine, Room 2a_68, Washington Hospital Center, 110 Irving Street, Northwest, Washington, DC 20010, USA
[d] Georgetown University School of Medicine, Washington, DC 20010, USA
* Corresponding author. EviMed Research Group, LLC, Post Office Box 303, Goshen, MA 01032.
E-mail address: marya@evimedgroup.org (M.D. Zilberberg).

Infect Dis Clin N Am 23 (2009) 625–642
doi:10.1016/j.idc.2009.04.008
0891-5520/09/$ – see front matter © 2009 Elsevier Inc. All rights reserved.

id.theclinics.com

formation, and chronic necrotizing aspergillosis (CNA). In these three conditions, the immune system is generally intact, and in select syndromes such as ABPA, it is the host response to infection that leads to a clinical syndrome. Invariably these three conditions are associated with local impairments of the intrapulmonary immune system as a result of local airway damage and destruction. Unless leading to hemoptysis that compromises the airway, patients who have these non-IPA syndromes usually do not require treatment in the ICU. Because of the disproportionate burden of IPA, the remainder of this discussion will focus on IPA.

Epidemiologically, the true incidence of IPA is unclear. Although certainly less common than infection with yeast, the frequency of IPA may be increasing. For example, Groll and colleagues[1] in examining autopsy data between 1978 and 1992 noted a rise in prevalence of all invasive mycoses from 0.4% to 3.1%, and Aspergillus as the causative organism increased from 17% to 60% over the same time period. Certainly one factor driving rates of IPA is the broadening use of immunosuppressive agents. Both the types of and duration of immunosuppression related to all forms of transplant are evolving. Attendant with more extensive immunosuppression is a greater risk for IPA. Not all forms of immunosuppression appear to carry similar risks for IPA. Both the extent and duration of neutropenia represent long recognized risk factors for IPA. More recently, use of select monoclonal antibody strategies for induction of immunosuppression has been thought to heighten the chance for IPA. In hematopoietic stem-cell transplant (HSCT) subjects, the development of graft versus host disease has been linked to a greater frequency of invasive mold infections. Following any type of transplant, cytomegalovirus (CMV) disease also amplifies the potential for IPA.

Recently, Patterson and Singh described the disproportionate distribution of IPA as a function of the type of transplant.[2] In a systematic review of over 20,000 cases of IPA, they reported that the incidence of IPA was greatest among those undergoing lung transplant, with 8.4% developing IPA.[2] Patients receiving kidney transplants face a substantially lower risk for IPA (0.7%).[2] The rate of IPA following either HSCT or heart transplant was approximately 6.0%. In part, this difference related to transplant type reflects both the difference in the agents used for immunosuppression (eg, renal transplant patients require much less immunosuppression) and also the fact that Aspergillus spores are inhaled. Hence, the lungs potentially are exposed to an excessive inoculum. The impact of IPA on post-transplant mortality was staggering: anywhere from 10% to 17% if all post-transplant deaths were attributed to IPA.[2]

More recent analyses suggest that the epidemiology of IPA in the ICU may be shifting away from those traditionally considered at risk. Several recent case series have described IPA in nonimmunocompromised critically ill subjects. Samarakoon and Soubani reported five cases of IPA among chronic obstructive pulmonary disease (COPD) patients from their medical center and performed a systematic review of literature on this topic.[3] These investigators found that among the 65 cases examined, clinical presentation was largely nonspecific, and in most (63%), radiological findings consisted of infiltrates. Although in 15 patients (23%) diagnosis was made with a bronchoalveolar lavage (BAL), in a plurality of cases (n=28, 43%) Aspergillus was recovered at autopsy. Despite treatment with antifungal agents in most cases, the mortality rate was 91%. The authors concluded that the likely risk factors in this cohort of COPD patients for IPA included chronic treatment with corticosteroids and advanced severe COPD.

Similarly, Vandewoude and colleagues[4] described 38 individuals (incidence 4 out of 1000 ICU admissions) who had IPA cared for between 1997 and 1999. Only 17 of them (45%) had traditional risk factors, while among the remaining 21 without evidence of immune compromise, invasive disease was a complication of their critical illness.[4] The authors noted that while in the presence of risk factors the actual mortality was similar to that predicted by Acute Physiology and Chronic Health Evaluation (APACHE) II, in those lacking the traditional risk factors for IPA, actual mortality exceeded that predicted by APACHE.[4] The same investigators in a case–control analysis calculated that the attributable mortality of IPA in the ICU approached 20%, finding the presence of this disease to be an independent predictor of hospital mortality among the critically ill.[5] Finally, Meerssemann and colleagues[6] described a 127-patient cohort of ICU patients who had IPA, of whom 89 did not have an underlying malignancy. Of these 89, 35 had COPD; nine had undergone a solid organ transplantation, and 17 were on immunosuppressive therapy. Observed mortality in this group (80%) was higher than that predicted by the Simplified Acute Physiology Score (SAPS) II (48%). Of particular interest, were five critically ill patients without any predisposition but with proven IPA. In an additional analysis addressing only critically ill patients colonized with Aspergillus (n = 172), Vandewoude and colleagues[7] concluded that nearly 50% of such subjects had invasive disease and not simply colonization. Again, despite the absence of typical risk factors for IPA, they detected the syndrome in patients, where before one might never have considered it a clinical possibility. Although thought-provoking, each of these analyses has major limitations because of essentially retrospective, single-center designs. Nonetheless, these findings, taken as a whole, suggest that the epidemiology of IPA in the ICU is shifting. In response, physicians need to remain vigilant and consider this syndrome in patients not significantly immunocompromised.

Diagnostically, IPA remains a challenge. Initially, the clinical manifestation of IPA may be nonspecific. As many as 30% of patients may be asymptomatic. Nonspecific symptoms such as dyspnea and fever are common. Radiographic manifestations of IPA also may be diverse. The classic description of cavitation associated with IPA is a late finding, and the absence of cavitation does not preclude a diagnosis of IPA. In some cases, the disease begins as small nodules that eventually coalesce. Alternatively, IPA can lead to peripheral, wedge-shaped opacities that resemble those seen after pulmonary infarction. The air crescent sign is a late finding in IPA and is caused by contraction of infarcted tissue surrounding the site of infection. Conversely, the halo sign, an area of low attenuation near the primary lesion, is an early finding that often is transient. These two signs are somewhat specific for invasive aspergillosis but lack sensitivity.[8]

To facilitate the diagnosis of IPA, two strategies have been proposed. The first addresses the risk for IPA based on airway colonization with Aspergillus. In many syndromes, colonization with a pathogen does not increase the subsequent risk for infection necessarily. With respect to IPA, this appears not to be the case. In the review by Paterson and Singh[2] described earlier, the authors estimated that colonization with Aspergillus correlated with an eventual risk for IPA ranging from 16% to 80%, depending on the type of transplantation. HSCT subjects faced a greater risk for IPA if they were known to be colonized (60% to 80%), while in lung recipients, a positive airway culture for Aspergillus conveyed a less than 20% chance of eventual IPA.[2] In unselected ICU patients, recovery of Aspergillus in apparently noninfected patients may also represent a harbinger of IPA. For example, Vandewoude and colleagues[7] performed a large cohort study of 172 patients (incidence 6.8/1000 ICU admissions) with a positive sputum culture for Aspergillus. Based on a predefined algorithm involving clinical presentation, radiographic signs, and BAL cultures, 83 cases were deemed to be IPA, while the remaining 89 were thought to be colonized with the organism. The algorithm was found to have good positive and negative predictive values for invasive disease in this population of patients.[7]

Serologically, ELISA-based testing for the presence of galactomanan (GM), a component of the mold cell wall, has held promise as a noninvasive tool in the approach to suspected IPA. Other areas of interest for noninvasive diagnosis address 1,3 beta-D-glucan and the presence of Aspergillus DNA. Initial reports suggested that the GM assay was fairly accurate and could suggest the presence of IPA days before it became clinically apparent.[9-11] These studies, however, were limited to mainly HSCT subjects. A meta-analysis of GM testing indicated that the assay was performed moderately well (approximate sensitivity and specificity 80%) but varied widely based on the cutoff used for defining a positive test.[12] The many agents that can confound the GM assays, along with the fact that the assay performs less well in people receiving antifungal prophylaxis further limit the utility of this diagnostic modality.[13,14]

Bronchoscopy remains a much-used tool in the approach to patients who have suspected IPA. Aggressive and early use of bronchoscopy has been shown to improve outcomes in mixed cohorts of immunosuppressed patients who have pulmonary infiltrates. Bronchoscopy, however, may not be reliable in suspected mold infections. Because Aspergillus may result in patchy involvement or be angioinvasive, BAL is only positive half the time in either known or probable IPA. The role for transbronchial biopsy (TBB) to increase the yield of bronchoscopy for suspected IPA remains controversial. First, many patients who have this condition are coagulopathic or thrombocytopenic, which may preclude TBB. Second, because it is patchy by nature, the bronchoscopist may simply fail to biopsy a site of involvement. In an effort to improve the diagnostic yield of bronchoscopy in IPA, Husain and colleagues[15] proposed measuring GM titers on BAL. In an analysis of over 100 patients, they determined that this approach was fairly specific and had modest sensitivity. Confirmatory studies are necessary before broad application of this strategy.

With respect to treatment, the number of trials exploring new agents and alternatives has exploded over the last decade. Treatment options for IPA consist of the polyene amphotericin B deoxycholate (D-AMB) or its less toxic lipid formulations (L-AMB), azoles, and echinocandins (Infectious Diseases Society of America [IDSA] guideline). In selected cases, surgery may be required.[16] The recommended first-line therapy for primary IPA is voriconazole, a broad-spectrum triazole, either intravenously or orally, depending on the underlying illness severity.[16] This recommendation is based on the results of a multinational multicenter randomized unblinded trial comparing the efficacy, safety, and tolerability of voriconazole with D-AMB in 277 immunocompromised patients who had definite or probable IPA.[17] Over one half of subjects randomized to voriconazole had either a complete or partial response, compared with 31.6% of the D-AMB group, meeting not only the noninferiority margin, but also showing superiority to D-AMB. More importantly, voriconazole was associated with an increased probability of intermediate-term survival. Although large and prospective, this trial has been criticized because of its open-label nature and because L-AMB was not employed as the comparator. Nonetheless, it represents the single largest randomized trial for Aspergillus and the only one suggesting a mortality benefit.

In the ICU, the main limitation with voriconazole has been the fact that the drug cannot be administered intravenously to patients who have impaired renal function. The carrier with the voriconazole can build up in those who have GFRs of less than 35% and lead to toxicity.[18] Moreover, because voriconazole is an azole and can lead rarely to hepatotoxicity, coupled with the fact that it is also prone to drug–drug interactions, there are alternative strategies for treating IPA. Because several studies document the equivalent efficacy of and better safety profile for L-AMB over D-AMB, only the former is recommended by the IDSA at the dosage of 3 to 5 mg/kg daily for treating IA.[16,19,20] For example, in a double-blind multicenter trial of immunocompromised patients who had proven invasive disease, 201 subjects were randomized to either a standard (3 mg/kg) or high (10 mg/kg) daily dose of L-AMB for 14 days followed by 3 mg/kg/d.[21] Although efficacy outcomes were similar in both groups, the high-dose group experienced higher rates of toxicity than observed with the standard dose.[21] Caspofungin, a member of the echinocandin family, represents an option for IA treatment among those who have refractory disease or for people unable to tolerate AMB or triazoles. Maertens and colleagues,[22] in an open-label noncomparative multicenter clinical trial in patients who had probable or proven IA intolerant of treatment with AMBs or triazoles, investigated the use of caspofungin at the dose of 50 mg daily following a 70 mg loading dose on day 1. A complete or partial clinical resolution was the primary outcome of the study. Among the 83 efficacy-evaluable patients, 45% responded favorably, and only two patients were forced to discontinue caspofungin because of drug-related toxicity. The authors concluded that caspofungin is a viable salvage treatment for IA, and it is recommended as such by the IDSA.[16,22]

Before trials with voriconazole, itraconazole, an older azole with activity against *Aspergillus*, was studied for IPA. Caillot and colleagues[23] reported the results of a trial of intravenous itraconazole followed by oral treatment for probable or definite IPA in 31 immunocompromised patients. In this single-arm open-label multicenter study, the primary outcome of complete or partial clinical resolution was met in 18 (58%) of the subjects, in the face of mostly mild-to-moderate toxicities.[23] The largest study of invasive *Aspergillus* was conducted by Patterson and colleagues[24] in North America and Western Europe and represented a naturalistic observational analysis examining case records of 595 patients who had IA, most of whom (56%) had IPA. This study was completed before the commercial availability of voriconazole. When looking at treatment regimens, 187 were treated with AMB alone, 58 with itraconazole alone, and 93 with a combination of the two (the remaining patients were treated with other various regimens).[24] Itraconazole resulted in a 57% rate of combined complete and partial response, similar to the combination therapy (54%) and higher than AMB alone (32%).[24] Although it boasts the largest study sample to date, rigorous randomized trials are lacking to compare the treatment of IA with itraconazole with either AMB or voriconazole. If using itraconazole, serum level measurements are needed to document adequate drug absorption.[16] Posaconazole is an additional extended- spectrum triazole available in the European Union for treating refractory disease. This monotherapy was investigated in an open-label prospective trial in 107 patients, the results of which were compared with 86 retrospectively collected historic controls.[25] Complete or partial response was achieved in 42% of posaconazole-treated patients versus only 26% of those on the comparator regimen.[25] In a logistic regression model, the authors noted that the adjusted odds ratio (OR) of response was 4.06 (95% CI, 1.50 to 11.04) for posaconazole over other salvage therapies.[25]

The final drug recommended as salvage therapy for IA is micafungin, a newer echinocandin.[16] Although a treatment dose has not been conclusively established, two trials indicate its efficacy in probable or definite IA. In a 225-patient open-label single-arm study, 35.6% of all patients treated with micafungin achieved a response, with the rates even higher in the primary (50%) and salvage (41%) groups.[26] An additional open-label study investigated the efficacy of micafungin alone or in combination for treating refractory or intolerant patients.[27] Of the 98 patients enrolled in the study, eight were treated singly with micafungin, of whom three (38%) achieved a response.[27] Clearly, the experience with micafungin is limited and not controlled well enough to render it a strongly recommended therapy. Similarly, because very little evidence exists for the efficacy and safety of combination regimens, these are not recommended for treating IA at this time.[16] Nonetheless, this is an active area of exploration. Two recent single-center analyses have promoted plans for large multi-center studies. First, in an observational analysis of 48 patients with IPA failing AMB, many of whom had undergone HSCT, Marr and colleagues[28] treated patients either with voriconazole alone or with voriconazole along with caspofungin. Cure rates and survival were greater in patients given combination therapy, and these differences persisted after controlling for multiple potential confounders. Second, Singh and colleagues[29] prospectively treated 40 solid organ transplant recipients with IPA with voriconazole and caspofungin and compared outcomes with a historical control cohort given AMB (n = 47). Survival was higher in patients given combination therapy, but this difference only approached statistical significance. Beyond anti-invectives, surgery may be required in selected cases of IPA. Generally, surgical resection is used in instances where invasion of great vessels is threatened or in patients who have hemoptysis in association with a solitary lesion amenable to resection.

CANDIDAL BLOODSTREAM INFECTIONS
Epidemiology

Unlike *Aspergillus*, epidemiologic data regarding bloodstream infection (BSI) caused by *Candida* are more abundant. First, candidal BSIs occur 7 to 15 times more frequently than do cases of IPA.[30] In fact, *Candida* represents the most common cause of invasive fungal disease.[30] According to surveillance data from the US Centers for Disease Control and Prevention, Candida now accounts for 12% of all hospital-acquired BSIs.[31] A major increase in candidal BSI initially was noted during the 1980s, with a more than quintupling in the rate of BSIs caused by this yeast.[32] More recently, rates of BSI caused by *Candida* have stabilized or declined. For example, Fridkin and colleagues[33] documented a fall in the incidence of candidal BSI among low birth weight neonates in the United States from 3.51 to 2.68 per 1000 patient days between 1995 and 2004. Similarly, a single-center pediatric study from Spain described that the incidence of candidemia had stabilized at a rate of 0.6 cases per 1000 hospitalizations between 1988 and 2000.[34] Contrary to this rise, Trick and colleagues[35] reviewed the National Nosocomial Surveillance System (NNIS) between 1989 and 1999 and noted that the rate of BSIs specifically caused by *C albicans* in critically ill adults with central venous catheters (CVCs) fell from approximately 8.1 cases per 1000 CVC days in 1989 to about 2.2 cases per 1000 CVC days in 1999. Strikingly, rates of non-*albicans* candidemia in aggregate remained stable during this period, although proportion of infections caused by *C glabrata* BSI increased significantly.[35] Other studies, both from the United States and abroad, however, have observed growth in the number of hospitalizations complicated by candidemia.[36–40] Martin and colleagues,[36] for instance, examined the epidemiology of sepsis in the United States between 1979 and 2000 and reported a tripling in the incidence of fungal sepsis. In an effort to gauge the burden of candidemia in patients presenting to the hospital as opposed to addressing a purely nosocomial process, Shorr and colleagues[37] reviewed over 60,000 admissions where the patient presented with a BSI. Although candidemia was infrequent (1.2%) relative to BSI with either a gram-positive of gram-negative pathogen, the prevalence of candidal BSIs rose from approximately 7.5 cases per 1000 BSIs in 2000 to 12 cases per 1000 BSIs in 2005.[37] Finally, a recent survey study reviewing United States hospital discharge data between 2000 and 2005 reported a 50% rise in the incidence of hospitalizations involving candidemia between 2000 and 2005.[38] Studies from Iceland and Finland have reported similar growth in candidemia incidence.[39,40] The differences in candidemia temporal trends documented in the previously mentioned studies likely reflect differing study methodologies and differing populations (eg, neonates) and geographic areas (eg, Spain).

From an economic perspective, patients who have candidal BSIs consume substantial resources. Estimates of the costs of care associated with this syndrome vary based on the methodology used, but unlike the discordance regarding the frequency of candidal BSIs, all reports examining outcomes in this condition suggest that costs of care range from $15,000 to $40,000 per case.[37,41,42] In one report, the excess costs of care for candidemia were more than $15,000 greater than for the costs related to treating other BSIs caused by bacterial pathogens.[37] Driving these greater costs was an accompanying 5-day excess length of stay in the setting of Candida.[37]

One evident epidemiologic trend has been a shift in the distribution of candidal species responsible for BSI. Over the last decade, the proportion of infections caused by C albicans has fallen. Presently, C albicans appears to account for only half of all BSIs caused by yeast.[43] More specifically, in 1990, 80% of all fungal BSIs were caused by C albicans.[43] In a large 3.5-year multicenter prospective observational study of candidemia within the United States, Nguyen and colleagues[44] demonstrated that nearly 50% of all candidal isolates were of non-albicans species, with C glabrata (6.3%) and C krusei (4.3%) representing over 10% of all cultures. In a study from Italy looking at 182 episodes of candidemia between 1999 and 2003, the investigators found an even lower proportion of C albicans, decreasing from 62% of all candidal isolates in 1999 to only 24% in 2003.[45] The opposite trend was detected for C glabrata, which went from 0% in 1999 to 26% in 2003.[45] The authors noted a strong correlation of the rise in non-albicans species with the use of fluconazole.[45] The prevalence of these non-albicans organisms is not restricted to the ICU. Shorr and colleagues[46] examined candidal BSIs at two large United States hospitals. They specifically focused on the microbiology of these infections and observed no difference in the proportion of non-albicans isolates recovered from ward patients and critically ill patients.[46] Interestingly, no clinical factors separated patients with C albicans from other forms of Candida. Finally, a large multinational microbiologic study by Pfaller and colleagues[47] detected a less dramatic shift in candidal species. In this study examining nearly 100,000 candidal isolates, the proportion represented by C albicans went from 68% between 1997 and 2000 to 63% in 2005, while the proportion of C glabrata remained stable between 10% and 11% during the same time frame. Interestingly, the prevalence of C tropicalis increased from 5.2% of all candidal isolates from 1997 to 2000 to 7.3% in 2005.[47] They also reported that in vitro resistance to fluconazole among C glabrata decreased from 19% to 15%, while that among C albicans increased from 0.9% to 1.6% and among C krusei from 66% to 79%.[47]

Risk Factors

Before considering treatment issues, clinicians must appreciate the risk factors for fungal BSIs. Through understanding the issues and variables that heighten the potential for candidemia, one can focus on efforts not only at prevention but also on prompt diagnosis and treatment. Common risk factors predisposing to candidemia include candidal colonization, prior exposure to antibiotics, renal failure, presence of a CVC, and need for total parenteral nutrition (TPN).[48–51] In a case–control study, Wey and colleagues[48] established that the number of antibiotics administered, candidal colonization, hemodialysis, and use of a Hickman catheter were strongly associated with the development of candidemia. A group of Swiss investigators led by Pittet in a study of 29 surgical ICU patients confirmed colonization to be a risk factor for candidal infection.[49] Additional risk factors consisted of length of previous antibiotic therapy and severity of illness.[49] Fraser and colleagues, in a 104-patient single-center cohort study, determined that sustained fungemia is more likely than transient fungemia among patients who have neutropenia, CVCs, and a need for mechanical ventilation (MV). They further reported that exposure to TPN independently heightened the chance for candidal BSI.[50] Blumberg and colleagues,[51] in a large multicenter cohort study, confirmed the importance of the CVC and TPN as risk factors for developing candidemia in the ICU. This group defined acute renal failure to be an additional strong predictor of candidemia development (relative risk [RR] 7.3, 95% CI, 2.5 to 8.8).[51] In the same cohort study, the incidence of candidemia was 9.8 cases per 1000 admissions; 55% of the cases were caused by non-*albicans* species, and over 10% of all isolates exhibited resistance to fluconazole.[51] Chow and colleagues[52] identified similar risk factors for *albicans* and non-*albicans* candidemia among ICU patients:

Major operations, particularly gastrointestinal (GI) procedures
Enteric source for bacteremia
Hemodialysis days
TPN duration and red blood cell transfusions

Specific to the ICU, several risk stratification schemes exist to facilitate identification of patients at high risk for candidemia.[53,54] A multicenter, prospective cohort study from Spain including 1699 adult ICU patients identified surgery, multifocal colonization, TPN, and severe sepsis to be strong predictors of candidal infection.[53] A key strength of this analysis was its multicenter nature and its systematic, prospective collection of information on colonization status. Assigning weighted points based on the β-coefficients for terms in a regression model, the investigators derived and validated a *Candida* score with good discriminative power.[53] The authors suggested that patients who have a score above 2.5 might benefit from early antifungal treatment, although this assertion requires validation in future trials.[53] Another large cohort study of nearly 3000 patients in United States and Brazilian ICUs determined that the presence of certain combinations of the following factors was highly predictive of subsequent development of invasive disease: antibiotics, CVC, TPN, dialysis, major surgery, pancreatitis, and steroids or other immunosuppressive agents.[54] The same team attempted to apply this rule in their ICU to reduce the incidence of BSIs.[55] In this study, the investigators stratified ICU patients using the previously developed rule, and, based on the presence of the required criteria, placed them on fluconazole prophylaxis.[55] In the year of implementation (2005) 36 patients met criteria for and received prophylaxis, and in the same year, only two candidal BSI cases were diagnosed, compared with nine cases in the previous year and before the rule implementation, corresponding to a reduction from 3.4 cases per 1000 CVC days to 0.8 cases per 1000 CVC days.[55] Because of the small sample size, no adjustment for confounding and other methodologic issues, it is difficult to draw conclusions about the effectiveness of this intervention, and the need for validating this approach remains.

Several substantial limitations remain associated with prior work regarding clinical prediction rules for risk of candidemia in the ICU. First, few of the risk stratification schemes have been validated prospectively. Second, although the presence of multiple risk factors may increase the chance for fungemia relatively, the absolute increase in risk may remain small. In other words, given the prevalence of MV, CVCs, broad-spectrum antibiotic use, and exposure to corticosteroids in critically ill patients, the currently available risk stratification schemes lack sufficient precision to allow for their broad application in identifying patients who might merit from either prophylaxis or presumptive therapy.

Because of frustration with risk stratification and diagnostic modalities, efforts recently have focused on developing surrogate markers to detect the presence of fungemia. Moreover, the sensitivity of blood cultures for this pathogen varies from 8% to 82%, depending on the population in question.[56] Additionally, cultures may take several days to become positive.[56] Similar to research addressing galctomannan for *Aspergillus*, the candidal cell wall has many components that can be detected with modern assays. The most promising target appears to be β-D-glucan. Unfortunately, diagnosis of candidemia remains a challenge. The β-D-glucan test has relatively high sensitivity, specificity, and positive and negative predictive values, although data in the ICU are lacking.[57] The mostly small studies conducted to date mainly have enrolled severely immunosuppressed patients. Molecular testing to detect *Candida* DNA is in early development, and it is not clear how useful it will be among the critically ill.[57] An additional challenge in the current environment is the proliferation of azole-resistant non-*albicans* species.

Prophylaxis and Presumptive Therapy

Because of the efficacy of prophylaxis in immunocompromised populations, some have advocated for a like strategy in high-risk critically ill patients. Garbino and colleagues[58] evaluated the role for fluconazole prophylaxis among 204 high-risk critically ill medical and surgical patients already undergoing a selective digestive decontamination regimen. In this double-blind randomized placebo-controlled trial, colonization rates with *Candida* were similar in both groups at entry into the study, and only 4 of 103 patients in the fluconazole group, compared with 10 of the 101 in the placebo group, developed candidal infections.[58] This study confirmed the results of an earlier randomized controlled trial by Eggimann and collegues.[59] In this randomized double-blind placebo-controlled trial, the efficacy of fluconazole prophylaxis against intra-abdominal candidiasis was tested in a cohort of surgical patients who had recurrent GI perforations or surgical anastomosis leakages. The rate of development of intra-abdominal *Candida* was 4% (1 of 23) in the fluconazole group and 35% (7 of 20) in the placebo group, corresponding to the relative risk of 0.12 (95% CI, 0.02 to 0.93).[59] A meta-analysis of fluconazole prophylaxis in surgical patients confirmed the effectiveness of this approach in reducing the incidence of invasive candidiasis, but did not find a survival advantage.[60] One concern with all of the trials of prophylaxis has been that they have defined candidal infection broadly, rather than specifically targeting BSI. In no study, has fluconazole prophylaxis been shown to reduce BSI with yeast. Admittedly, each study has been underpowered to address this question. Nonetheless, given that broader use of fluconazole could promote either the emergence of resistance or lead to an accelerated shift in microbiology toward organisms like *C glabrata*, this is not recommended routinely. Randomized prevention trials are ongoing with other nonfluconazole alternatives.

Beyond either prophylactic therapy or treatment when a candidal BSI is documented, the role for presumptive treatment is evolving. As with many bacterial infections, delay in initiation of treatment for fungemia independently increases the risk for mortality. An analysis by the Spanish group for fungal Infection in the ICU found that a delay in starting antifungal treatment increased the risk of hospital death by more than 60%, although this impact on death did not reach statistical significance because of the analysis' small sample size.[61] Others have provided more conclusive evidence of how a delay in treatment adversely affects outcomes. Morrell and colleagues[62] performed a single-center retrospective cohort study investigating the impact of treatment delay on mortality among 157 consecutive patients with *Candida* blood stream infection. In this study most of the isolates (53.5%) were *C albicans,* and the cumulative proportion of *C glabrata* and *C krusei* was 14%. The investigators found that only 5 of the 157 patients received prompt, appropriate empiric therapy for candidemia. In a multivariate analysis, they reported that a delay of as little as 12 hours from when the eventually positive blood cultures were drawn more than doubled the risk for death (OR 2.09, 95% CI, 1.53 to 2.84).[62] Readers should note that the delay was defined, not as time from when the laboratory contacted the provider and reported yeast in the cultures, but the time from which the initial evaluation for infection commenced. Garey and colleagues[63] confirmed the Morrel group's observation. In this multicenter cohort, investigators noted increasing mortality based on the delay, measured in days from when the culture was drawn to antifungal treatment. Similarly, a recent study by Labelle and colleagues[64] expanded the definition of inappropriate therapy for fungemia to encompass more than just the time to treatment. In their analysis, they also defined the inadequate dosing of fluconazole as inappropriate. This, along with a delay in therapy independently raised the risk of death ninefold.[64] All four of these studies underscore the importance of prompt appropriate treatment of candidemia to impact survival. They also reveal the need for an emphasis on prevention and an urgent need for rapid diagnostic strategies.

Embracing the need to be prompt in treatment of suspected candidemia should not lead intensivists to endorse presumptive therapy. In this case, presumptive therapy represents the administration of antifungals purely based on the presence of several risk factors for candidal infection and the development of a new fever. This approach represents a standard strategy for prolonged neutropenic fever. For critically ill subjects, however, a large multicenter, randomized trial demonstrated the futility of this paradigm.[65] In this study, ICU patients who had persistent fever were assigned randomly to empiric fluconazole or placebo. To enrich the population as to their risk for fungemia, the protocol required patients to concurrently be receiving broad-spectrum antibiotics and have CVCs in place. Additionally, most subjects had been undergoing MV for several days. Overall, outcomes including mortality and fever resolution were similar.[65] The main reason for these negative findings was that the rate of eventually documented fungemia was low; approximately 7% of subjects subsequently were diagnosed with a candidal BSI. This fact underscores the need for better risk stratification schemes. Also, the list of causes of fever in the ICU is extensive. Because the investigators did not require an effort to exclude other possible causes for fever, such as the presence of a new pneumonia, one limitation of the trial may have been that the entry criteria simply did not reflect the way clinical decision making takes place at the bedside in the ICU.[65] In other words, the potential for fungemia is not simply a function of the number of risk factors present, but more properly reflects whether an alternative diagnosis for the nonspecific signs and symptoms that can be seen in with this condition is more or less likely.

Treatment

A key step in the approach to fungemia, irrespective of the antifungal used, remains management of the CVC. In many instances, the CVC represents the portal of entry for the fungus into the patient. Alternatively, the CVC may become seeded as a secondary point in the disease process. Current guidelines strongly advocate prompt CVC removal.[66] This in part is based on the observation that the biofilm evolving on a CVC represents a relatively protected site for fungus. Older-generation antifungals (eg, fluconazole) penetrate biofilm very poorly. Moreover, older analyses have identified that CVC retention may be an independent predictor of mortality.[67,68]

Some have criticized this approach of uniform CVC removal, because the initial reports addressing CVC removal failed to address confounding issues such as severity of illness and why the CVC was not removed.[69] Patients in whom the CVC is not removed in fact may be described better as subjects for whom the CVC cannot be removed given comorbid issues, the need for continued central access, and risks associated with replacing the CVC. For example, Rodriguez and colleagues[70] determined that severity of illness was the most important predictor of mortality in candidemic patients and that assessments of timing of removal were confounded by this overriding issue. They concluded that decisions regarding CVC removal must be individualized. Similarly, in a qualitative review of the topic, Pasqualotto and Severo observed that many analyses were too flawed to allow one to draw meaningful conclusions.[71] They advocated for a randomized trial to determine appropriate practice. More careful and up-to-date analyses, however, clearly show the risks related to failing to remove the CVC in persons with fungemia. Raad and colleagues[72] explored predictors of mortality in over 400 patients with cancer and candidemia. After adjusting for severity of illness, immune system status, and the source of the candidemia, failure to remove the CVC increased the probability of death more than fourfold. Labelle and colleagues[64] reached similar conclusions. In addition to taking many variables into consideration that included severity of illness, comorbid illness, and most importantly the timing and appropriateness of antifungal treatment, they observed that catheter retention independently heightened the risk for death more than sixfold.[64]

The past decade has witnessed a proliferation of commercially available antifungals. At present, the clinician must consider various forms of amphotericin, azoles, and echinocandins. For many years, amphotericin (AMB) represented the standard of care for candidemia. Although the utility of AMB is limited by its multiple toxicities, the newer liposomal AMB (L-AMB) formulations are tolerated better. In general, the L-AMB options lead to less nausea, vomiting, and fever. They clearly cause less nephrotoxicity. Unfortunately, L-AMB preparations still may result in substantial potassium wasting as is seen with AMB deoxycholate. Clinical trials document that L-AMB has similar but not better, efficacy relative to conventional AMB preparations.[73]

Fluconazole represents a well-tolerated alternative for candidemia. In a randomized trial, fluconazole was shown to result in similar outcomes when compared with AMB.[74] In this study, evaluating 206 non-neutropenic patients evenly divided between the two treatment regimens, mortality rates with fluconazole and AMB were 33% and 40%, respectively. This difference was not statistically different. Notably, the rates of blood culture clearance were also similar. The authors concluded that in patients without neutropenia, fluconazole and AMB had similar effectiveness.[74] A similar trial from Canada confirmed these findings.[75] One major limitation of studies employing fluconazole is that they were completed in an era when the prevalence of C glabrata and C krusei were much lower. For example, in the initial report by Rex and colleagues,[74] these pathogens accounted for less than 15% of all isolates, while in modern settings, the proportion of candidal BSIs caused by these yeast species may be increasing. Furthermore, dosing of fluconazole can be confusing. Current guidelines recommend treatment with a greater dose of fluconazole. This theoretically allows one to potentially overcome the dose-dependent resistance seen in some candidal isolates. Unfortunately, observational analyses document that clinicians often underdose this agent.[64]

Voriconazole, a triazole with excellent activity against *Aspergillus*, also has been examined as an alternative to AMB in non-neutropenic patients who have candidemia.[76] In a randomized, noninferiority trial enrolling over 400 patients, voriconazole was found to be similar in effectiveness to AMB.[76] Interestingly, despite more adverse event-related treatment discontinuations in the voriconazole group, there were fewer reports of toxicities with voriconazole than with AMB.[76] Again, the limitation of voriconazole for many critically ill patients arises because of the carrier molecule for the compound. One unique aspect of the trial reported by Kullberg and colleagues was the systematic analysis of transitioning to oral therapy. Those given voriconazole could step down to the oral form, while those treated with AMB could switch to oral fluconazole. Before this trial, patients infected with yeast who were not likely to respond to fluconazole had no oral alternative. Now those infected with C glabrata and C krusei can be switched to an oral agent, which may facilitate more rapid hospital discharge or help prevent the need of placement of a new CVC for continued antifungal treatment. Other azole compounds, itraconazole and posaconazole, exist. At present, these agents have not been well-evaluated as alternative treatments for invasive candidal infection.

A newer class of compounds, echinocandins, comprises three commercially available alternatives: caspofungin, micafungin, and anidulafungin. Echinocandins target the fungal cell wall. In general, these agents are tolerated well and come only as intravenous formulations.[77–79] As a class, they tend to have few drug–drug interactions. Two of the three (caspofungin and anidulafungin) require a loading dose.[77,78] With respect to pharmacokinetics, anidulafungin has the longest half-life and greatest volume of distribution. Caspofungin must be dose-reduced in patients who have impaired liver function.[77] This may have implications for use in the ICU, where occult liver disease caused by either hepatitis C infection or alcohol abuse can be an issue. Anidulafungin has been studied in patients with various ranges of liver impairment, and because the drug is not metabolized by the liver, dose reduction is not required.[78] Similarly, micafungin does not appear to require dose reduction in people who have mild-to-moderate liver disease; this issue has not been worked out in patients who have severe hepatic impairment.[79] Anidulafungin also does not interact with the cytochrome P450 system, which reduces the potential for many serious drug–drug interactions that can be encountered in patients in the ICU.[78]

Four clinical trials have evaluated the various echinocandins. The first, by Mora-Duarte and colleagues,[80] compared caspofungin with AMB as a treatment for candidemia in 224 patients who had invasive candidal infections, 80% of which represented candidemia. In this noninferiority trial stratifying patients based on the presence of neutropenia, caspofungin performed as well as AMB in terms of the primary outcome of favorable response, regardless of the presence or absence of neutropenia.[80] In an analysis of a predefined subpopulation of per-protocol subjects, caspofungin led to more favorable responses. This, however, was due to the fact that the number of patients having to discontinue therapy because of tolerability issues was higher in the AMB arm. Importantly, AMB deoxycholate was employed in this trial, so differences in tolerability are not surprising. Caspofungin has not been compared with either L-AMB or fluconazole in a randomized study.

Micafungin, in turn, has been compared with both L-AMB[81] and caspofungin.[82] Kuse and colleagues[81] randomly assigned over 500 individuals who had disseminated candidiasis to treatment with either micafungin or liposomal AMB. Micafungin proved noninferior to L-AMB, regardless of neutropenia status, and once again its toxicity profile was favorable compared with L-AMB.[81] In this trial, the starting dose of micafungin was 100 mg daily, but investigators could increase the dose to 150 mg daily. The study protocol did not prespecify criteria for dose escalation, raising concern that in some instances a 100 mg dose may be inadequate. A more recent study directly compared micafungin with caspofungin for candidemia.[82] The study population (n = 600) was randomized to one of three arms: caspofungin, micafungin 100 mg daily, or micafungin 150 mg daily. Outcomes were the same with all three strategies. In general, it therefore appears that the 100 mg dose of micafungin is adequate. Nonetheless, clinicians must note that among the patients given either dose of micafungin, the number of infections caused by C glabrata and C krusei was quite small.[82]

Anidulafungin is the only echinocandin to be compared directly with fluconazole. Reboli and colleagues[83] randomized 245 subjects to either anidulafungin or fluconazole. As with other studies, most patients suffered from candidemia, and few were neutropenic. Because of the innate resistance of C krusei to fluconazole, patients found to be infected with this pathogen were dropped from the trial. Overall, 40% of infections were caused by non-albicans species, including C glabrata. Clinical success rates were significantly higher at end of therapy in patients treated with anidulafungin. This 15.4% difference in response rates did not arise because of fluconazole resistance, as few isolates displayed this. Anidulafungin, however, did not lead to higher survival rates.[83] This report has been criticized, because one site in the study enrolled a disproportionate number of subjects. Additionally, concern has been expressed about a potential center effect. Statistical tests for an interaction between study site and outcome did not confirm this to be an issue.

SUMMARY

Mold and yeast infections remain diagnostic and therapeutic challenges. The prevalence of both of these types of infections is likely to grow over the next decade. Unfortunately, mortality rates with either process are exceedingly high. Coupled with the economic burden of these illness, physicians must remain vigilant when approaching patients at risk for these fungal diseases. Fortunately, newer diagnostic modalities are being developed and tested. Likely some combination of sero-diagnosis testing along with clinical risk stratification will evolve in the coming years. For both conditions, prompt diagnosis and treatment remain the keys to ensuring favorable outcomes. Newer agents for treatment are now commercially available. The literature on these therapies, as is the research into many aspects of fungal infection, is changing rapidly. Hence clinicians caring for the critically ill must strive to remain abreast of this information.

REFERENCES

1. Groll AH, Shah PM, Mentzel C, et al. Trends in the postmortem epidemiology of invasive fungal infections at a university hospital. J Infect 1996;33:23–32.
2. Paterson DL, Singh N. Invasive aspergillosis in transplant recipients. Medicine (Baltimore) 1999;78:123–38.
3. Samarakoon P, Soubani AO. Invasive pulmonary aspergillosis in patients with COPD: a report of five cases and systematic review of the literature. Chron Respir Dis 2008;5:19–27.
4. Vandewoude K, Blot S, Benoit D, et al. Invasive aspergillosis in critically ill patients: analysis of risk factors fro acquisition and mortality. Acta Clin Belg 2004;59:251–7.
5. Vandewoude KH, Blot SI, Benoit D, et al. Invasive aspergillosis in critically ill patients: attributable mortality and excesses in length of ICU stay and ventilator dependence. J Hosp Infect 2004;56:269–76.
6. Meersseman W, Vandecasteele SJ, Wilmer A, et al. Invasive aspergillosis in critically ill patients without malignancy. Am J Respir Crit Care Med 2004;170:621–5.
7. Vandewoude KH, Blot SI, Depuydt P, et al. Clinical relevance of Aspergillus isolation from respiratory tract samples in critically ill patients. Crit Care 2006;10:31.

8. Buckingham SJ, Hansell DM. Aspergillus in the lung: diverse and coincident forms. Eur Radiol 2003;13:1786–800.

9. Maertens J, Verhaegen J, Lagrou K, et al. Screening for circulating galacto-mannan as a noninvasive diagnostic tool for invasive aspergillosis in prolonged neutropenic patients and stem cell transplantation recipients: a prospective validation. Blood 2001;97:1604–10.

10. Sulahian A, Tabouret M, Ribaud P, et al. Comparison of an enzyme immunoassay and latex agglutination test for detection of galactomannan in the diagnosis of aspergillosis. Eur J Clin Microbiol Infect Dis 1996;15:139–45.

11. Swanink CM, Meis JF, Rijs AJ, et al. Specificity of a sandwich enzyme-linked immunosorbent assay for detecting *Aspergillus galactomannan.* J Clin Microbiol 1997;35:257–60.

12. Pfeiffer CD, Fine JP, Safdar N. Diagnosis of invasive aspergillosis using a galac-tomannan assay: a meta-analysis. Clin Infect Dis 2006;42:1417–27.

13. Herbrecht R, Letscher-Bru V, Oprea C, et al. *Aspergillus galactomannan* detection in the diagnosis of invasive aspergillosis in cancer patients. J Clin Oncol 2002;20:1898–906.

14. Pinel C, Fricker-Hidalgo H, Lebeau B, et al. Detection of circulating *Aspergillus fumigatus* galactomannan: value and limits of the Platelia test for diagnosing invasive aspergillosis. J Clin Microbiol 2003;41:2184–6.

15. Husain S, Paterson DL, Studer SM, et al. *Aspergillus galactomannan* antigen in the bronchoalveolar lavage fluid for the diagnosis of invasive aspergillosis in lung transplant recipients. Transplantation 2007;83:1330–6.

16. Walsh TJ, Anaissie EJ, Denning DW, et al. Treatment of aspergillosis: clinical practice guidelines of the Infectious Diseases Society of America. Clin Infect Dis 2008;46:327–60.

17. Herbrecht R, Denning DW, Patterson TF, et al. Voriconazole versus amphotericin B for primary therapy of invasive aspergillosis. N Engl J Med 2002;347:408–15.

18. Hope WW, Billaud EM, Lestner J, et al. Therapeutic drug monitoring for triazoles. Curr Opin Infect Dis 2008;21:580–6.

19. Bowden R, Chandrasekar P, White MH, et al. A double-blind, randomized, controlled trial of amphotericin B colloidal dispersion versus amphotericin B for treatment of invasive aspergillosis in immunocompromised patients. Clin Infect Dis 2002;35:359–66.

20. Leenders AC, Daenen S, Jansen RLH, et al. Liposomal amphotericin B compared with amphotericin B deoxycholate in the treatment of documented and suspected neutropenia-associated invasive fungal infections. Br J Haematol 1998;103: 205–12.

21. Cornley OA, Maertens J, Bresnik M, et al. Liposomal amphotericin B as initial therapy for invasive mold infection: a randomized trial comparing a high-loading dose regimen with standard dosing (AmBiLoad trial). Clin Infect Dis 2007;44: 1289–97.

22. Maertens J, Raad I, Petrikkos G, et al. Efficacy and safety of caspofungin for treatment of invasive aspergillosis in patients refractory to or intolerant of conventional antifungal therapy. Clin Infect Dis 2004;39:1563–71.

23. Caillot D, Bassaris H, McGeer A, et al. Intravenous itraconazole followed by oral itraconazole I. The treatment of invasive pulmonary aspergillosis in patients with hematologic malignancies, chronic granulomatous disease, or AIDS. Clin Infect Dis 2001;33:e83–90.

24. Patterson TF, Kirkpatrick WR, White M, et al. Invasive aspergillosis: disease spectrum, treatment practices, and outcomes. Medicine 2000;79:250–60.

25. Walsh TJ, Raad I, Patterson TF, et al. Treatment of invasive aspergillosis with posaconazole in patients who are refractory to or intolerant of conventional therapy: an externally controlled trial. Clin Infect Dis 2007;44:2–12.
26. Denning DW, Marr KA, Lau WM, et al. Micafungin (FK463), alone or in combination with other systemic antifungal agents, for the treatment of acute invasive aspergillosis. J Infect 2006;53:337–49.
27. Kontoyiannis DP, Ratanatharathorn V, Young JA, et al. Micafungin alone or in combination with other systemic antifungal therapies in hematopoietic stem cell transplant recipients with invasive aspergillosis. Transpl Infect Dis 2009;11: 89–93.
28. Marr KA, Boeckh M, Carter RA, et al. Combination antifungal therapy for invasive aspergillosis. Clin Infect Dis 2004;39:797–802.
29. Singh N, Limaye AP, Forrest G, et al. Combination of voriconazole and caspofungin as primary therapy for invasive aspergillosis in solid organ transplant recipients: a prospective, multicenter, observational study. Transplantation 2006;15: 320–6.
30. Pfaller MA, Diekema DJ. Epidemiology of invasive candidiasis: a persistent public health problem. Clin Microbiol Rev 2007;20:133–63.
31. Hidron AI, Edwards JR, Patel J, et al. Antimicrobial-resistant pathogens associated with healthcare-associated infections: annual summary of data reported to the National Healthcare Safety Network at the Centers for Disease Control and Prevention, 2006–2007. Infect Control Hosp Epidemiol 2008;29:996–1011.
32. Banerjee SN, Emori TG, Culver DH. Secular trends in nosocomial primary bloodstream infections in the United States, 1980–1989. National Nosocomial Infections Surveillance System. Am J Med 1991;91:86S–9S.
33. Fridkin SK, Kaufman D, Edwards JR, et al. Changing incidence of *Candida* bloodstream infections among NICU patients in the United States: 1995–2004. Pediatrics 2006;117:1680–7.
34. San Miguel LG, Cobo J, Otheo E, et al. Secular trends of candidemia in a large tertiary-care hospital from 1988 to 2000: emergence of *Candida parapsilosis*. Infect Control Hosp Epidemiol 2005;26:548–52.
35. Trick WE, Fridkin SK, Edwards JR, et al. Secular trend of hospital-acquired candidemia among intensive care unit patients in the United States during 1989–1999. Clin Infect Dis 2002;35:627–30.
36. Martin GS, Mannino DM, Eaton S, et al. The epidemiology of sepsis in the United States from 1979 through 2000. N Engl J Med 2003;348:1546–54.
37. Shorr AF, Shorr AF, Tabak YP, et al. Burden of early-onset candidemia: analysis of culture-positive bloodstream infections from a large US database. Crit Care Med, in press.
38. Zilberberg MD, Shorr AF, Kollef MH. Secular trends in candidemia-related hospitalizations in the US, 2000–2005. Infect Control Hosp Epidemiol 2008;29:978–80.
39. Sandven P, Bevanger L, Digranes A, et al. Candidemia in Norway (1991 to 2003): results from a nationwide study. J Clin Microbiol 2006;44:1977–81.
40. Poikonen E, Lyytikamen O, Anttila VJ, et al. Canididemia in Finland, 1995–1999. Emerg Infect Dis 2003;9:985–90.
41. Smith PB, Morgan J, Benjamin JD, et al. Excess costs of hospital care associated with neonatal candidemia. Pediatr Infect Dis J 2007;26:197–200.
42. Zaoutis TE, Argon J, Chu J, et al. The epidemiology and attributable outcomes of candidemia in adults and children hospitalized in the United States: a propensity analysis. Clin Infect Dis 2005;41:1232–9.

43. Snydman DR. Shifting patterns in the epidemiology of nosocomial *Candida* infections. Chest 2003;123:500–3.
44. Nguyen MH, Peacock JE Jr, Morris AJ, et al. The changing face of candidemia: emergence of non-*Candida albicans* species and antifungal resistance. Am J Med 1996;100:617–23.
45. Bassetti M, Righi E, Costa A, et al. Epidemiological trends in nosocomial candidemia in intensive care. BMC Infect Dis 2006;6:21.
46. Shorr AF, Lazarus DR, Sherner JH, et al. Do clinical features allow for accurate prediction of fungal pathogenesis in bloodstream infections? Potential implications of the increasing prevalence of non-*albicans* candidemia. Crit Care Med 2007;35:1077–83.
47. Pfaller MA, Diekema DJ, Gibbs DL, et al. Results from the ARTEMIS DISK Global Antifungal Surveillance study, 1997 to 2005: an 8.5-year analysis of susceptibilities of *Candida* species and other yeast species to fluconazole and voriconazole determined by CLSI standardized disk diffusion testing. J Clin Microbiol 2007;45: 1735–45.
48. Wey SB, Mori M, Pfaller MA, et al. Risk factors for hospital-acquired candidemia. A matched case–control study. Arch Intern Med 1989;149:2349–53.
49. Pittet D, Monod M, Suter PM, et al. *Candida* colonization and subsequent infections in critically ill surgical patients. Ann Surg 1994;220:751–8.
50. Fraser VJ, Jones M, Dunkel J, et al. Candidemia in a tertiary care hospital: epidemiology, risk factors, and predictors of mortality. Clin Infect Dis 1992;15:414–21.
51. Blumberg HM, Jarvis WR, Soucie JM, et al. Risk factors for candidal bloodstream infections in surgical intensive care unit patients: the NEMIS prospective multicenter study. The National Epidemiology of Mycosis Survey. Clin Infect Dis 2001;33:177–86.
52. Chow JK, Golan Y, Ruthazer R, et al. Risk factors for *albicans* and non-*albicans* candidemia in the intensive care unit. Crit Care Med 2008;36:1993–8.
53. Leon C, Ruiz-Santana S, Saavedra P, et al. A bedside scoring system (*Candida* score) for early antifungal treatment in non-neutropenic critically ill patients with *Candida* colonization. Crit Care Med 2006;34:730–7.
54. Ostrosky-Zeichner L, Sable C, Sobel J, et al. Multicenter retrospective development and validation of a clinical prediction rule for nosocomial invasive candidiasis in the intensive care setting. Eur J Clin Microbiol Infect Dis 2007;26:271–6.
55. Faiz S, Neale B, Rios E, et al. Risk-based fluconazole prophylaxis of *Candida* bloodstream infection in a medical intensive care unit. Eur J Clin Microbiol Infect Dis 2008; in press.
56. Reiss E, Morrison CJ. Nonculture methods for diagnosis of disseminated candidiasis. Clin Microbiol Rev 1993;6:311–23.
57. Mean M, Marchetti O, Calandra T. Bench-to-bedside review: *Candida* infections in the intensive care unit. Crit Care 2008;12:204.
58. Garbino J, Lew DP, Romand JA, et al. Prevention of severe *Candida* infections in non-neutropenic, high-risk, critically ill patients: a randomized, double-blind, placebo-controlled trial in patients treated by selective digestive decontamination. Intensive Care Med 2002;28:1708–17.
59. Eggimann P, Francioli P, Bille J, et al. Fluconazole prophylaxis prevents intraabdominal candidiasis in high-risk surgical patients. Crit Care Med 1999;27: 1066–72.
60. Shorr AF, Chung K, Jackson WL, et al. Fluconazole prophylaxis in critically ill surgical patients: a meta-analysis. Crit Care Med 2005;33:1928–35.

61. Nolla-Salas J, Sitges-Serra A, Leon-Gil C, et al. Candidemia in non-neutropenic critically ill patients: analysis of prognostic factors and assessment of systemic antifungal therapy. Study Group of Fungal Infection in the ICU. Intensive Care Med 1997;23:23–30.

62. Morrell M, Fraser VJ, Kollef MH. Delaying the empiric treatment of Candida bloodstream infection until positive blood culture results are obtained: a potential risk factor for hospital mortality. Antimicrobial Agents Chemother 2005;49:3640–5.

63. Garey KW, Rege M, Pai MP, et al. Time to initiation of fluconazole therapy impacts mortality in patients with candidemia: a multi-institutional study. Clin Infect Dis 2006;43:25–31.

64. Labelle AJ, Micek ST, Roubinian N, et al. Treatment-related risk factors for hospital mortality in Candida bloodstream infections. Crit Care Med 2008;36:2967–72.

65. Shuster MG, Edwards JE, Sobel JD, et al. Empirical fluconazole versus placebo for intensive care unit patients: a randomized trial. Ann Intern Med 2008;149: 83–90.

66. Pappas PG, Rex JH, Sobel JD, et al. Guidelines for treatment of candidiasis. Clin Infect Dis 2004;38:161–89.

67. Nucci M, Colombo AL, Silveira F, et al. Risk factors for death in patients with candidemia. Infect Control Hosp Epidemiol 1998;19:846–50.

68. Pasqualotto AC, de Moraes AB, Zanini RR, et al. Analysis of independent risk factors for death among pediatric patients with candidemia and a central venous catheter in place. Infect Control Hosp Epidemiol 2007;28:799–804.

69. Walsh TJ, Rex JH. All catheter-related candidemia is not the same: assessment of the balance between the risks and benefits of removal of vascular catheters. Clin Infect Dis 2002;34:600–2.

70. Rodriguez D, Park BJ, Almirante B, et al. Impact of early central venous catheter removal on outcome in patients with candidaemia. Clin Microbiol Infect 2007;13: 788–93.

71. Pasqualotto AC, Severo LC. The importance of central venous catheter removal in patients with candidaemia: time to rethink our practice? Clin Microbiol Infect 2008;14:2–4.

72. Raad I, Hanna H, Boktour M, et al. Management of central venous catheters in patients with cancer and candidemia. Clin Infect Dis 2004;38:1119–27.

73. Walsh TJ, Finberg RW, Arndt C, et al. Liposomal amphotericin B for empirical therapy in patients with persistent fever and neutropenia. National Institute of Allergy and Infectious Diseases Mycoses Study Group. N Engl J Med 1999; 340:764–71.

74. Rex JH, Bennett JE, Sugar AM, et al. A randomized trial comparing fluconazole with amphotericin B for the treatment of candidemia in patients without neutropenia. Candidemia Study Group and the National Institute. N Engl J Med 1994;331: 1325–30.

75. Phillips P, Shafran S, Garber G, et al. Multicenter randomized trial of fluconazole versus amphotericin B for treatment of candidemia in non-neutropenic patients. Canadian Candidemia Study Group. Eur J Clin Microbiol Infect Dis 1997;16: 337–45.

76. Kullberg BJ, Sobel JD, Ruhnke M, et al. Voriconazole versus a regimen of amphotericin B followed by fluconazole for candidaemia in non-neutropenic patients: a randomised noninferiority trial. Lancet 2005;366:1435–42.

77. Caspofungin prescribing information. Available at: http://www.merck.com/ product/usa/pi_circulars/c/cancidas/cancidas_pi.pdf. Accessed January 18, 2009.

78. Anidulafungin prescribing information. Available at: http://media.pfizer.com/files/products/uspi_eraxis.pdf. Accessed January 18, 2009.
79. Micafungin prescribing information. Available at: http://www.astellas.us/docs/mycamine-ic.xml. Accessed January 18, 2009.
80. Mora-Duarte J, Betts R, Rotstein C, et al. Comparison of caspofungin and amphotericin B for invasive candidiasis. N Engl J Med 2002;347:2020–9.
81. Kuse ER, Chetchotosakd P, da Cunha CA, et al. Micafungin versus liposomal amphotericin B for candidaemia and invasive candidosis: a phase III randomised double-blind trial. Lancet 2007;369:1519–27.
82. Pappas PG, Rotstein CM, Betts RF, et al. Micafungin versus caspofungin for treatment of candidemia and other forms of invasive candidiasis. Clin Infect Dis 2007; 45:883–93.
83. Reboli AC, Rotstein C, Pappas PG, et al. Anidulafungin versus fluconazole for invasive candidiasis. N Engl J Med 2007;356:2472–82.

Acute Infective Endocarditis

Jay R. McDonald, MD[a,b,]*

KEYWORDS

- Endocarditis • Critical care • Antimicrobial agents
- Thoracic surgery • Heart valves

Despite advances in medical and surgical therapy, infective endocarditis (IE) remains a highly morbid and deadly infection. Endocarditis is an inflammation of the endocardium, the inner lining of the heart and heart valves. While such inflammation can be caused by a variety of disease states, infectious agents cause most cases of endocarditis.

In his Gulstonian lectures of 1885, Sir William Osler drew a distinction between "simple" and "malignant" forms of endocarditis.[1] The "simple" form described by Osler correlates to what has become known as subacute bacterial endocarditis. Subacute IE typically presents with subtle constitutional symptoms and is frequently not diagnosed until it has been present for months. The "malignant" form described by Osler, characterized by an acute onset and fulminant course, correlates to what is now known as acute IE. The focus of this review is acute IE, though many studies of diagnosis and treatment do not differentiate between acute and subacute disease, and indeed many principles of diagnosis and management of IE for acute and subacute disease are identical.

PATHOGENESIS

Vegetation formation is a multistep process. The first step is endocardial injury, which may occur by many mechanisms. The most common mechanism is injury by turbulent blood flow from an acquired or congenital intracardiac abnormality. The most common site of such injury, and thus the most common site of vegetation formation, is on the line of closure of a valve surface, typically on the atrial surface of atrioventricular valves or on the ventricular surface of semilunar valves.[2] Alternatively, an

This work was supported by grant number K12RR023249 and KL2RR024994 from the National Institutes of Health.
[a] Infectious Disease Section, Specialty Care Service, St. Louis VA Medical Center, 915 N Grand Boulevard, Mailcode 151/JC, St. Louis, MO 63106, USA
[b] Division of Infectious Diseases, Department of Internal Medicine, Washington University School of Medicine, 660 N Euclid Avenue, St. Louis, MO 63110, USA
* St. Louis VA Medical Center, 915 N Grand Boulevard, Mailcode 151/JC, St. Louis, MO 63106.
E-mail address: jay.mcdonald1@va.gov

intravascular catheter or other device may directly abrade the endocardium. In injection drug users, direct injection of contaminating debris may damage the tricuspid valve surface.

The endothelial damage triggers sterile thrombus formation, which occurs by deposition of fibrin and platelets. Though mechanical endocardial damage usually precedes sterile thrombus formation, a sterile thrombus can be induced without direct trauma.[3] Physiologic stresses, such as hypersensitivity states, hormonal changes, and high altitude, can also induce sterile endocardial thrombosis.[3] Clinical states associated with sterile thrombus formation in humans include malignancy, rheumatic diseases, and uremia.

Once a sterile thrombus is present, transient bacteremia can seed the thrombus. Bacteria are introduced into the bloodstream when a body surface heavily colonized by bacteria (oral cavity, gut lumen, genitourinary mucosa) is traumatized. Routine daily activities, such as chewing food and brushing teeth, lead to frequent low-level, transient bacteremias in healthy adults.[4] Blood-borne bacteria may adhere to the damaged endocardial surface. Bacteria have different adhesive capacities based on bacterial surface characteristics and virulence factors, called *adhesins*. For example, the adhesive properties of viridans streptococci are related to the amount of dextran present in the streptococcal cell wall, as well as specific surface proteins, such as FimA.[5,6]

Once bacteria have attached to the endocardium, the vegetation "matures" through additional deposition of fibrin and bacterial proliferation. Histologically, the vegetation consists primarily of fibrin, platelets, and bacteria; the absence of vasculature makes penetration by phagocytic cells rare. The majority of bacteria in mature vegetation are found below the surface of the vegetation, protected from phagocytes and high concentrations of antibiotics.

EPIDEMIOLOGY
Demographics and Risk Factors

The incidence of IE is between 2 and 10 episodes per 100,000 person-years in most population-based studies,[7–9] and as high as 20 episodes per 100,000 person-years in the elderly.[10] There are approximately 15,000 new cases of IE diagnosed each year in the United States, and it accounts for about 1 in 1000 admissions to the hospital.[11]

Most studies demonstrate that the rate of IE has been stable over time,[12,13] though changes in diagnostic tools and criteria make temporal comparisons difficult. Despite a relatively stable rate, the nature of IE has changed dramatically over the past several decades. IE is more commonly associated with invasive medical procedures and old age, and less associated with rheumatic heart disease and poor dentition.[14,15] These epidemiologic trends support the observation that acute IE is increasing in frequency relative to subacute and chronic IE: In the pre-antibiotic era, approximately 20% of IE was acute, while more recent studies show that about 33% of IE is acute.[12,16]

IE is more common in men than women,[11] and is more common with increasing age.[10] The mean age of IE patients has increased over time, from under 30 years in the pre-antibiotic era[17] to nearly 60 years in the 1990s.[18] In the elderly, IE is more often associated with intracardiac prosthetic devices and bacteria from the gastrointestinal tract.[19] In a large observational cohort study, IE most commonly involved the mitral valve only (approximately 40% of patients), followed by the aortic valve only (36% of patients), followed by multivalvular disease.[18,20] Right-sided valves are rarely affected except among injection drug users. The pulmonic valve is least likely to be involved in IE.

Structural heart disease is a risk factor for IE because it results in turbulent blood flow. About 75% of patients who develop IE have underlying structural heart disease.[13] In the past, rheumatic heart disease with mitral stenosis was the most common valvular defect in patients with IE. Recently, the most common predisposing lesions have been mitral regurgitation, aortic valve disease (stenosis and regurgitation), and congenital heart disease.[21,22] Mitral valve prolapse is a risk factor for IE, primarily when regurgitation is present.[23]

The presence of a prosthetic cardiac valve is a strong risk factor for IE. The risk is highest in the first year after valve implantation. Mechanical valves are associated with higher risk than bioprosthetic valves in the first years after surgery, but that relationship reverses in later years after surgery.[2] Implanted valve rings are associated with lower risk of IE than prosthetic valves.[24]

In addition to structural heart disease and prosthetic valves, established risk factors for IE include prior episodes of IE, invasive medical procedures, and injection drug use. Some studies have demonstrated that diabetes mellitus and kidney disease may be risk factors as well.[25]

Nosocomial IE is increasing in frequency and importance. Between 14% and 31% of all IE is nosocomial in recent case series.[26–28] In a longitudinal single-center study in Spain, the proportion of IE acquired in the hospital increased almost 10-fold in a 15-year period. Compared with community-acquired IE, nosocomial IE was associated with threefold higher mortality, and was most commonly caused by *Staphylococcus aureus*, coagulase-negative staphylococci, and enterococci.[27]

Infective Endocarditis in Critical Care

Because IE often occurs in patients with multiple comorbid illnesses and those who have undergone recent invasive procedures, it is commonly diagnosed and treated in the intensive care unit (ICU).

From 1993 to 2000, IE was diagnosed in 3% of ICU patients in two medical ICUs in France.[29] Among 228 cases of IE in this study, 64% of cases were native valve endocarditis (NVE), of which 21% were nosocomial. *S aureus* was the causative agent in half of all IE cases. Complications were frequent: Neurologic events complicated 40% of cases, congestive heart failure (CHF) 29%, and septic shock 26%. In-hospital mortality was 45%. Septic shock, neurologic complications, and immunocompromise predicted in-hospital mortality.[29]

In another study, which took place between 1994 and 1999, IE was identified in 0.8% of all ICU patients in four medical ICUs in Vienna, Austria.[30] Just over half of the 33 patients came to the ICU with the diagnosis of IE, while 45% were first diagnosed in the ICU. The majority (79%) had NVE, and *S aureus* was the most common pathogen, causing 36% of IE. Severity of illness was high, with 79% of patients receiving mechanical ventilation, 73% receiving vasopressors, and 54% dying during their hospital stay. Acute renal failure occurred in 39% of patients, and was the only independent predictor of mortality.[30]

Nosocomial IE in the ICU can usually be attributed to a hospital-acquired infection at another primary site. Of 31 nosocomial cases of IE described by Mourvillier and colleagues,[29] 21 were related to intravenous catheter infection and three to surgical site infection. In another study, among 22 nosocomial IE cases in an ICU, 11 were related to an intravascular device and eight to a surgical site infection. Fifteen of these 22 patients had no predisposing cardiac lesion. *S aureus* was the causative pathogen in 68% of patients, and 68% of the patients died.[31]

Wolff and colleagues[32] described 122 cases of prosthetic valve endocarditis (PVE) in a French ICU from 1978 to 1992. *S aureus* accounted for 61% of disease occurring in the first 2 months after valve implantation, and streptococci and *S aureus* were the most common causes of late disease. Heart failure was seen in half of cases, and mortality was 34% at 4 months. Predictors of mortality among *S aureus* cases were septic shock, heart failure, mediastinitis, and elevated prothrombin time.[32]

APPROACH TO THE PATIENT
Diagnosis

Diagnostic criteria
The Duke criteria incorporate information from echocardiography, history and physical examination, microbiology, and pathology to diagnose IE (**Box 1**). They were originally proposed in 1994,[33] and were subsequently shown to be superior to previous diagnostic criteria.[34,35] The criteria were modified in 2000 to revise the definition of "possible IE," add criteria for microbiologic diagnosis of Q fever IE, eliminate echocardiographic minor criteria, and include recommendations for choosing between transthoracic echocardiography (TTE) and transesophageal echocardiography (TEE).[36]

History and physical examination
The clinical presentation of subacute IE is variable, but the presentation of acute IE is more straightforward. Unlike patients with subacute IE who typically report longstanding constitutional symptoms, patients with acute IE typically describe the abrupt onset of fever and rigors, and may present with symptoms of embolism. The history should include specific inquiry about known risk factors for IE, including invasive procedures, injection drug use, structural heart disease, and prior endocarditis. Symptoms referable to other organ systems may indicate a primary source of bacteremia. Complications of IE may be apparent from the history, including heart failure, conduction disturbances, or embolism.

The physical examination must be comprehensive, with special attention to examination of the heart, dentition, all sites of invasive devices and recent procedures, and potential destinations of embolism. Heart murmur is present in 85% of patients with IE, but a changing murmur is only apparent in 5% to 10% of cases. About half of patients with IE have evidence of embolic phenomena on physical examination.[2,11] When clinical suspicion is present, a lack of clinical findings does not rule out the diagnosis of IE.

Laboratory tests
At least three blood cultures should be drawn when IE is suspected, with the first and last drawn at least 1 hour apart. If fastidious organisms are suspected, the microbiology laboratory should be informed that IE is on the differential diagnosis. Electrocardiogram, chest radiograph, urinalysis, and rheumatoid factor may assist in making the diagnosis or identifying complications of IE.

Echocardiography
Diagnosis of IE is made in part by echocardiographic findings. The presence of an oscillating intracardiac mass, either on a valve, in the path of a regurgitant jet, or on implanted material, is the classic finding, though abscess or new partial dehiscence of a prosthetic valve also meets diagnostic criteria.[36] Other findings associated with IE include aneurysm, fistula, and leaflet perforation.[37]

The use of echocardiography to rule out IE should be based on the clinician's pretest probability of disease. Pretest probability, in turn, is based on the presence of clinical and microbiologic features unique to each patient, including the likelihood of alternative diagnoses. Studies have proposed algorithms for use of echocardiography to diagnose IE.[38,39] While these studies cannot substitute for the judgment of an experienced clinician, they highlight some of the features that affect pretest

---

Box 1
Modified Duke criteria for diagnosis of infective endocarditis[a]

Major criteria

Microbiologic evidence of IE

Typical organisms cultured from two separate blood cultures:

Viridans streptococci, *S aureus*, HACEK (*Haemophilus, Actinobacillus, Cardiobacterium, Eikenella,* or *Kingella*) organism, or *Streptococcus bovis*; or community-acquired enterococcus in the absence of an alternative primary site of infection

Persistently positive blood cultures with other organism

At least two positives drawn more than 12 hours apart; or all of three or majority of four, with first and last drawn more than 1 hour apart

One culture (or phase 1 IgG > 1:800) for *Coxiella burnetii*

Evidence of endocardial involvement

Echocardiogram showing oscillating intracardiac mass without alternative explanation, or abscess, or new partial dehiscence of prosthetic valve, or new valvular regurgitation

Minor criteria

Predisposition to infective endocarditis

Previous IE, injection drug use, prosthetic heart valve, or cardiac lesion causing turbulent blood flow

Fever over 38° C

Vascular phenomenon

Arterial embolism, pulmonary infarct, mycotic aneurysm, intracranial or conjunctival hemorrhage, or Janeway lesions

Immunologic phenomenon

Glomerulonephritis, Osler nodes, Roth spots, or positive rheumatoid factor

Microbiologic finding not meeting major criteria

[a] Definite endocarditis requires two major criteria, or one major and three minor criteria, or five minor criteria. Possible endocarditis requires one major and one minor criterion, or three minor criteria.

Data from Li JS, Sexton DJ, Mick N, et al. Proposed modifications to the Duke criteria for the diagnosis of infective endocarditis. Clin Infect Dis 2000;30:633–8.

---

probability of IE: presence of bacteremia, type of organism, presence of known IE risk factors, and clinical examination.

TTE and TEE both have a role in the diagnosis and evaluation of IE. TTE has low sensitivity compared with TEE (46% versus 93%), though both are highly specific (95% versus 96%).[2] TTE is a reasonable first test in patients with low pretest probability of IE despite its sensitivity of less than 50%.[40] In some patients who undergo TTE and are found to have IE, subsequent TEE may be advisable to evaluate perivalvular extension of disease, vegetation size, and other factors that may inform surgical decision-making. In patients with higher pretest probability for disease, or in whom TTE is rendered less sensitive by obesity, lung hyperinflation, or valve prosthesis, TEE is the initial echocardiographic modality of choice in IE.[40] Several studies have demonstrated that TTE alone will miss a significant number of cases of IE in patients with medium to high pretest probability of disease, including those meeting Duke criteria for "possible" IE, and patients with S aureus bacteremia.[41,42]

Alternative imaging modalities

Cardiac CT and MRI have been reported to diagnose complications of IE, including aortic root abscesses and arteriovenous fistulae.[37] Current limitations to these modalities include difficulties in evaluating valve motion, spatial resolution, and time required to acquire images.[37] A recent study of cardiac multislice CT showed that its test characteristics were similar to those for TEE for the diagnosis of IE in 37 patients, 29 of whom underwent cardiac surgery, though all four leaflet perforations were missed with CT.[43] While CT and MRI may be useful as an adjunct to echocardiography in selected cases at centers with expertise in these techniques, they are not part of the current standard of care in the routine diagnosis of IE. The technology involved in cardiac CT and MRI is evolving rapidly, and at some point in the future cardiac CT and MRI may be useful in IE diagnosis.

Antibiotic Therapy: General Principles

All patients with IE should receive antibiotic therapy, and more than half of cases are managed with antibiotic therapy alone.[40] Some organism-specific recommendations for treatment are discussed below in the section on specific organisms. A recent scientific statement by the American Heart Association provides an excellent summary of evidence and antibiotic recommendations, and should be consulted for IE cases that are beyond the scope of this review.[40]

Though treatment must be individualized, some general principles of antibiotic therapy apply to all patients. Because the vegetation structure sequesters bacteria from the bloodstream, long durations of therapy are necessary. Parenteral antibiotics are preferred over oral regimens because of the need for sustained and reliable blood levels of antibiotic. Blood cultures should be drawn every 24 to 48 hours after initiation of antibiotics, until they are negative. Duration of treatment should be counted from the time of the first negative blood cultures. If vancomycin or an aminoglycoside is used, drug levels should be monitored to ensure adequate dosing and to prevent toxicity.[11,40]

Aminoglycosides are often used in combination with a cell wall–active agent (β-lactam or vancomycin) for synergy in the treatment of IE caused by staphylococci, streptococci, and enterococci. Cell wall–active agents increase aminoglycoside entry into bacteria, and therefore synergy requires dosing in close temporal proximity to one another. The use of combination therapy is supported by in vitro and animal studies, but clinical data in humans are scarce.[44] A recent meta-analysis of clinical trials of combination therapy included 261 patients with IE due to S aureus or viridans streptococci in five separate studies. There was no benefit of combination therapy in terms of mortality or treatment success.[45] However, in a single study, combination therapy for S aureus IE did reduce the duration of bacteremia, though it did not improve clinical outcomes.[46] Because of the small size of these studies, it is possible that a meaningful clinical benefit does exist, but studies have not been adequately powered to detect it.

Surgical Therapy

Decisions regarding surgical therapy for patients with IE are multifactorial and complex, and the need for surgery should be individualized to each patient. For these reasons, early input from an experienced cardiothoracic surgeon can be invaluable in managing a patient with IE. Among all patients with IE, 40% to 45% eventually undergo surgery, and rates of surgery are similar for NVE and PVE. Predictors of surgery include younger age, CHF, abscess, and coagulase-negative staphylococcal IE.[47,48] The majority of surgery for IE is performed for hemodynamic indications, such as CHF.[49]

Because there have been no randomized controlled trials of surgical plus medical therapy versus medical therapy alone in the treatment of IE, current guidelines for surgical treatment of IE are based primarily on observational data, which are prone to biases, such as confounding by indication and survival treatment selection bias.[50] Because of these biases, careful adjustment for factors associated with risk of death and likelihood of receiving surgery is necessary.

Several recent studies have attempted to account for these factors, and results have been conflicting regarding the benefit of surgery. In a study reporting a 10-year experience at seven United States hospitals, 230 of 513 adults with NVE underwent cardiac surgery. After propensity analyses to account for differences in treatment assignment and prognostic factors, surgery was associated with reduced mortality (15% versus 28%, $P = .01$), especially in patients with moderate to severe heart failure (14% versus 51%, $P = .001$).[51] In contrast, a study that matched 27 surgical and 27 nonsurgical ICU patients with IE by propensity score found no benefit of surgery (odds ratio 0.96).[29] A study of NVE from the International Collaboration on Endocarditis Merged Database, which included patients from seven centers in five countries, showed a survival benefit from surgery only in patients in the highest quintile of surgical likelihood (11.2% in the surgery group versus 38.0% in the no-surgery group, $P<.001$).[52] A study of PVE from the same study group found a statistically nonsignificant benefit of surgery (22.1% in the surgery group versus 32.4% in the no-surgery group, $P = .18$) in patients with PVE matched on propensity score.[48] Finally, in an analysis of an 18-year experience with left-sided IE at a single center in the United States, after matching by propensity score, decade of diagnosis, and follow-up time, surgery was not significantly associated with mortality (adjusted hazard ratio (HR) 1.3, 95% CI 0.5–3.1).[53] Thus, the benefit of surgery is unclear, and is likely restricted to specific subgroups of patients.

There are several subgroups of patients in which early surgery should be strongly considered. Patients with CHF or severe valvular dysfunction likely to precipitate acute CHF should be considered for surgery, particularly when the aortic valve is involved.[51,54–57] Patients with intracardiac abscess should be strongly considered for surgery, in light of decreased penetration of antibiotics to the site of infection,[58] and the possibility of the abscess causing heart block acute valvular dysfunction.[54,57,58] Patients with IE caused by organisms known to be refractory to medical management, including *Pseudomonas*, *Candida*, and multidrug-resistant organisms, may benefit from surgical management, as well as those at highest risk for embolism.[40,54,55]

Patients with PVE should be carefully considered for surgery,[47,48,55] though low-risk patients with PVE may be adequately managed with medical therapy alone.[59,60] Characteristics that suggest lower risk include absence of heart failure, abscess, or valve dehiscence, and those whose IE is caused by less virulent organisms, such as viridans streptococci.[59]

Right-Sided Infective Endocarditis

Right-sided IE, which accounts for about 10% of cases of IE, occurs most commonly in injection drug users, and has different clinical characteristics and outcomes compared with left-sided IE.[61,62] Patients with right-sided IE are typically younger and have fewer comorbid medical conditions and less underlying valve disease than patients with left-sided IE.[14,61] *S aureus* is responsible for about 70% of right-sided IE.[61–63] Patients with right-sided IE often present with signs and symptoms of septic pulmonary emboli, including pleuritic chest pain, dyspnea, and hemoptysis. More than half present with chest radiograph consistent with septic pulmonary emboli.[64] The mortality rate among patients with right-sided IE is typically less than 10%.[14,61,62]

In a study of 1529 episodes of IE in injection drug users in Spain, 79% had right-sided IE, 16% had left-sided IE, and 5% had both.[61] Only 1% of the right-sided IE was of the pulmonic valve. It has not been definitively established why the tricuspid valve is so frequently involved in IE in injection drug users. While it may be related to valve damage caused by bombardment of the tricuspid valve by impurities in injected material, this damage has not always been apparent in autopsy studies of injection drug users. Other theories include drug-induced microthrombi on the valve, drug-induced pulmonary hypertension, and increased right-sided expression of molecules that bind bacteria.[61,63]

Carefully selected cases of tricuspid valve IE may be managed with short courses of parenteral antibiotics, or with oral regimens.[40,61,62,65,66] Patients with factors associated with poor prognosis, including concurrent left-sided IE, metastatic infection, heart failure, large vegetation, or immune compromise should not be considered for shorter course therapy or oral regimens.[40]

Prosthetic Valve Endocarditis

The risk of PVE is 1% to 5% in the first year after implantation, and decreases to about 1% per year thereafter.[67,68] The risk of PVE is similar overall among mechanical and bioprosthetic valves, though early IE risk may be higher and late IE risk lower among mechanical valves compared with bioprosthetic valves.[68–70] PVE risk is comparable among valves in the aortic and mitral positions.[68–70] PVE occurring in the first 12 months after surgery is most often caused by coagulase-negative staphylococci or S aureus,[69] while late-onset PVE has similar microbiology to NVE.[70,71] Mortality in PVE is predicted by heart failure, S aureus, and the presence of intracardiac abscess or fistula.[32,60,72,73]

Surgical therapy for PVE is frequently indicated, as discussed above, and is performed in about half of all cases of PVE.[73] Recommendations for medical therapy in the treatment of PVE are generally similar to those for treatment of NVE, though they differ substantially for staphylococcal PVE. For PVE caused by oxacillin-susceptible strains of staphylococci, duration of nafcillin or oxacillin should be at least 6 weeks, rifampin should be added for the same duration, and low-dose gentamicin should be given for 2 weeks.[40]

Cardiovascular Device–Related Infective Endocarditis

Use of intracardiac pacemakers and implantable cardioverter-defibrillators (ICDs) has been steadily increasing, but infection of these devices has been increasing even more rapidly.[74] Most infections of pacemakers and ICDs occur only at the pocket, but 10% of pacemaker-associated infections include IE.[75] Pacemaker/ICD IE is best diagnosed with TEE, as TTE has sensitivity of less than 30% for lead vegetations.[76,77] However, it may be impossible to definitively distinguish a sterile thrombus from an infected thrombus on a lead.[2] An intracardiac oscillating mass on a pacemaker/ICD lead qualifies as a major criterion in the Duke criteria for IE diagnosis.[36]

There have been no randomized studies of device removal plus antibiotics versus antibiotics alone in the treatment of pacemaker/ICD IE, but optimal management includes removal of the device, at a minimum until bacteremia clears, but longer if possible. One retrospective study of any pacemaker/ICD infection showed a relapse rate of less than 1% among 117 patients who underwent device removal, and 50%

among 6 patients in whom the device was retained.[77] If a pacemaker/ICD must be replaced before completion of therapy, it may be advisable to treat as PVE.

SPECIFIC ORGANISMS

For IE caused by organisms not addressed below or in **Tables 1** and **2**, the American Heart Association's Scientific Statement on Infective Endocarditis should be consulted for treatment recommendations.[40]

Staphylococcus aureus

S aureus is the leading cause of acute IE. The incidence of S aureus IE has been steadily increasing in recent decades, becoming the predominant organism in IE in most reports.[40,78,79] Increasing use of intravenous catheters and implanted prosthetic devices has led to higher rates of health care–associated staphylococcal bacteremia, placing more patients at risk for IE.[79]

S aureus IE tends to involve the mitral valve more often than the aortic, and is the most common cause of IE among injection drug users.[18] IE caused by community-associated strains of methicillin-resistant S aureus, compared with strains of hospital-acquired methicillin-resistant S aureus, occurs in a younger population with a higher prevalence of injection drug use.[80] S aureus IE is associated with higher rates of embolism and mortality compared with IE caused by other organisms.[18,81,82] In a large cohort study of S aureus IE, embolism occurred in 60% of cases of S aureus IE versus 31% of cases caused by other organisms.[18]

NVE caused by methicillin-susceptible strains of S aureus should be treated with 6 weeks of intravenous nafcillin or oxacillin (see **Table 1**). Gentamicin can be added for 3 to 5 days at 1 mg/kg every 8 hours, though its use is considered optional based on existing studies and potential toxicities.[44–46] Methicillin-resistant S aureus IE should be treated with vancomycin alone for 6 weeks, with goal vancomycin troughs of 10 to 15 µg/dL.[40] Antibiotic therapy for PVE caused by S aureus is shown in **Table 2**.

Coagulase-Negative Staphylococci

While coagulase-negative staphylococci cause about 6% of NVE, they cause very little acute IE.[83] Coagulase-negative staphylococcal IE is more indolent than IE caused by other organisms. One significant exception is the species Staphylococcus lugdunensis, a coagulase-negative staphylococcus that behaves clinically like S aureus, and has been described to cause acute IE with an aggressive clinical course.[84] In the first year after prosthetic valve implantation, coagulase-negative staphylococci are the second most common cause of PVE, after S aureus.[71] IE caused by coagulase-negative staphylococci should be treated with antibiotic regimens similar to those used to treat S aureus (see **Tables 1** and **2**).

Streptococci

Streptococcal IE comprises about 30% of all IE, though it is less prevalent among acute IE.[18] Most streptococcal IE is caused by viridans streptococci, which are oral flora and include S mitis, S mutans, S salivarius, S sanguis, and the S intermedius group (S intermedius, S anginosus, and S constellatus).[11]

Streptococcus bovis, a group D streptococcal species, is the most common nonviridans streptococcal species to cause IE.[85] S bovis bacteremia is strongly associated with colon polyps and cancer.[86] S bovis accounts for 5% to 15% of cases of IE in the United States.[85] Other streptococci account for less than 5% of cases of definite IE.[18] Treatment of IE caused by viridans streptococci or by S bovis depends on the degree

Table 1
Selected NVE treatment regimens

Organism	Drug	Duration	Notes
Oxacillin-sensitive *Staphylococcus*	Oxacillin/nafcillin 2 g IV q 4 h **WITH OR WITHOUT**	6 wk	For nonanaphylactoid penicillin allergy, substitute cefazolin 2 g IV q 8 h for oxacillin/nafcillin; for anaphylactoid penicillin allergy, substitute vancomycin 15 mg/kg IV q 12 h[b] for oxacillin/nafcillin, and do not use gentamicin
	Gentamicin 1 mg/kg IV/IM q 8 h[a]	3–5 d	
Oxacillin-resistant *Staphylococcus*	Vancomycin 15 mg/kg IV q 12 h[b]	6 wk	—
Viridans streptococci/*S bovis* with penicillin MIC ≤ 0.12 μg/mL	Penicillin G 12–18 million U IV per 24 h[c] **OR**	4 wk	For penicillin/ceftriaxone allergy, vancomycin 15 mg/kg IV q 12 h[b]
	Ceftriaxone 2 g IV/IM q24 h	4 weeks	
Viridans streptococci/*S bovis* with penicillin MIC > 0.12 to ≤ 0.5 μg/mL	Penicillin G 24 million U IV per 24 h[c] **PLUS**	4 wk	For penicillin/ceftriaxone allergy, vancomycin 15 mg/kg IV q 12 h[b]
	Gentamicin 3 mg/kg IV/IM q 24 h **OR**	2 wk	
	Ceftriaxone 2 g IV/IM q 24 h **PLUS**	4 wk	
	Gentamicin 3 mg/kg IV/IM q 24 h	2 wk	

Viridans streptococci/*S bovis* or nutritionally variant streptococci with penicillin MIC > 0.5 µg/mL	See treatment regimen for penicillin/ampicillin-resistant enterococcal endocarditis	—	—
Enterococcus spp susceptible to penicillin, ampicillin, gentamicin, and vancomycin	Ampicillin 2 g IV q 4 h **PLUS** Gentamicin 1 mg/kg IV/IM q 8 h[a] **OR** Penicillin G 18–30 million U IV per 24 h[c] **PLUS** Gentamicin 1 mg/kg IV/IM q 8 h[a]	4–6 wk / 4–6 wk / 4–6 weeks / 4–6 wk	For penicillin/ampicillin allergy, vancomycin 15 mg/kg IV q 12 h[b] for 6 wk **PLUS** gentamicin 1 mg/kg IV/IM q 8 h[a] for 6 wk
Enterococcus spp resistant to penicillin/ampicillin; susceptible to vancomycin and gentamicin	Vancomycin 15 mg/kg IV q 12 h[b] **PLUS** Gentamicin 1 mg/kg IV/IM q 8 h[a]	6 wk / 6 wk	If β-lactamase production, ampicillin-sulbactam 3 g IV q 6 h **PLUS** gentamicin 1 mg/kg IV/IM q 8 h[a] for 6 wk

All doses based on normal renal function.

Abbreviations: IM, intramuscularly; IV, intravenously; MIC, minimum inhibitory concentration.

[a] Target gentamicin peak 3–4 µg/mL; target trough <1 µg/mL.

[b] Target vancomycin peak 30–45 µg/mL; target trough 10–15 µg/mL.

[c] Penicillin dosing can be by continuous infusion, or dosed q 4–6 h in equal divided doses.

Data from Baddour LM, Wilson WR, Bayer AS, et al. Infective endocarditis: diagnosis, antimicrobial therapy, and management of complications. A statement for healthcare professionals from the Committee on Rheumatic Fever, Endocarditis, and Kawasaki Disease, Council of Cardiovascular Disease in the Young, and the Councils on Clinical Cardiology, Stroke, and Cardiovascular Surgery and Anesthesia, American Heart Association. Circulation 2005;111:e394–434.

Table 2
Selected PVE treatment regimens

Organism	Drug	Duration	Alternative/Comments
Oxacillin-sensitive *Staphylococcus*	Oxacillin/nafcillin 2 g IV q 4 h **PLUS**	≥6 wk	For nonanaphylactoid penicillin allergy, substitute cefazolin 2 g IV q 8 h for oxacillin/nafcillin; for anaphylactoid penicillin allergy, substitute vancomycin 15 mg/kg IV q 12 h[b] for oxacillin/nafcillin
	Rifampin 300 mg IV/PO q 8 h[a] **PLUS**	≥6 wk	
	Gentamicin 1 mg/kg IV/IM q 8 h[a]	2 wk	
Oxacillin-resistant *Staphylococcus*	Vancomycin 15 mg/kg IV q 12 h[b] **PLUS**	≥6 wk	—
	Rifampin 300 mg IV/po q 8 h[a] **PLUS**	≥6 wk	
	Gentamicin 1 mg/kg IV/IM q 8 h[a]	2 wk	
Viridans streptococci/ *S bovis* with penicillin MIC ≤ 0.12 μg/mL	Penicillin G 24 million U IV per 24 h[c] **WITH OR WITHOUT**	6 wk	For penicillin/ceftriaxone allergy, vancomycin 15 mg/kg q 12 h[b] for 6 wk without gentamicin
	Gentamicin 3 mg/kg IV/IM q 24 h **OR**	2 wk	
	Ceftriaxone 2 g IV/IM q 24 h **WITH OR WITHOUT**	6 wk	
	Gentamicin 3 mg/kg IV/IM q 24 h	2 wk	

Viridans streptococci/ S bovis with penicillin MIC > 0.12	Penicillin G 24 million U IV per 24 h[c] **PLUS**	6 wk	For penicillin/ceftriaxone allergy, vancomycin 15 mg/kg q 12 h[b] for 6 wk without gentamicin
	Gentamicin 3 mg/kg IV/IM q 24 h **OR**	6 wk	
	Ceftriaxone 2 g IV/IM q 24 h **PLUS**	6 wk	
	Gentamicin 3 mg/kg IV/IM q 24 h	6 wk	
Enterococcus spp	PVE treatment regimens identical to NVE treatment regimens; see **Table 1**	—	—

All doses based on normal renal function.

Abbreviations: IM, intramuscularly; IV, intravenously; MIC, minimum inhibitory concentration.

[a] Target gentamicin peak 3–4 μg/mL; target trough <1 μg/mL.

[b] Target vancomycin peak 30–45 μg/mL; target trough 10–15 μg/mL.

[c] Penicillin dosing can be by continuous infusion, or dosed q 4–6 h in equal divided doses.

Data from Baddour LM, Wilson WR, Bayer AS, et al. Infective endocarditis: diagnosis, antimicrobial therapy, and management of complications. A statement for healthcare professionals from the Committee on Rheumatic Fever, Endocarditis, and Kawasaki Disease, Council of Cardiovascular Disease in the Young, and the Councils on Clinical Cardiology, Stroke, and Cardiovascular Surgery and Anesthesia, American Heart Association. Circulation 2005;111:e394–434.

of penicillin resistance of the infecting organism. Aminoglycosides are recommended in some settings for synergistic effects, though clinical data in humans is incomplete.[40,44,45] See **Tables 1** and **2** for treatment recommendations.

Enterococci

After staphylococci and streptococci, enterococci are the third leading cause of IE, causing about 10% of cases.[20,79] Enterococcal IE tends to occur in older men with many comorbid medical conditions.[20,87] It occurs disproportionally on the aortic valve, and is less commonly associated with embolic events compared with IE caused by other organisms.[20]

Enterococci were formerly designated as a member of genus *Streptococcus*, but now are a genus unto themselves. Unlike streptococci, enterococci are relatively resistant to penicillin, ampicillin, and vancomycin, and killing of susceptible strains often requires the addition of gentamicin or streptomycin for synergy. For this reason, all enterococcal isolates in IE cases should be tested for high-level resistance to gentamicin and streptomycin. Current guidelines suggest 4 to 6 weeks of aminoglycoside in combination with a cell wall–active agent for IE caused by appropriately susceptible isolates,[40] but observational data suggest that outcomes may be similar when the aminoglycoside is given for a shorter duration.[88] In cases where aminoglycoside is contraindicated because of toxicities, or when high-level resistance is present, there is in vitro data[89] but limited clinical data[90] suggesting that the combination of ampicillin and ceftriaxone achieve synergistic killing of susceptible enterococci, and may be a reasonable therapeutic alternative when aminoglycosides cannot be used. See **Tables 1** and **2** for treatment recommendations.

Gram-Negative Bacilli

Gram-negative bacilli account for approximately 5% of IE diagnoses. These can be divided into HACEK and non-HACEK IE. The acronym HACEK stands for *Haemophilus*, *Actinobacillus*, *Cardiobacterium*, *Eikenella*, and *Kingella*. IE due to HACEK organisms is rarely acute.[11] Older literature suggest that these fastidious organisms require prolonged incubation periods to grow in the microbiology lab, but with modern culture techniques, most HACEK organisms grow within 5 days.[91]

In a recent international cohort including 2761 cases of IE from 2000 to 2005, only 1.8% of cases were caused by non-HACEK gram-negative organisms, most commonly *Escherichia coli* and *Pseudomonas aeruginosa*.[92] Unlike older case series in which injection drug use was strongly implicated in the majority of cases,[93,94] most cases in this cohort (57%) were health care–acquired, and mortality was high (24%).[92]

COMPLICATIONS
Congestive Heart Failure

CHF is the most common complication of both NVE and PVE, occurring in over half of all cases of IE.[2] It is usually caused by valvular dysfunction, not myocardial failure,[54] and is most commonly associated with aortic valve dysfunction.[56,57] In retrospective studies of IE patients with CHF, medical management alone is associated with higher mortality than surgical and medical management combined,[56] even after adjustment for propensity to receive surgical therapy.[51]

Intracardiac Abscess

Intracardiac abscesses occur in approximately 10% to 40% of cases of IE,[58,95,96] and are particularly common in PVE and aortic valve disease.[56,58] Abscess related to the aortic valve can extend into the conduction system, causing heart block.[54,56,58]

S aureus is the organism most commonly associated with intracardiac abscess.[58,95,96] Diagnosis usually requires TEE, though even TEE has a sensitivity of only about 50% compared with intraoperative examination.[97] Surgical intervention is usually necessary to achieve cure of abscess.[54,95]

Embolism

Embolic events occur in 20% to 50% of patients with IE.[98,99] The central nervous system is the most common destination of embolism, followed by the spleen, kidneys, lungs, and liver.[55,98] Risk of embolism is highest in the time immediately following diagnosis, and risk decreases once antibiotic therapy has been initiated.[100,101] Vegetations most likely to embolize are those measuring greater than 10 mm and those on the anterior mitral valve leaflet.[55]

Central nervous system embolism accounts for 40% to 65% of all embolic events in IE, and the middle cerebral artery is the most common site.[98,100] In a study of 60 patients with left-sided IE who underwent brain MRI, cerebrospinal fluid analyses, and structured neurologic examinations, 35% of patients had a symptomatic cerebrovascular event, and another 30% had an asymptomatic event, for a total incidence of 65%.[102] The risk of central nervous system embolism declines after initiation of antimicrobial therapy.[102,103] In a prospective study of 1437 patients with left-sided IE at 61 medical centers, the risk of central nervous system embolism declined by 65% between the first and second week of antibiotics.[104]

Mortality

Mortality among IE patients has been estimated at 15% to 20% during the index hospitalization, and 20% to 30% at 1 year.[20,99,104–106] Mortality is similar between NVE and PVE, and between mitral and aortic IE.[55] Right-sided IE has lower mortality than left-sided disease.[55] In NVE, viridans streptococci and enterococci are associated with lower mortality compared with S aureus.[20] IE caused by gram-negative bacilli and fungi has greater than 50% mortality.[55] Nosocomial acquisition of IE,[107] older age,[99] immunocompromise,[29] diabetes mellitus,[104] Acute Physiology and Chronic Health Evaluation Score II (APACHE II) score,[104] hemodynamic instability,[29] altered mental status,[29,106,107] and renal failure[99,106,107] are significant predictors of mortality. IE complications predictive of mortality include CHF,[18,99] intracardiac abscess,[18] embolism,[29,106,107] and large mobile vegetation.[27,99,106]

PREVENTION

Though there have been no randomized controlled trials that prove the effectiveness of IE prophylaxis around the time of dental, gastrointestinal, or genitourinary (GU) procedures, it has been common practice since the 1950s.[4] Recent literature, however, has shown that only a small percentage of IE cases are attributable to dental procedures, and that a huge amount of prophylaxis would be needed to prevent only a small number of cases.[4,108,109]

The most recent practice guideline from the American Heart Association for the Prevention of Infective Endocarditis, published in 2007, calls into question many of the long-held assumptions about IE prevention, and contains many new and revised recommendations.[4] Prophylaxis solely for IE prevention is recommended only in patients undergoing a high-risk procedure, and with a high-risk cardiac lesion. A high-risk procedure is defined as (1) any dental procedure that involves manipulation of gum tissue, or the periapical region of teeth, or perforation of oral mucosa; (2) invasive respiratory tract procedure involving breaks in the respiratory mucosa; or (3) invasive procedure involving infected skin or soft tissue. A high-risk cardiac lesion is defined as one of the following: (1) prosthetic heart valve or prosthetic material used in a valve repair; (2) previous IE; (3) unrepaired cyanotic heart disease; (4) completely repaired congenital heart defect in the first 6 months after repair only; (5) repaired congenital heart defect with residual defect adjacent to prosthetic material; or (6) cardiac transplant recipient with cardiac valvulopathy. Prophylaxis is no longer recommended for those undergoing gastrointestinal or GU procedures.[4]

SUMMARY

Acute IE is a complex disease with changing epidemiology and a rapidly evolving knowledge base. To consistently achieve optimal outcomes in the management of IE, the clinical team must have an understanding of the epidemiology, microbiology, and natural history of IE, as well as a grasp of the guiding principles of diagnosis and medical and surgical management.

REFERENCES

1. Osler W. Gulstonian lectures on malignant endocarditis. Br Med J 1885;1: 467–70, 522–6, 577–9.
2. Bashore TM, Cabell C, Fowler VJ Jr. Update on infective endocarditis. Curr Probl Cardiol 2006;4:274–352.
3. Tunkel AR, Scheld WM. Experimental models of endocarditis. In: Kaye D, editor. Infective endocarditis. New York: Raven Press; 1992. p. 37–61.
4. Wilson W, Taubert KA, Gewitz PB, et al. Prevention of infective endocarditis: guidelines from the American Heart Association: a guideline from the American Heart Association Rheumatic Fever, Endocarditis, and Kawasaki Disease Committee, Council on Cardiovascular Disease in the Young, and the Council on Clinical Cardiology, Council on Cardiovascular Surgery and Anesthesia, and the Quality of Care and Outcomes Research Interdisciplinary Working Group. Circulation 2007;116:1736–54.
5. Scheld WM, Valvone JA, Sande MA. Bacterial adherence in the pathogenesis of endocarditis. Interaction of bacterial dextran, platelets, and fibrin. J Clin Invest 1978;61:1394–403.
6. Burnette-Curley D, Wells V, Viscount H, et al. FimA, a major virulence determinant associated with Streptococcus parasanguis endocarditis. Infect Immun 1995;63:4669–74.
7. Berlin JA, Abrutyn E, Strom BL, et al. Incidence of infective endocarditis in the Delaware Valley, 1988–1990. Am J Cardiol 1995;76(12):933–6.
8. Delahaye F, Goulet V, Lacassin F, et al. Characteristics of infective endocarditis in France 1991: a one year survey. Eur Heart J 1995;16:394–401.
9. Moreillon P, Que Y-A. Infective endocarditis. Lancet 2004;363:139–49.
10. Cabell CH, Fowler VG Jr, Engemann JJ, et al. Endocarditis in the elderly: incidence, surgery, and survival in 16,921 patients over 12 years. Circulation 2002;106(19):547.
11. Fowler VG, Scheld WM, Bayer AS. Endocarditis and intravascular infections. In: Mandell GL, Bennett JE, Dolin R, editors. Mandell, Douglas and Bennett's principles and practice of infectious diseases. 6th edition. Philadelphia: Churchill Livingstone; 2005. p. 975–1021.
12. Durack DT, Petersdorf RG. Changes in the epidemiology of endocarditis. In: Kaplan EL, Taranta AV, editors. Infective endocarditis. An American Heart Association symposium. Dallas: American Heart Association; 1977. p. 3–23.

13. Griffin MR, Wilson WR, Edwards WD, et al. Infective endocarditis. Olmsted County, Minnesota, 1950 through 1981. JAMA 1985;254:1199–202.
14. Hoen B, Alla F, Selton-Suty C, et al. Changing profile of infective endocarditis: results of a 1-year survey in France. JAMA 2002;288:75–81.
15. Tleyjeh IM, Abdel-Latif A, Rahbi H, et al. A systematic review of population-based studies of infective endocarditis. Chest 2007;132(3):1025–35.
16. Harris SL. Definitions and demographic characteristics. In: Kaye D, editor. Infective endocarditis. New York: Raven Press; 1992. p. 1–30.
17. Thayer WS. Studies on bacterial (infective) endocarditis. Johns Hopkins Hosp Rep 1926;22:1–8.
18. Miro JM, Anguera I, Cabell CH, et al. *Staphylococcus aureus* native valve infective endocarditis: report of 566 episodes from the International Collaboration on Endocarditis Merged Database. Clin Infect Dis 2005;41:507–14.
19. Selton-Suty C, Hoen B, Grentzinger A, et al. Clinical and bacteriological characteristics of infective endocarditis in the elderly. Heart 1997;77(3):260–3.
20. McDonald JR, Olaison L, Anderson DJ, et al. Enterococcal native valve endocarditis: report of 107 episodes from the International Collaboration on Endocarditis Merged Database. Am J Med 2005;11:759–66.
21. Michel PL, Acar J. Native cardiac disease predisposing to infective endocarditis. Eur Heart J 1995;16(Supp I B):2–9.
22. Weinberger I, Rotenberg Z, Zacharovitch D, et al. Native valve infective endocarditis in the 1970s versus 1980s: underlying cardiac lesions and infecting organisms. Clin Cardiol 1990;13:94–8.
23. Clemens JD, Horwitz RI, Jaffe CC, et al. A controlled evaluation of the risk of bacterial endocarditis in persons with mitral-valve prolapse. N Engl J Med 1982;307:776–80.
24. Gordon SM, Serkey JM, Longworth DL, et al. Early onset prosthetic valve endocarditis: the Cleveland clinic experience 1992–1997. Ann Thorac Surg 2000; 69(5):1388–92.
25. Strom BL, Abrutyn E, Berlin JA, et al. Risk factors for infective endocarditis: oral hygiene and nondental exposures. Circulation 2000;102:2842–8.
26. Pelletier LL, Petersdorf RG. Infective endocarditis: a review of 125 cases from the University of Washington hospitals, 1963–72. Medicine (Baltimore) 1977; 56:287–99.
27. Martín-Dávila P, Fortún J, Navas E, et al. Nosocomial endocarditis in a tertiary hospital: an increasing trend in native valve cases. Chest 2005;128:772–9.
28. Terpenning MS, Buggy BP, Kaufmann CA. Hospital-acquired infective endocarditis. Arch Intern Med 1988;148:1601–3.
29. Mourvillier B, Trouillet JL, Timsit JF, et al. Infective endocarditis in the intensive care unit: clinical spectrum and prognostic factors in 228 consecutive patients. Intensive Care Med 2004;30:2046–52.
30. Karth GD, Koreny M, Binder T, et al. Complicated infective endocarditis necessitating ICU admission: clinical course and prognosis. Crit Care 2002;6:149–54.
31. Gouello JP, Asfar P, Brenet O, et al. Nosocomial endocarditis in the intensive care unit: an analysis of 22 cases. Crit Care Med 2000;28:377–82.
32. Wolff M, Witchitz S, Chastang C, et al. Prosthetic valve endocarditis in the ICU. Prognostic factors of overall survival in a series of 122 cases and consequences for treatment decision. Chest 1995;108:688–94.
33. Durack DT, Lukes AS, Bright DK. New criteria for diagnosis of infective endocarditis: utilization of specific echocardiographic findings. Duke endocarditis service. Am J Med 1994;96:200–7.

34. Bayer AS, Ward JL, Ginzton LE, et al. Evaluation of new clinical criteria for the diagnosis of infective endocarditis. Am J Med 1994;96:211–5.
35. Hoen B, Selton-Suty C, Danchin N, et al. Evaluation of the Duke criteria versus the Beth Israel criteria for the diagnosis of infective endocarditis. Clin Infect Dis 1995;21:905–11.
36. Li JS, Sexton DJ, Mick N, et al. Proposed modifications to the Duke criteria for the diagnosis of infective endocarditis. Clin Infect Dis 2000;30:633–8.
37. Sachdev M, Peterson GE, Jollis JG. Imaging techniques for diagnosis of infective endocarditis. Infect Dis Clin North Am 2002;16:319–37.
38. Kuruppu JC, Corretti M, Mackowiak P, et al. Overuse of transthoracic echocardiography in the diagnosis of native valve endocarditis. Arch Intern Med 2002;162:1715–20.
39. Greaves K, Mou D, Patel A, et al. Clinical criteria and the appropriate use of transthoracic echocardiography for the exclusion of infective endocarditis. Heart 2003;89:273–5.
40. Baddour LM, Wilson WR, Bayer AS, et al. Infective endocarditis: diagnosis, antimicrobial therapy, and management of complications. A statement for healthcare professionals from the Committee on Rheumatic Fever, Endocarditis, and Kawasaki Disease, Council of Cardiovascular Disease in the Young, and the Councils on Clinical Cardiology, Stroke, and Cardiovascular Surgery and Anesthesia, American Heart Association. Circulation 2005;111:e394–434.
41. Roe MT, Abramson MA, Li J, et al. Clinical information determines the impact of transesophageal echocardiography on the diagnosis of infective endocarditis by the Duke criteria. Am Heart J 2000;139:945–51.
42. Fowler VG, Li J, Corey GR, et al. Role of echocardiography in evaluation of patients with Staphylococcus aureus bacteremia: experience in 103 patients. J Am Coll Cardiol 1997;30:1072–8.
43. Feuchtner GM, Stolzmann P, Dichtl W, et al. Multislice computed tomography in infective endocarditis. J Am Coll Cardiol 2009;53:436–44.
44. Leibovici L, Vidal L, Paul M. Aminoglycoside drugs in clinical practice: an evidence-based approach. J Antimicrob Chemother 2009;63:246–51.
45. Falagas ME, Matthaiou DK, Bliziotis IA. The role of aminoglycosides in combination with a beta-lactam for the treatment of bacterial endocarditis: a meta-analysis of comparative trials. J Antimicrob Chemother 2006;57:639–47.
46. Korzeniowski O, Sande MA. Combination antimicrobial therapy for Staphylococcus aureus endocarditis in patients addicted to parenteral drugs and in nonaddicts: a prospective study. Ann Intern Med 1982;97:496–503.
47. Vlessis AA, Hovaguimian H, Jaggers J, et al. Infective endocarditis: Ten-year review of medical and surgical therapy. Ann Thorac Surg 1996;61:1217–22.
48. Wang A, Pappas P, Anstrom KJ, et al. The use and effect of surgical therapy for prosthetic valve infective endocarditis: a propensity analysis of a multicenter, international cohort. Am Heart J 2005;150:1086–91.
49. Tornos P, Iung B, Permanyer-Miralda G, et al. Infective endocarditis in Europe: lessons from the Euro-Heart Survey. Heart 2005;91:571–5.
50. Tleyjeh IM, Kashour T, Zimmerman V, et al. The role of valve surgery in infective endocarditis management: a systematic review of observational studies that included propensity score analysis. Am Heart J 2008;156:901–9.
51. Vikram HR, Buenconsejo J, Hasbun R, et al. Impact of valve surgery on 6-month mortality in adults with complicated, left-sided native valve endocarditis. JAMA 2003;290:3207–14.

52. Cabell CH, Abrutyn E, Fowler VG, et al. Use of surgery in patients with native valve infective endocarditis: results from the International Collaboration on Endocarditis Merged Database. Am Heart J 2005;150:1092-8.
53. Tleyjeh IM, Ghomrawi HM, Steckelberg JM, et al. The impact of valve surgery on 6-month mortality in left-sided infective endocarditis. Circulation 2007;115: 1721-8.
54. Sexton DJ, Spelman D. Current best practices and guidelines: assessment and management of complications in infective endocarditis. Cardiol Clin 2003;21: 273-82.
55. Mylonakis E, Calderwood SB. Infective endocarditis in adults. N Engl J Med 2001;345:1318-30.
56. Moon MR, Stinson EB, Miller DC. Surgical treatment of endocarditis. Prog Cardiovasc Dis 1997;40:239-64.
57. Mills J, Utley J, Abbott J. Heart failure in infective endocarditis: predisposing factors, course, and treatment. Chest 1974;66:151-7.
58. Graupner C, Vilacosta I, San Román JA, et al. Periannular extension of infective endocarditis. J Am Coll Cardiol 2002;39:1204-11.
59. Akowuah EF, Davies W, Oliver S, et al. Prosthetic valve endocarditis: early and late outcome following medical or surgical treatment. Heart 2003;89:269-72.
60. Habib G, Tribouilloy C, Thuny F, et al. Prosthetic valve endocarditis: who needs surgery? A multicentre study of 104 cases. Heart 2005;91:954-9.
61. Moss R, Munt B. Injection drug use and right sided endocarditis. Heart 2003;89: 577-81.
62. Miro JM, del Rio A, Mestres CA. Infective endocarditis and cardiac surgery in intravenous drug abusers and HIV-1 infected patients. Cardiol Clin 2003;21: 167-84.
63. Jain V, Yang M-H, Kovacicova-Lezcano G, et al. Infective endocarditis in an urban medical center: association of individual drugs with valvular involvement. J Infect 2008;57:132-8.
64. Hecht S, Berger M. Right-sided endocarditis in intravenous drug users. Prognostic features in 102 episodes. Ann Intern Med 1992;117:560-6.
65. DiNubile MJ. Short-course antibiotic therapy for right-sided endocarditis caused by Staphylococcus aureus in injection drug users. Ann Intern Med 1994;121: 873-6.
66. Heldman AW, Hartert TV, Ray SC, et al. Oral antibiotic treatment of right-sided staphylococcal endocarditis in injection drug users: prospective randomized comparison with parenteral therapy. Am J Med 1996;101:68-76.
67. Mahesh B, Angelini G, Caputo M, et al. Prosthetic valve endocarditis. Ann Thorac Surg 2005;80:1151-8.
68. Stanbridge TN, Isalska BJ. Aspects of prosthetic valve endocarditis. J Infect 1997;35:1-6.
69. Piper C, Körfer R, Horstkotte D. Prosthetic valve endocarditis. Heart 2001;85: 590-3.
70. Karchmer AW, Longworth DL. Infections of intracardiac devices. Cardiol Clin 2003;21:253-71.
71. Baddour LM, Wilson WR. Prosthetic valve endocarditis and cardiovascular device-related infections. In: Mandell GL, Bennett JE, Dolin R, editors. Mandell, Douglas and Bennett's principles and practice of infectious diseases. 6th edition. Philadelphia: Churchill Livingstone; 2005. p. 1022-44.
72. Sampedro MF, Patel R. Infections associated with long-term prosthetic devices. Infect Dis Clin North Am 2007;21:785-819.

73. Wang A, Athan E, Pappas PA, et al. Contemporary clinical profile and outcome of prosthetic valve endocarditis. JAMA 2007;297:1354–61.
74. Cabell C, Heidenreich P, Chu V, et al. Increasing rates of cardiac device infections among Medicare beneficiaries: 1990–1999. Am Heart J 2004;147:582–6.
75. Arber N, Pras E, Copperman Y, et al. Pacemaker endocarditis: report of 44 cases and review of the literature. Medicine 1994;73:299–305.
76. Baddour LM, Bettmann MA, Bolger AF, et al. Nonvalvular cardiovascular device-related infections. Circulation 2003;108:2015–31.
77. Chua JD, Wilkoff BL, Lee I, et al. Diagnosis and management of infections involving implantable electrophysiologic cardiac devices. Ann Intern Med 2000;133:604–8.
78. Tleyjeh IM, Steckelberg JM, Murad HS, et al. Temporal trends in infective endocarditis: a population-based study in Olmsted County, Minnesota. JAMA 2005; 293:3061–2.
79. Fowler VG, Miro JM, Hoen B, et al. *Staphylococcus aureus* endocarditis: a consequence of medical progress. JAMA 2005;293:3012–21.
80. Millar BC, Prendergast BD, Moore JE. Community-associated MRSA (CA-MRSA): an emerging pathogen in infective endocarditis. J Antimicrob Chemother 2008;61:1–7.
81. Cabell CH, Jollis JG, Peterson GE, et al. Changing patient characteristics and the effect on mortality in endocarditis. Arch Intern Med 2002;162:90–7.
82. Chirouze C, Cabell CH, Fowler VG, et al. Prognostic factors in 61 cases of *Staphylococcus aureus* prosthetic valve infective endocarditis from the International Collaboration on Endocarditis Merged Database. Clin Infect Dis 2004;38: 1323–7.
83. Chu VH, Cabell CH, Abrutyn E, et al. Native valve endocarditis due to coagulase-negative staphylococci: report of 99 episodes from the International Collaboration on Endocarditis Merged Database. Clin Infect Dis 2004;39: 1527–30.
84. Anguera I, Del Rio A, Miró JM, et al. *Staphylococcus lugdunensis* infective endocarditis: description of 10 cases and analysis of native valve, prosthetic valve, and pacemaker lead endocarditis clinical profiles. Heart 2005;91:e10.
85. Hoen B, Chirouze C, Cabell CH, et al. Emergence of endocarditis due to group D streptococci: findings derived from the merged database of the International Collaboration on Endocarditis. Eur J Clin Microbiol Infect Dis 2005;24: 12–6.
86. Tripodi MF, Adinolfi LE, Ragone E, et al. *Streptococcus bovis* endocarditis and its association with chronic liver disease: an underestimated risk factor. Clin Infect Dis 2004;38:1394–400.
87. Anderson DJ, Olaison L, McDonald JR, et al. Enterococcal prosthetic valve infective endocarditis: report of 45 episodes from the International Collaboration on Endocarditis Merged Database. Eur J Clin Microbiol Infect Dis 2005;24: 665–70.
88. Olaison L, Schadewitz K. Enterococcal endocarditis in Sweden, 1995–1999: can shorter therapy with aminoglycosides be used? Clin Infect Dis 2002;34: 159–66.
89. Gavalda J, Onrubia PL, Gonez MT, et al. Efficacy of ampicillin combined with ceftriaxone and gentamicin in the treatment of experimental endocarditis due to *Enterococcus faecalis* with no high-level resistance to aminoglycosides. J Antimicrob Chemother 2003;52:514–7.

90. Gavalda J, Len O, Miro JM, et al. Brief communication: treatment of *Enterococcus faecalis* endocarditis with ampicillin plus ceftriaxone. Ann Intern Med 2007;146:574–9.

91. Baron EJ, Scott JD, Tompkins LS. Prolonged incubation and extensive subculturing do not increase recovery of clinically significant microorganisms from standard automated blood cultures. Clin Infect Dis 2005;41:1677–80.

92. Morpeth S, Murdoch D, Cabell CH, et al. Non-HACEK gram-negative bacillus endocarditis. Ann Intern Med 2007;147:829–35.

93. Wieland M, Lederman MM, Kline-King C, et al. Left-sided endocarditis due to *Pseudomonas aeruginosa*. A report of 10 cases and review of the literature. Medicine (Baltimore) 1986;65:180–9.

94. Levine DP, Crane LR, Zervos MJ. Bacteremia in narcotic addicts at the Detroit Medical Center. II. Infectious endocarditis: a prospective comparative study. Rev Infect Dis 1986;8:374–96.

95. Daniel WG, Mugge A, Martin RP, et al. Improvement in the diagnosis of abscesses associated with endocarditis by transesophageal echocardiography. N Engl J Med 1991;324:795–800.

96. Anguera I, Mire JM, Cabell CH, et al. Clinical characteristics and outcome of aortic endocarditis with periannular abscess in the International Collaboration on Endocarditis Merged Database. Am J Cardiol 2005;96:976–81.

97. Hill EE, Herijgers P, Claus P, et al. Abscess in infective endocarditis: the value of transesophageal echocardiography and outcome: a 5-year study. Am Heart J 2007;154:923–8.

98. Mouly S, Ruimy R, Launay O, et al. The changing clinical aspects of infective endocarditis: descriptive review of 90 episodes in a French teaching hospital and risk factors for death. J Infect 2002;45:246–56.

99. Thuny F, Disalvo G, Belliard O, et al. Risk of embolism and death in infective endocarditis: prognostic value of echocardiography, a prospective multicenter study. Circulation 2005;112:69–75.

100. Heiro M, Nikoskelainen J, Engblom E, et al. Neurologic manifestations of infective endocarditis: a 17-year experience in a teaching hospital in Finland. Arch Intern Med 2000;160:2781–7.

101. Steckelberg JM, Murphy JG, Ballard D, et al. Emboli in infective endocarditis: the prognostic value of echocardiography. Ann Intern Med 1991;114:635–40.

102. Snygg-Martin U, Gustafsson L, Rosengren L, et al. Cerebrovascular complications in patients with left-sided infective endocarditis are common: a prospective study using magnetic resonance imaging and neurochemical brain damage markers. Clin Infect Dis 2008;47:23–30.

103. Dickerman SA, Abrutyn E, Barsic B, et al. The relationship between the initiation of antimicrobial therapy and the incidence of stroke in infective endocarditis: an analysis from the ICE Prospective Cohort Study (ICE-PCS). Am Heart J 2007;154:1086–94.

104. Chu VH, Cabell CH, Benjamin DK Jr, et al. Early predictors of in-hospital death in infective endocarditis. Circulation 2004;110:1745–9.

105. Wallace SM, Walton BI, Kharbanda RK, et al. Mortality from infective endocarditis: clinical predictors of outcome. Heart 2002;88:53–60.

106. Leblebicioglu H, Yilmaz H, Tasova Y, et al. Characteristics and analysis of risk factors for mortality in infective endocarditis. Eur J Epidemiol 2006;21:25–31.

107. Hsu CN, Wang JY, Tseng CD, et al. Clinical features and predictors for mortality in patients with infective endocarditis at a university hospital in Taiwan from 1995 to 2003. Epidemiol Infect 2006;134:589–97.

108. Duval X, Alla F, Hoen B, et al. Estimated risk of endocarditis in adults with predisposing cardiac conditions undergoing dental procedures with or without antibiotic prophylaxis. Clin Infect Dis 2006;42:e102–7.

109. Agha Z, Lofgren RP, VanRuiswyk JV. Is antibiotic prophylaxis for bacterial endocarditis cost-effective? Med Decis Making 2005;25:308–20.

New Antimicrobial Agents for Use in the Intensive Care Unit

David J. Ritchie, PharmD, BCPS, FCCP[a,b,*], Bryan T. Alexander, PharmD[a],
Patrick M. Finnegan, PharmD, BCPS[b]

KEYWORDS

- New antimicrobials • Intensive care unit • Infection
- Antimicrobial resistance • Investigational agents

Timely provision of adequate antimicrobial coverage in an initial anti-infective treatment regimen results in optimal outcomes for bacterial and fungal infections.[1-7] However, selection of appropriate antimicrobial regimens for treatment of infections in the intensive care unit (ICU) can be challenging due to expansion of resistance, which typically requires use of multidrug anti-infective regimens to provide adequate coverage of important pathogens commonly seen in the ICU setting. Indeed, a recent additional call to action by the Infectious Diseases Society of America (IDSA) has enforced the impact that antimicrobial-resistant pathogens can have on patient care.[8] The term *ESKAPE* has been coined by this IDSA group to refer to *Enterococcus faecium, Staphylococcus aureus, Klebsiella pneumoniae, Acinetobacter baumanii, Pseudomonas aeruginosa*, and *Enterobacter* species, the etiologic causes of the majority of hospital-acquired infections in the United States that are able to effectively "escape" our antibiotic arsenal and that also mandate discovery of new antimicrobial agents. This article reviews select antibacterial agents and an antifungal agent in late stages of clinical development that appear to have potential for treatment of infections in the ICU.

CEFTAROLINE

Ceftaroline fosamil is a fifth-generation cephalosporin prodrug, so named because of its spectrum of activity against a broad range of gram-positive and gram-negative bacteria. The active agent, ceftaroline, is active against methicillin-resistant *Staphylococcus aureus* (MRSA) with an MIC_{90} (minimum inhibitory concentration required to

---

[a] Barnes-Jewish Hospital, Mailstop 90-52-411, 216 S. Kingshighway Boulevard, St. Louis, MO 63110, USA
[b] St. Louis College of Pharmacy, 4588 Parkview Place, St. Louis, MO 63110, USA
* Corresponding author. Barnes-Jewish Hospital, Mailstop 90-52-411, 216 S. Kingshighway Boulevard, St. Louis, MO 63110.
E-mail address: dritchie@stlcop.edu (D.J. Ritchie).

Infect Dis Clin N Am 23 (2009) 665–681
doi:10.1016/j.idc.2009.04.010
0891-5520/09/$ – see front matter © 2009 Elsevier Inc. All rights reserved.
id.theclinics.com

inhibit the growth of 90% of organisms) of 1 to 2 μg/mL because of its enhanced binding to penicillin-binding protein 2a as compared with other β-lactam antibiotics.[9–12] The drug is also active against penicillin- and cephalosporin-resistant *Streptococcus pneumoniae*, β-hemolytic streptococci, *Enterococcus faecalis* (variable activity), but has little to no activity against vancomycin-resistant *E faecium*.[9–11,13,14] Against relevant gram-negative pathogens, ceftaroline has broad-spectrum activity similar to that of ceftriaxone. However, MICs are generally higher than those of cefepime against most nonfermenting gram-negative bacteria and Enterobacteriaceae, and the drug is expected to be inactive against *Pseudomonas* and *Acinetobacter* spp.[9,11] Ceftaroline appears to be a weak inducer of AmpC β-lactamases and, like other clinically available cephalosporins (besides cefepime), is labile to AmpC and expected to be clinically ineffective against such isolates.[10] As with other advanced-generation cephalosporins, ceftaroline is not reliably active against extended-spectrum β-lactamase–producing strains of Enterobacteriaceae.[10,11]

Early phase clinical trials established a ceftaroline dosing regimen of 600 mg intravenous (IV) every 12 hours (as 1-hour infusions) as the preferred dosing regimen for future study.[15] Ceftaroline is less than 20% protein bound in serum, and has a volume of distribution similar to extracellular fluid volume at about 16 to 17 L.[16,17] The drug is primarily eliminated by renal excretion, and multiple-dose pharmacokinetic studies identified the half-life at about 2.5 to 3 hours.[15,18] Ceftaroline does exhibit an extended half-life and area under the curve under conditions of mild-to-moderate renal impairment, and would be expected to require dose adjustment in these populations.[18,19] There are no currently available data on ceftaroline clearance in dialysis. In support of potential pneumonia indications, lung tissue penetration was measured in rabbits at the end of drug infusion at 42% of serum concentrations.[20]

One phase II clinical trial comparing 7 to 14 days of ceftaroline to vancomycin 1 g IV every 12 hours with or without aztreonam 1 g IV every 8 hours for complicated skin and skin structure infections (cSSSIs) has been conducted. Clinical cure rates were similar between the ceftaroline (96.7%) and standard therapy (88.9%) groups.[21] Phase III clinical trials for this indication are now complete; however, data were not yet in print at the time of this writing.[22] Perhaps more interesting for ICU practitioners, phase III trials are currently ongoing to compare 5 to 7 days of ceftaroline with ceftriaxone 1 g IV daily for treatment of community-acquired pneumonia.[22]

Adverse effects in all ceftaroline studies to date have been minor, and include headache, nausea, insomnia, and abnormal body odor.[15,19,21] It appears safe to assume that ceftaroline is likely to have an adverse effect profile consistent with currently available cephalosporins, until proven otherwise.

Pending phase III trials confirming its efficacy and safety, ceftaroline appears to be a promising new alternative in the treatment of gram-positive infections in general, and serious MRSA infections specifically. Despite possessing broad gram-negative coverage, ceftaroline is not active against *Pseudomonas* or *Acinetobacter* spp, which will limit the ability of the agent to be used as empiric monotherapy for serious infections in the ICU. This fact, along with potential competition from another investigational fifth-generation cephalosporin, ceftobiprole, and other investigational anti-MRSA agents, may limit use of the agent in the ICU setting.

CEFTOBIPROLE

Ceftobiprole medocaril is another fifth-generation cephalosporin prodrug, with a broad spectrum of activity similar to ceftaroline. As with ceftaroline, this agent was designed to maximize binding to penicillin-binding protein 2a and yield potent anti-MRSA activity with an MIC_{90} of 2 μg/mL.[23–25] Ceftobiprole is active against cephalosporin-resistant *S pneumoniae* and ampicillin-sensitive *E faecalis*, but not *E faecium*.[23,24] Ceftobiprole has broader gram-negative activity than ceftaroline, and appears to have a gram-negative spectrum of activity intermediate between ceftriaxone and cefepime, largely due to its increased stability to AmpC β-lactamases as compared with ceftriaxone and ceftaroline.[23,26–28] Ceftobiprole also has activity against *P aeruginosa*, and MICs against this pathogen are generally similar to those of cefepime and ceftazidime.[23–25,29] Activity against *Acinetobacter* spp appears to be highly variable.[23,29] As with other advanced-generation cephalosporins, ceftobiprole is not reliably active against extended-spectrum β-lactamase–producing bacteria.[27,28]

The volume of distribution is similar to extracellular fluid volume at about 18 L, although this value may be doubled in patients with ventilator-associated pneumonia (VAP).[30,31] There are currently no data on the epithelial lining fluid penetration of ceftobiprole; however, a pharmacokinetic study is ongoing to evaluate bronchoalveolar lavage fluid concentrations of ceftobiprole following IV infusion.[32] The drug is 16% plasma protein bound, is primarily eliminated in the urine, and has a half-life of about 3 to 4 hours.[30,33,34] Due to its extensive renal clearance, dose adjustments have been proposed for patients with mild-to-moderate renal impairment.[30,35] Ceftobiprole appears to be removed effectively by some hemodialysis modalities.[36]

Results of early phase clinical trials and Monte Carlo simulations suggested two dosing regimens for ceftobiprole: 500 mg IV every 12 hours (as 1-hour infusions) for treatment of gram-positive infections and 500 mg IV every 8 hours (as 2-hour infusions) for empiric treatment of mixed gram-positive and gram-negative infections.[35] Two phase III clinical trials have been completed with ceftobiprole for cSSSIs. The first study enrolled patients with suspected gram-positive infection, and used the 500-mg-every-12-hour ceftobiprole regimen, compared with vancomycin 1 g IV every 12 hours for 7 to 14 days. Clinical cure rates were similar between the ceftobiprole (93.3%) and vancomycin (93.5%) groups.[37] The second study included patients with diabetic foot and mixed bacterial cSSSIs, and compared ceftobiprole 500 mg IV every 8 hours with vancomycin 1 g IV every 12 hours plus ceftazidime 1 g IV every 8 hours for 7 to 14 days. Clinical cure rates in this trial were also similar between the ceftobiprole (90.5%) and standard therapy (90.2%) groups.[38] Ceftobiprole 500 mg IV every 8 hours was also compared with a combination of ceftazidime plus linezolid for treatment of nosocomial pneumonia. While demonstrating noninferiority versus the combination regimen, ceftobiprole was unexpectedly associated with lower cure rates in patients with VAP, particularly in those under age 45 and with high creatinine clearance.[39]

The adverse effect profile of ceftobiprole is minor and similar to other cephalosporins. Those identified thus far in phase III clinical trials were nausea, diarrhea, and taste disturbances at rates of less than 15%.[37,38] It appears safe to assume that ceftobiprole is likely to have an adverse effect profile consistent with currently available cephalosporins, until proven otherwise.

Ceftopibrole is a unique agent with broad-spectrum activity, including both MRSA and *P aeruginosa*. However, ceftobiprole's long-term potency and ability to withstand resistance development with *Pseudomonas* spp and MRSA over time are uncertain, and its efficacy and safety for infections other than cSSSI have not yet been established.[39–41] Nonetheless, ceftobiprole is the only agent currently in phase III clinical trials that is active against both *Pseudomonas* spp and MRSA, and therefore has potential for use as empiric monotherapy for serious infections in the ICU. However, the question of whether dose escalation beyond 500 mg IV every 8 hours will improve the performance of the drug for VAP remains unanswered.

DALBAVANCIN

Dalbavancin is an investigational lipoglycopeptide with a bactericidal mechanism of action similar to other glycopeptides in that it complexes with the D-alanyl-D-alanine (D-Ala-D-Ala) terminal of peptidoglycan precursors and inhibits transglycosylation and transpeptidation. Like teicoplanin, dalbavancin possesses a lipophilic side chain that leads to both high protein binding and an extended half-life, which allows for a unique once-weekly dosing of the drug.[42–44]

Dalbavancin is more potent than vancomycin against staphylococci, and is highly active against both methicillin-susceptible S aureus (MSSA) and MRSA with $MIC_{90}s$ of less than 0.13 and 0.25 mg/L, respectively.[45] Dalbavancin is also active against vancomycin-intermediate Staphylococcus aureus (VISA), although MIC_{90} ranges are higher at 1 to 2 μg/mL.[46–48] Streptococci, including penicillin-resistant S pneumoniae, are inhibited by dalbavancin, as are enterococci with the VanB or VanC phenotype. However, dalbavancin is not active against enterococci with the VanA phenotype.[45–47]

Dalbavancin is administered IV, and the most commonly used dose in clinical trials has been 1000 mg on day 1 and 500 mg weekly thereafter. This dose achieves a maximum serum concentration of 312 μg/mL with mean serum concentrations of greater than 35 μg/mL maintained for a 7-day dosing period. The drug has a volume of distribution (Vd) of 0.11 L/kg and a half-life of 147 to 258 hours, supporting once-weekly dosing. The drug is only 40% eliminated by the kidneys, with no apparent need for dose adjustments in the setting of either moderate renal or hepatic impairment.[42,43] The drug does not appear to interact with any of the P450 cytochromes, and is not known to possess any clinically relevant drug interactions.[42,49]

Clinical data for dalbavancin include phase II and III trials in both uncomplicated and cSSSI, and catheter-related bloodstream infections. Dalbavancin 1000 mg IV on day 1 followed by 500 mg IV on day 8 was compared with linezolid 600 mg twice daily for 14 days in a randomized, double-blind, phase III trial for treatment of cSSSIs. The overall success rates at the test of cure visit were similar for both daptomycin and linezolid at 88.4% and 86.8%, respectively (P value not given).[50] Dalbavancin has been compared with β-lactams, clindamycin, vancomycin, and linezolid in other SSSI trials, and was shown to be at least noninferior in each trial.[48,51] Another phase II study evaluated dalbavancin versus vancomycin for treatment of bloodstream infections. This trial used the same weekly dalbavancin dosing regimen as above and compared it to vancomycin 1 g twice daily for 7 days. Dalbavancin had a statistically higher overall success rate of 87% versus vancomycin at 50% success (P<.05) in this trial.[52]

Dalbavancin has been well tolerated throughout clinical trials, with the most commonly seen adverse effects being fever, headache, and nausea. No significant nervous, auditory, vestibular, or cardiac adverse effects have been noted in either dose escalation or clinical trials.[49,53]

Dalbavancin provides coverage for both glycopeptide-sensitive and -resistant MRSA. However, coverage of vancomycin-resistant enterococci (VRE) is limited. The drug has the convenience of once-weekly dosing, which should allow for simplified in-hospital and at-home regimens. However, whether this infrequent dosing scheme is value-added in the ICU setting is unknown. The clinical data are limited to cSSSI and bacteremia. Pfizer pharmaceuticals, the current owner of dalbavancin, has released a statement indicating that it plans on conducting additional phase III trials in cSSSI, upon recommendations from regulatory authorities.[54] It remains to be seen if dalbavancin will be studied for treatment of pneumonia, meningitis, or endocarditis, and this uncertainty will likely limit applicability in the intensive care environment.

ORITAVANCIN

Oritavancin, another investigational glycopeptide, contains novel structural modifications that allow it to dimerize and anchor itself in the bacterial membrane. These modifications also confer an enhanced spectrum of activity over traditional glycopeptide antibiotics.[43,55] Ortivancin has similar in vitro activity as vancomycin against staphylococci and is equipotent against both MSSA and MRSA.[45,46] Oritavancin also has activity against VISA and vancomycin-resistant S Aureus (VRSA), but MICs are increased to 1 mg/L and 0.5 mg/L, respectively.[46,56,57] Oritivancin is active against enterococci, including VRE; however, MICs are significantly higher against VRE versus vancomycin-sensitive strains. The drug is also active against penicillin-sensitive and penicillin-resistant S pneumoniae.[45,46]

Oritavancin has been typically dosed at 1.5–3 mg/kg IV once daily as well as a flat 200 mg daily.[55] Although the drug is 90% bound to plasma proteins, it exhibits rapid tissue distribution. However, the propensity for oritavancin binding to pulmonary surfactant warrants careful assessment, based on some evidence of an effect noted in a murine pneumonia model.[58] Approximately 60% of the administered dose is retained in the liver, but there is no evidence to indicate that oritavancin undergoes hepatic metabolism.[59] In vitro studies of cultured macrophages show intracellular levels up to 400 times those seen in the serum, the clinical significance of which is unknown.[60] The drug is predominantly eliminated by the kidneys; however, high protein binding and extensive tissue distribution leads to a very slow renal clearance, with only 5% unchanged drug recovered at 7 days postdose.[59]

Clinical data for oritavancin are limited. Two phase III trials evaluating oritavancin for cSSSI have been completed. In the first study, oritavancin 1.5 mg/kg and 3 mg/kg daily met criteria for noninferiority versus vancomycin plus cephalexin. Patients receiving either dose of oritavancin showed a shorter mean duration of therapy (5.3 or 5.7 days, respectively) than those in the vancomycin group (11.9 days).[55] A second cSSSI trial of a fixed oritavancin dose of 200 mg IV daily versus vancomycin plus cephalexin found clinical cure rates of 78.6% for oritavancin and 76.2% for vancomycin plus cephalexin (95% CI −3.4–7.8). Again the average days of therapy were shorter for oritavancin than with vancomycin (5.3 versus 10.9 days, $P<.0001$). An additional study (SIMPLIFI [A Study for Patients with Complicated Skin and Skin Structure Infections]) designed to assess novel oritavancin dosing regimens in the treatment of cSSSI compared oritavancin as a single large dose, oritavancin dosed on day 1 with an optional dose on day 5, and oritavancin 200 mg once daily for 3 to 7 days. The study has been completed, but, at the time of this writing, results were not yet available.[61] Oritavancin has also showed equivalence to vancomycin or an active β-lactam for treatment of S aureus bloodstream infection when administered at 5 to 10 mg/kg daily.[62] Data evaluating oritavancin for treatment of meningitis and cardiac infections exist only in animal models. In these models, oritavancin successfully treated meningitis caused by S pneumoniae and endocarditis caused by MRSA and VRE.[63–66]

Oritavancin has been well tolerated in clinical trials, with the most predominant adverse effects being headache, nausea, vomiting, sleep disorders, and injection-site reactions. Elevated transaminases seen in early trials of oritavancin were not seen in either of the phase III clinical trials in patients with cSSSI.[55,59]

Oritavancin is highly active against both S aureus and Enterococcus spp, covering the most resistant strains of both species. However, clinical data are very limited, and it is unclear if future studies are planned for more critical infections. The potential for oritavancin to bind to pulmonary surfactant may significantly limit utility for treatment of pulmonary infections. The very high intracellular concentration profile will also need to be carefully assessed. At the time of this writing, oritavancin had not yet secured US. Food and Drug Administration (FDA) approval due to a lack of adequate efficacy and safety data.[67]

TELAVANCIN

Telavancin is an investigational glycopeptide derivative of vancomycin. Like oritavancin, telavancin has the ability to anchor itself in the bacterial membrane, which disrupts polymerization and cross-linking of peptidoglycan. Telavancin also interferes with the normal function of the bacterial membrane, leading to a decrease in the barrier function of the membrane. This dual mechanism helps to explain its high potency and rapidly bactericidal activity.[68,69]

Telavancin is bactericidal against staphylococci, including MRSA, VISA, and VRSA with MIC_{90} ranges of 0.25 to 1, 0.5 to 2, and 2 to 4 mg/L, respectively.[69–72] Telavancin, like oritavancin, is potent against both penicillin-susceptible and -resistant strains of S pneumoniae. Telavancin is also active against vancomycin-susceptible E faecium and E faecalis. However, MICs are increased against vancomycin-resistant E faecium and E faecalis.[68–70]

The usual dose of telavancin is 7.5 to 10 mg/kg/d. The drug is highly protein bound and has a volume of distribution of 0.1 L/kg. Telavancin has a half-life of 7 to 9 hours, is predominately eliminated by the kidneys, and will likely require dose adjustments in patients with renal impairment.[42,68,69]

Of the investigational glycopeptides and lipoglycopeptides, telavancin has the richest set of clinical data to support its use. A set of two phase III trials of telavancin for cSSSIs was conducted. The two identical trials, ATLAS (Assessment of Telavancin in Complicated Skin and Skin Structure Infections) I and II, compared telavancin 10 mg/kg/d to vancomycin 1 g every 12 hours and found telavancin to be noninferior to vancomycin with a combined clinical cure rate in patients with MRSA infection of 90.6% and 86.4% for telavancin and vancomycin, respectively ($P = .06$).[42,73] Telavancin has also been studied in hospital-acquired pneumonia (HAP). The ATTAIN (Comparison of Telavancin and Vancomycin for Hospital-Acquired Pneumonia Due to Methicillin-Resistant Staphylococcus Aureus) one and two trials were both randomized, double-blind trials with a combined population of 1503 patients, of which 464 had documented MRSA infections. Patients were randomized to receive telavancin 10 mg/kg IV once daily or vancomycin 1g IV every 12 hours. Telavancin was shown to be noninferior to vancomycin in these studies. In addition, preliminary results showed that clinical cure rates were 82% for telavancin and 74% for vancomycin in patients infected with MRSA (P not significant). Also of interest was the finding that a subset of patients with VAP showed a cure rate of 80% for telavancin and 68% for vancomycin (P not given).[74]

Telavancin has been well tolerated in clinical trials, with the most common adverse effects being taste disturbances, headache, and dizziness. Other potentially serious adverse effects include elevations in serum creatinine, microalbuminuria, and decreased platelet counts, each of which occurred at rates similar to comparator agents.[42,68,69] Of potential concern is an apparent risk of low birth weight and limb defects seen in pregnant animals receiving telavancin. The FDA has recommended that the benefits of this drug should outweigh the risk when used in pregnant women.[75]

Telavancin is a potent agent against resistant gram-positive organisms. To date, four phase III trials have shown telavancin to be similar to comparator agents in both skin and skin structure infections and HAP. The agent would appear to be a viable treatment for MRSA HAP and VAP, based on supporting in vitro and clinical data. In clinical trials, telavancin exhibited similar adverse effect profiles as comparator agents. In light of these favorable efficacy and safety data, and at the time of this writing, the US FDA Anti-Infective Drugs Advisory Committee granted telavancin a favorable review.[75]

ICLAPRIM

Iclaprim (formerly AR-100 and Ro 48-2622) is an investigational IV diaminopyrimidine antibacterial agent that, like trimethoprim, selectively inhibits dihydrofolate reductase of both gram-positive and gram-negative bacteria and exerts bactericidal effects.[76,77] Iclaprim is active against MSSA, community- and nosocomial-MRSA, VISA, VRSA, groups A and B streptococci, and pneumococci, and is variably active against entero-cocci.[78–82] Iclaprim appears to have similar gram-negative activity to that of trimeth-oprim, including activity against Escherichia coli, K pneumoniae, Enterobacter, Citrobacter freundii, and Proteus vulgaris.[83,84] Iclaprim also appears to have activity against the atypical respiratory pathogens Legionella and Chlamydia pneumoniae, but is not active against P aeruginosa or anaerobes.[78,83,85,86] Although the possible effect of thymidine release from bacteria and infected host tissues on the activity of iclaprim in vivo is unknown, the activity of the drug did appear to be rendered bacte-riostatic in vitro against a wild-type isolate of S aureus in the presence of increasing concentrations of thymidine.[87,88]

Iclaprim achieves a maximum serum concentration of 0.85 μg/mL following a dose of 0.8 mg/kg by IV infusion over 30 minutes and appears to have linear pharmacoki-netics.[89,90] The drug is 93% plasma protein bound, has a Vd of 1.15 L/kg, and achieves concentrations in epithelial lining fluid that exceed plasma concentrations by 2.7- to 12-fold.[91] The drug is primarily metabolized to phase I metabolites, and subsequently to glucuronide metabolites. The half-life is 2.5 to 4.1 hours, and clear-ance is reduced in moderate hepatic insufficiency to the extent that dosage adjust-ments appear warranted. Iclaprim clearance is unaffected by renal insufficiency.[89,92]

A new drug application for iclaprim was submitted to the FDA for treatment of cSSSIs on the basis of combined results from two similar randomized, multicenter, double-blind phase III trials (Assist-1 and Assist-2) versus linezolid.[93] Based on revised analyses by FDA reviewers, iclaprim 0.8 mg/kg every 12 hours failed to achieve non-inferiority versus linezolid for treatment of cSSSI, and was potentially inferior to linezolid in Assist-1.[89] These findings cast doubt on the feasibility of iclaprim for treat-ment of cSSSIs. However, at the time of this writing, a clinical trial comparing iclaprim to vancomycin for treatment of HAP, VAP, or health care–associated pneumonia (HCAP) was currently recruiting.[94]

Overall, iclaprim appears to be fairly well tolerated, but has been associated with gastrointestinal disturbances, including elevations in hepatic transaminases, anemia, pyrexia, headache, and pruritis. Iclaprim also prolongs the QTc interval, but was not associated with any known cases of torsades de pointes or other ventricular arrhyth-mias in phase III studies. The drug may inhibit CYP3A4 and P-glycoprotein, but the clinical significance of any potential resultant drug interactions is uncertain.[89]

The possible role of iclaprim for treatment of infections in the ICU is unclear. Recent FDA advisory committee deliberations suggest that the drug may not have a role for cSSSIs. However, at the time of this writing, iclaprim was undergoing study for HAP/VAP/HCAP, and, pending results, may prove useful as a component of a multi-drug treatment of HAP/VAP/HCAP as a result of its activity against MRSA. However, the absence of P aeruginosa coverage will likely limit the utility of iclaprim as empiric monotherapy for many infections in the ICU setting.

ISAVUCONAZOLE

Isavuconazole (BAL4815 converted from BAL8557) is an investigational IV and oral systemic triazole antifungal agent with broad-spectrum activity against clinically important yeasts and molds. The agent is currently under investigation for treatment of candidemia and other invasive *Candida* infections, as well as invasive aspergillosis.[95] Isavuconazole is active against a wide range of *Candida* species, including *C krusei* and *C glabrata*, and appears to maintain activity against fluconazole-resistant strains.[96,97] As with other azole antifungals, there have been strains of *C glabrata* with elevated MICs reported to isavuconazole.[96] The drug is broadly active against *Aspergillus* (including *A fumigatus, A terreus, A niger*, and *A flavus*), *Cryptococcus* species, and the dimorphic fungi *Histoplasma* and *Blastomyces*.[98–101] However, isavuconazole appears to have limited activity against zygomycetes, with MIC values exceeding those of posaconazole's.[97,102]

Isavuconazole is under investigation in oral and IV dosage forms. The oral formulation has excellent bioavailability that is unaffected by food, and the IV dosage formulation does not require addition of cyclodextrin.[103–106] The compound is rapidly converted by plasma esterases to active isavuconazole, and linear pharmacokinetics are observed.[104] The drug is widely distributed with a Vd of 308 to 542 L, and is 98% protein bound. The drug is slowly eliminated by CYP-mediated hepatic metabolism with a half-life of 85 to 117 hours that is extended in patients with mild-moderate liver impairment.[104,107] The drug is subsequently eliminated primarily in the feces, with only less than 0.4% excreted unchanged in the urine.[104,106]

Results of clinical trials of isavuconazole for treatment of invasive candidiasis or aspergillosis are not yet available. However, isavuconazole has been shown to be effective in neutropenic murine models of invasive candidiasis and aspergillosis.[108,109] Isavuconazole 50 to 100 mg daily as well as a 400 mg weekly regimen has been shown to be noninferior to fluconazole 100 mg/d for treatment of esophageal candidiasis.[110]

Isavuconazole appears to be well tolerated. The most frequent adverse effects are headache, nasopharyngitis, and rhinitis, all of mild-moderate intensity. Reversible elevation in hepatic transaminases has also been reported, as have intercurrent infections, but no ECG abnormalities have been noted.[103,104,110,111] Preliminary data indicate that isavuconazole had no significant impact on the pharmacokinetics of cyclosporine or warfarin, but did significantly increase tacrolimus exposure.[112–114] Rifampin appears to significantly reduce isavuconazole maximum serum concentration (Cmax) and area under the curve, while ketoconazole increases isavuconazole exposure.[115,116] Definitive published data assessing isavuconazole drug interaction potential are not yet available, but the compound may be associated with fewer CYP450-mediated drug interactions than voriconazole or itraconazole.[104,117]

The potential role of isavuconazole for treatment of fungal infections in the ICU setting is not yet clear. Based on in vitro data, as well as some animal model data, the drug does appear to have potential for treatment of invasive candidiasis as well as invasive aspergillosis. Whether isavuconazole can be successfully used for treatment of zygomycete infections is unclear, and its potency against these organisms is inferior to posaconazole's. Its absence of cyclodextrin as an accompanying vehicle removes concern over use in patients with compromised renal function who are at risk for cyclodextrin accumulation and toxicity, which represents a potential advantage over voriconazole in this patient population. Preliminary data suggesting a lower propensity of isavuconazole to cause CYP450-mediated drug interactions than some other azoles may also represent an advantage for the drug in the ICU.

SUMMARY

Emerging antimicrobial resistance has made treatment of infections in the ICU increasingly difficult. A need exists for new antimicrobial agents with activity against resistant gram-positive, gram-negative, and fungal organisms to provide adequate empiric and definitive therapy. Unfortunately, none of the agents discussed in this article are therapeutic advances for treatment of infections caused by the gram-negative ESKAPE pathogens. Due to its combined activity against nosocomial gram-positive and gram-negative pathogens, ceftobiprole appears to be the only agent discussed to have a potential role as empiric monotherapy for some suspected mixed infections in the ICU. Dalbavancin, oritavancin, telavancin, iclaprim, ceftaroline, and ceftobiprole are active against MRSA and some other resistant gram-positive pathogens and appear to have potential for treatment of some serious infectious caused by these organisms. However, data are very limited. For treatment of HAP, VAP, and HCAP, favorable efficacy data had been released only for telavancin and ceftobiprole (non-VAP) at the time of this writing.

Isavuconazole is an antifungal triazole that is broadly active against *Candida* and *Aspergillus*. Whether its absence of cyclodextrin in the formulation and projected favorable drug interaction profile ultimately prove to be clinically significant advantages in the ICU setting remains to be seen.

At the time of this writing, each new agent discussed in this paper was still investigational in the United States, with their ultimate fates on the United States market not yet established.

REFERENCES

1. Kollef MH, Sherman G, Ward S, et al. Inadequate antimicrobial treatment of infections: a risk factor for hospital mortality among critically ill patients. Chest 1999;115:462–74.
2. Ibrahim EH, Sherman G, Ward S, et al. The influence of inadequate antimicrobial treatment of bloodstream infections on patient outcomes in the ICU setting. Chest 2000;118:146–55.
3. Micek ST, Lloyd AE, Ritchie DJ, et al. *Pseudomonas aeruginosa* bloodstream infection: importance of appropriate initial antimicrobial treatment. Antimicrob Agents Chemother 2005;49(4):1306–11.
4. Schramm GE, Johnson JA, Doherty JA, et al. Methicillin-resistant *Staphylococcus aureus* sterile-site infection: the importance of appropriate initial antimicrobial treatment. Crit Care Med 2006;34(8):2069–74.
5. Micek ST, Kollef KE, Reichley RM, et al. Health care-associated pneumonia and community-acquired pneumonia: a single-center experience. Antimicrob Agents Chemother 2007;51(10):3568–73.
6. Morrell M, Fraser VJ, Kollef MH. Delaying the empiric treatment of *Candida* bloodstream infection until positive blood culture results are obtained: a potential risk factor for hospital mortality. Antimicrob Agents Chemother 2005;49(9): 3640–5.
7. Garey KW, Rege M, Pai MP, et al. Time to imitation of fluconazole therapy impacts mortality in patients with candidemia: a multi-institutional study. Clin Infect Dis 2006;43:25–31.
8. Boucher HW, Talbot GH, Bradley JS, et al. Bad bugs, no drugs: no ESKAPE! An update from the Infectious Diseases Society of America. Clin Infect Dis 2009;48: 1–12.

9. Sader HS, Fritsche TR, Kaniga K, et al. Antimicrobial activity and spectrum of PPI-0903M (T-91825), a novel cephalosporin, tested against a worldwide collection of clinical strains. Antimicrob Agents Chemother 2005;49(8):3501–12.

10. Mushtaq S, Warner M, Ge Y, et al. In vitro activity of ceftaroline (PPI-0903M, T-91825) against bacteria with defined resistance mechanisms and phenotypes. J Antimicrob Chemother 2007;60:300–11.

11. Ge Y, Biek D, Talbot GH, et al. In vitro profiling of ceftaroline against a collection of recent bacterial clinical isolates from across the United States. Antimicrob Agents Chemother 2008;52(9):3398–407.

12. Iizawa Y, Nagai J, Ishikawa T, et al. In vitro antimicrobial activity of T-91825, a novel anti-MRSA cephalosporin, and in vivo anti-MRSA activity of its prodrug, TAL-599. J Infect Chemother 2004;10:146–56.

13. Fenoll A, Aguilar L, Robledo O, et al. In vitro activity of ceftaroline against *Streptococcus pneumoniae* isolates exhibiting resistance to penicillin, amoxicillin, and cefotaxime. Antimicrob Agents Chemother 2008;52(11):4209–10.

14. McGee L, Biek D, Ge Y, et al. In vitro evaluation of the antimicrobial activity of ceftaroline against cephalosporin-resistant isolates of *Streptococcus pneumoniae*. Antimicrob Agents Chemother 2009;53(2):552–6.

15. Ge Y, Redman R, Floren L, et al. The pharmacokinetics (PK) and safety of ceftaroline (PPI-0903) in healthy subjects receiving multiple-dose intravenous (IV) infusions. (abstract A-1937). In: abstracts of the 46th Annual Interscience Conference on Antimicrobial Agents and Chemotherapy. San Francisco: September 27–30, 2006.

16. Ge Y, Hubbel A. In vitro evaluation of plasma protein binding and metabolic stability of ceftaroline (PPI-0903). (abstract A-1935). In: abstracts of the 46th Annual Interscience Conference on Antimicrobial Agents and Chemotherapy. San Francisco: September 27–30, 2006.

17. Ge Y, Liao S, Talbot GH. Population pharmacokinetics (PK) analysis of ceftaroline (CPT) in volunteers and patients with complicated skin and skin structure infection (cSSSI). (abstract A-34). In: abstracts of the 47th Annual Interscience Conference on Antimicrobial Agents and Chemotherapy. Chicago: September 17–20, 2007.

18. Ge Y, Thye D, Liao S, et al. Pharmacokinetics (PK) of ceftaroline (PPI-0903) in subjects with mild or moderate renal impairment (RI). (abstract A-1939). In: abstracts of the 46th Annual Interscience Conference on Antimicrobial Agents and Chemotherapy. San Francisco: September 27–30, 2006.

19. Ge Y, Floren L, Redman R, et al. Single-dose pharmacokinetics (PK) of ceftaroline (PPI-0903) in healthy subjects. (abstract A-1936). In: abstracts of the 46th Annual Interscience Conference on Antimicrobial Agents and Chemotherapy. San Francisco: September 27–30, 2006.

20. Jacqueline C, Caillon J, Miegeville A, et al. Penetration of ceftaroline (PPI-0903), a newcephalosporin, into lung tissues: measurement of plasma and lung tissue concentrations after a short IV infusion in the rabbit. (abstract A-1938). In: abstracts of the 46th Annual Interscience Conference on Antimicrobial Agents and Chemotherapy. San Francisco: September 27–30, 2006.

21. Talbot GH, Thye D, Das A, et al. Phase 2 study of ceftaroline versus standard therapy in the treatment of complicated skin and skin structure infections. Antimicrob Agents Chemother 2007;51(10):3612–6.

22. Available at: http://www.clinicaltrials.gov/ct2/results?term=ceftaroline. Accessed February 2, 2009.

23. Fritsche TR, Sader HS, Jones RN. Antimicrobial activity of ceftobiprole, a novel anti-methicillin-resistant *Staphylococcus aureus* cephalosporin, tested against contemporary pathogens: results from the SENTRY antimicrobial surveillance program (2005-2006). Diagn Microbiol Infect Dis 2008;61:86–95.

24. Amsler KM, Davies TA, Shang W, et al. In vitro activity of ceftobiprole against pathogens from two phase 3 clinical trials of complicated skin and skin structure infections. Antimicrob Agents Chemother 2008;52(9):3418–23.

25. Amsler K, Jacobs M, Sahm D, et al. Ceftobiprole activity against baseline pathogens from recent pneumonia trials. (abstract C1-159). In: abstracts of the 48th Annual Interscience Conference on Antimicrobial Agents and Chemotherapy. Washington, DC: October 25–28, 2008.

26. Hebeisen P, Heinze-Krauss I, Angehrn P, et al. In vitro and in vivo properties of Ro-63-9141, a novel broad-spectrum cephalosporin with activity against methicillin-resistant staphylococci. Antimicrob Agents Chemother 2001;45(3):825–36.

27. Queenan AM, Shang W, Kania M, et al. Interactions of ceftobiprole with ß-lactamases from molecular classes A to D. Antimicrob Agents Chemother 2007; 51(9):3089–95.

28. Livermore DM, Hope R, Brick G, et al. Non-susceptibility trends among Enterobacteriaceae from bacteraemias in the UK and Ireland, 2001-06. J Antimicrob Chemother 2008;62(suppl 2):ii41 51.

29. Livermore DM, Hope R, Brick G, et al. Non-susceptibility trends among *Pseudomonas aeruginosa* and other non-fermentative gram-negative bacteria from bacteraemias in the UK and Ireland, 2001-06. J Antimicrob Chemother 2008; 62(suppl 2):ii55–63.

30. Murthy B, Schmitt-Hoffmann A. Pharmacokinetics and pharmacodynamics of ceftobiprole, an anti-MRSA cephalosporin with broad-spectrum activity. Clin Pharmacokinet 2008;47(1):21–33.

31. Kimko H, Murthy B, Balis D, et al. Pharmacokinetics of ceftobiprole (BPR) in patients with ventilator-associated pneumonia (VAP). (abstract A-1881). In: abstracts of the 48th Annual Interscience Conference on Antimicrobial Agents and Chemotherapy. Washington, DC: October 25–28, 2008.

32. Available at: http://www.clinicaltrials.gov/ct2/results?term=ceftobiprole. Accessed February 2, 2009.

33. Schmitt-Hoffmann, Roos B, Schleimer M, A et al. Single-dose pharmacokinetics and safety of a novel broad-spectrum cephalosporin (BAL5788) in healthy volunteers. Antimicrob Agents Chemother. 2004;48(7):2570–5.

34. Schmitt-Hoffmann A, Nyman L, Roos B, et al. Multiple-dose pharmacokinetics and safety of a novel broad-spectrum cephalosporin (BAL5788) in healthy volunteers. Antimicrob Agents Chemother 2004;48(7):2576 80.

35. Lodise TP Jr, Pypstra R, Kahn JB, et al. Probability of target attainment for ceftobiprole as derived from a population pharmacokinetic analysis of 150 subjects. Antimicrob Agents Chemother 2007;51(7):2378–87.

36. Murthy B, Skee D, Vaccaro N, et al. An open-label pharmacokinetic study of ceftobiprole in healthy subjects and subjects with end-stage renal disease receiving hemodialysis. (abstract A-1896). In: abstracts of the 48th Annual Interscience Conference on Antimicrobial Agents and Chemotherapy. Washington, DC: October 25–28, 2008.

37. Noel GJ, Strauss RS, Amsler K, et al. Results of a double-blind, randomized trial of ceftobiprole treatment of complicated skin and skin structure infections caused by gram-positive bacteria. Antimicrob Agents Chemother 2008;52(1): 37–44.

38. Noel GJ, Bush K, Bagchi P, et al. A randomized, double-blind trial comparing ceftobiprole medocaril with vancomycin plus ceftazidime for the treatment of patients with complicated skin and skin structure infections. Clin Infect Dis 2008;46:647–55.

39. Noel GJ, Strauss RS, Shah A, et al. Ceftobiprole versus ceftazidime combined with linezolid for treatment of patients with nosocomial pneumonia. (abstract K-486). In: abstracts of the 48th Annual Interscience Conference on Antimicrobial Agents and Chemotherapy. Washington, DC: October 25–28, 2008.

40. Baum EZ, Crespo-Carbone SM, Foleno BD, et al. MexXY expression in *Pseudomonas aeruginosa* (PsA) and susceptibility to cephalosporins, including ceftobiprole. (abstract C1-158). In: abstracts of the 48th Annual Interscience Conference on Antimicrobial Agents and Chemotherapy. Washington, DC: October 25–28, 2008.

41. Queenan AM, Shang W, Crespo-Carbone S, et al. Mechanisms of ceftobiprole and ceftazidime resistance development in gram-negative clinical isolates from cSSSI subjects. (abstract C1-154). In: abstracts of the 48th Annual Interscience Conference on Antimicrobial Agents and Chemotherapy. Washington, DC: October 25–28, 2008.

42. Zhanel GG, Trapp S, Gin AS, et al. Dalbavancin and telavancin: novel lipoglycopeptides for the treatment of gram-positive infections. Expert Rev Ant Infect Ther 2008;6(1):67–81.

43. Van Bambeke F, Van Laethem YV, Courvalin P, et al. Glycopeptide antibiotics from conventional molecules to new derivatives. Drugs 2004;64(9):913–36.

44. Malabarba A, Goldstein BP. Origin, structure, and activity in vitro and in vivo of dalbavancin. J Antimicrob Chemother 2005;55(suppl S2):ii15–20.

45. Candiani G, Abbondi M, Borgonovi M, et al. In-vitro and in-vivo antibacterial activity of BI 397, a new semi-synthetic glycopeptide antibiotic. J Antimicrob Chemother 1999;44:179–92.

46. Van Bambeke F. Glycopeptides and glycodepsipeptides in clinical development: a comparative review of their antibacterial spectrum, pharmacokinetics, and clinical efficacy. Curr Opin Investig Drugs 2006;7(8):740–9.

47. Goldstein BP, Draghi DC, Sheehan DJ, et al. Bactericidal activity and resistance development profiling of dalbavancin. Antimicrob Agents Chemother 2007; 51(4):1150–4.

48. Chen AY, Zervos MJ, Vazquez JA. Dalbavancin: a novel antimicrobial. Int J Clin Pract 2007;61(5):853–63.

49. Lin S-W, Carver PL, DePestel DD. Dalbavancin: a new option for the treatment of gram-positive infections. Ann Pharmacother 2006;40:449–60.

50. Jauregui LE, Babazadeh S, Seltzer E, et al. Randomized, double-blind comparison of once-weekly dalbavancin versus twice-daily linezolid therapy for the treatment of complicated skin and skin structure infections. Clin Infect Dis 2005;41:1407–15.

51. Seltzer E, Dorr M, Goldstein BP, et al. Once-weekly dalbavancin versus standard-of-care antimicrobial regimens for treatment of skin and soft-tissue infections. Clin Infect Dis 2003;37:1298–303.

52. Raad I, Darouiche R, Vazquez J, et al. Efficacy and safety of weekly dalbavancin therapy for catheter-related bloodstream infection caused by gram-positive pathogens. Clin Infect Dis 2005;40:374–80.

53. Leighton A, Gottlieb A, Dorr M, et al. Tolerability, pharmacokinetics, and serum bactericidal activity of intravenous dalbavancin in healthy volunteers. Antimicrob Agents Chemother 2004;48(3):940–5.

54. Available at: http://mediaroom.pfizer.com/news/pfizer/20080909005943/en. Accessed January 6, 2009.
55. Mercier R-C, Hrebickova L. Oritavancin: a new avenue for resistant gram-positive bacteria. Expert Rev Anti Infect Ther 2005;3(3):325–32.
56. Tenover FC, Lancaster MV, Hill BC, et al. Characterization of staphylococci with reduced susceptibilities to vancomycin and other glycopeptides. J Clin Microbiol 1998;36(4):1020–7.
57. Judice JK, Pace JL. Semi-synthetic glycopeptide antibacterials. Bioorg Med Chem Lett 2003;13:4165–8.
58. Lehoux D, McKay G, Fadhil I, et al. Efficacy of oritavancin in a mouse model of *Streptococcus pneumoniae* pneumonia. (abstract P1781). In: Program and abstracts of the European Society of Clinical Microbiology and Infectious Diseases 25th ICC. Munich: March 31–April 3, 2007.
59. Bhavnani SM, Owen JS, Loutit JS, et al. Pharmacokinetics, safety, and tolerability of ascending single intravenous doses of oritavancin administered to healthy human subjects. Diagn Microbiol Infect Dis 2004;50:95–102.
60. Van Bambeke F, Saffran J, Mingeot-Leclercq M-P, et al. Mixed-lipid storage disorder induced in macrophages and fibroblasts by oritavancin (LY333328), a new glycopeptide antibiotic with exceptional cellular accumulation. Antimicrob Agents Chemother 2005;49(5):1695–700.
61. A study for patients with complicated skin and skin structure infections (SIMPLIFI). Available at: http://clinicaltrials.gov/ct2/show/NCT00514527?term=oritavancin& rank=1. Accessed February 1, 2009.
62. Loutit JS, O'Riordan W, San Juan J, et al. Phase 2 trial comparing four regimens of oritavancin vs. comparator in the treatment of patients with *S. aureus* bacteraemia. (abstract P541). Clin Microbiol Infect 2004;10(issue s3):122.
63. Kaatz GW, Seo SM, Aeschlimann JR, et al. Efficacy of LY333328 against experimental methicillin-resistant *Staphylococcus aureus* endocarditis. Antimicrob Agents Chemother 1998;42(4):981–3.
64. Lefort A, Saleh-Mghir A, Garry L, et al. Activity of LY333328 combined with gentamicin in vitro and in rabbit experimental endocarditis due to vancomycin-susceptible or -resistant *Enterococcus faecalis*. Antimicrob Agents Chemother 2000;44(11):3017–20.
65. Gerber J, Smirnov A, Wellmer A, et al. Activity of LY333328 in experimental meningitis caused by a *Streptococcus pneumoniae* strain susceptible to penicillin. Antimicrob Agents Chemother 2001;45(7):2169–72.
66. Cabellos C, Fernandez A, Maiques JM, et al. Experimental study of LY333328 (oritavancin), alone and in combination, in therapy of cephalosporin-resistant pneumococcal meningitis. Antimicrob Agents Chemother 2003;47(6):1907–11.
67. Available at: http://www.investorcalendar.com/IC/GenRelease.asp?ID=138672. Accessed February 1, 2009.
68. Leonard SN, Rybak MJ. Telavancin: an antimicrobial with a multifunctional mechanism of action for the treatment of serious gram-positive infections. Pharmacotherapy 2008;28(4):458–68.
69. Attwood RJ, LaPlante KL. Telavancin: a novel lipoglycopeptide antimicrobial agent. Am J Health Syst Pharm 2007;64:2335–48.
70. King A, Phillips I, Kaniga K. Comparative in vitro activity of telavancin (TD-6424), a rapidly bactericidal, concentration-dependent anti-infective with multiple mechanisms of action against gram-positive bacteria. J Antimicrob Chemother 2004;53:797–803.

71. Gander S, Kinnaird A, Finch R. Telavancin: in vitro activity against staphylococci in a biofilm model. J Antimicrob Chemother 2005;56:337–43.

72. Leuthner KD, Cheung CM, Rybak MJ. Comparative activity of the new lipoglycopeptide telavancin in the presence and absence of serum against 50 glycopeptide non-susceptible staphylococci and three vancomycin-resistant Staphylococcus aureus. J Antimicrob Chemother 2006;58:338–43.

73. Dunbar LM, Tang DM, Manausa RM. A review of telavancin in the treatment of complicated skin and skin structure infections (cSSSI). Ther Clin Risk Manag 2008;4(1):235–44.

74. Available at: http://ir.theravance.com/ReleaseDetail.cfm?ReleaseID=279919. Accessed January 6, 2009.

75. Available at: http://ir.theravance.com/ReleaseDetail.cfm?ReleaseID=348983. Accessed January 24, 2009.

76. Schneider P, Hawser S, Islam K. Iclaprim, a novel diaminopyrimidine with potent activity on trimethoprim sensitive and resistant bacteria. Bioorg Med Chem Lett 2003;13:4217–21.

77. Hawser S, Lociuro S, Islam K. Dihydrofolate reductase inhibitors as antibacterial agents. Biochem Pharmacol 2006;71:941–8.

78. Laue H, Weiss L, Bernardi A, et al. In vitro activity of the novel diaminopyrimidine, iclaprim, in combination with folate inhibitors and other antimicrobials with different mechanisms of action. J Antimicrob Chemother 2007; 60:1391–4.

79. Bozdogan B, Esel D, Whitener C, et al. Antibacterial susceptibility of a vancomycin-resistant Staphylococcus aureus strain isolated at the Hershey Medical center. J Antimicrob Chemother 2003;52:864–8.

80. Mason E, Lamberth L, Hawser S, et al. In-vitro activity of iclaprim against community-acquired and nosocomial clinical isolates of Staphylococcus aureus (abstract E-904). In: abstracts of the 47th Annual Interscience Conference on Antimicrobial Agents and Chemotherapy. Chicago: September 17–20, 2007.

81. Sader HS, Jones RN, Rhomberg P, et al. Comparativeevaluation of iclaprim potency and bactericidal activity tested against enterococci; results from the International Study of Iclaprim Susceptibility (ISIS) (abstract E-910). In: abstracts of the 47th Annual Interscience Conference on Antimicrobial Agents and Chemotherapy. Chicago: September 17–20, 2007.

82. Jones RN, Fritsche TR, Hawser S, et al. In vitro activityof iclaprim, a novel diaminopyrimidine, tested against ß-hemolytic streptococci from the USA and Europe: results from the International Study of Iclaprim Susceptibility (ISIS) (abstract E-911). In: abstracts of the 47th Annual Interscience Conference on Antimicrobial Agents and Chemotherapy. Chicago: September 17–20, 2007.

83. Hawser S, Lociuro S, Islam K. In vitro spectrum of activity of iclaprim against various Gram-positive and Gram-negative pathogens (poster CPLA-32). Presented at: The third International Symposium on Resistant Gram-positive Infections. Niagara-on-the-Lake, Ontario: October 9–11, 2006.

84. Jones RN, Fritsche TR, Islam K, et al. Antimicrobial activity of a novel dihydrofolate reductase, iclaprim, tested against clinical strains of Enterobacteriaceae: results from the International Study of Iclaprim Susceptibility (ISIS) (abstract E-909). In: abstracts of the 47th Annual Interscience Conference on Antimicrobial Agents and Chemotherapy. Chicago: September 17–20, 2007.

85. Kohlhoff SA, Roblin PM, Reznik T, et al. In vitro activity of a novel diaminopyrimidine compound, iclaprim, against Chlamydia trachomatis and C. pneumoniae. Antimicrob Agents Chemother 2004;48(5):1885–6.

86. Morrissey I, Hawser S. Activity of iclaprim against Legionella pneumophila. J Antimicrob Chemother 2007;60:905–6.
87. Proctor RA. Role of folate antagonists in the treatment of methicillin-resistant Staphylococcus aureus infection. Clin Infect Dis 2008;46:584–93.
88. Haldimann A, Hawser S, Bihr M, et al. Effect of thymidine on the activity of diaminopyrimidine antibacterial agents: generation and characterization of thymidine kinase-deficient Staphylococcus aureus mutants (abstract C1-940). In: abstracts of the 46th Annual Interscience Conference on Antimicrobial Agents and Chemotherapy. San Francisco: September 27–30, 2006.
89. Food and Drug Administration (FDA). FDA briefing document for Anti-infective Drugs Advisory Committee Meeting, November 20, 2008 (Iclaprim for the treatment of complicated skin and skin structure infection). Available at: http://fda.gov/ohrms/dockets/ac/08/briefing/2008-4394b3-01-FDA.pdf. Accessed December 23, 2008.
90. Brandt R, Neuenhofer D, Thomsen T, et al. Pharmacokinetics and bioavailability of iclaprim oral and intravenous formulations in humans. (abstract A-806). In: abstracts of the 47th Annual Interscience Conference on Antimicrobial Agents and Chemotherapy. Chicago: September 17–20, 2007.
91. Andrews J, Honeybourne D, Ashby J, et al. Concentrations in plasma, epithelial lining fluid, alveolar macrophages and bronchial mucosa after a single intravenous dose of 1.6 mg/kg of Iclaprim (AR-100) in healthy men. J Antimicrob Chemother 2007;60:677–80.
92. Hadvary P, de la Motte S, Klinger J, et al. Pharmacokinetics of iclaprim in subjects with varying degree of hepatic or renal insufficiency or obesity. (poster 448). In: abstracts of the 45th Annual Meeting of the Infectious Diseases Society of America. San Diego: October 4–7, 2007.
93. Hadvary P, Stevens D, Solonets M, et al. Clinical efficacy of iclaprim in complicated skin and skin structure infection (cSSSI): results of combined ASSIST phase III studies. (abstract L-1512). In: abstracts of the 48th Annual Interscience Conference on Antimicrobial Agents and Chemotherapy. Washington, DC: October 25–28, 2008.
94. Clinical efficacy of intravenous iclaprim versus vancomycin in the treatment of hospital-acquired, ventilator-associated, or health-care-associated pneumonia. http://www.clinicaltrials.gov/ct2/show/NCT00543608?term=iclaprim&rank=1. Accessed January 2, 2009.
95. Available at: http://www.clinicaltrials.gov/ct2/results?term=isavuconazole. Accessed January 2, 2009.
96. Seifert H, Aurbach U, Stefanik D, et al. In vitro activities of isavuconazole and other antifungal agents against Candida bloodstream isolates. Antimicrob Agents Chemother 2007;51(5):1818–21.
97. Guinea J, Pelaez T, Recio S, et al. In vitro activities of isavuconazole (BAL4815), voriconazole, and fluconazole against 1,007 isolates of zygomycete, Candida, Aspergillus, Fusarium, and Scedosporium species. Antimicrob Agents Chemother 2008;52(4):1396–400.
98. Warn PA, Sharp A, Denning DW. In vitro activity of a new triazole BAL4815, the active component of BAL8557 (the water-soluble prodrug), against Aspergillus spp. J Antimicrob Chemother 2006;57:135–8.
99. Illnait-Zaragozi M-T, Martinez GF, Curfs-Breuker I, et al. In vitro activity of the new azole isavuconazole (BAL4815) compared with six other antifungal agents against 162 Cryptococcus neoformans isolates from Cuba. Antimicrob Agents Chemother 2008;52(4):1580–2.

100. Martin de la Escalera C, Aller AI, Lopez-Oviedo E, et al. Activity of BAL 4815 against filamentous fungi. J Antimicrob Chemother 2008;61:1083–6.

101. Gonzalez GM. In vitro activities of isavuconazole against opportunistic filamentous and dimorphic fungi. Med Mycol 2009;47(1):71–6.

102. Perkhofer S, Lechner V, Lass-Florl C. The in vitro activity of isavuconazole against Aspergillus species and zygomycetes according to EUCAST methodology (abstract M-1526). In: abstracts of the 48th Annual Interscience Conference on Antimicrobial Agents and Chemotherapy. Washington, DC: October 25–28, 2008.

103. Schmitt-Hoffmann A, Roos B, Heep M, et al. Single-ascending-dose pharmacokinetics and safety of the novel broad-spectrum antifungal triazole BAL4815 after intravenous infusions (50, 100, and 200 milligrams) and oral administrations (100, 200, and 400 milligrams) of its prodrug, BAL8557, in healthy volunteers. Antimicrob Agents Chemother 2006;50(1):279–85.

104. Schmitt-Hoffmann A, Roos B, Maares J, et al. Multiple-dose pharmacokinetics and safety of the new antifungal triazole BAL4815 after intravenous infusion and oral administration of its prodrug, BAL8557, in healthy volunteers. Antimicrob Agents Chemother 2006;50(1):286–93.

105. Schmitt-Hoffmann A, Roos B, Roehrle M, et al. No relevant food effect in man on isavuconazole oral pharmacokinetics preliminary data (abstract A-008). In: abstracts of the 48th Annual Interscience Conference on Antimicrobial Agents and Chemotherapy. Washington, DC: October 25–28, 2008.

106. Ohwada J, Tsukazaki M, Hayase T, et al. Design, synthesis and antifungal activity of a novel water soluble prodrug of antifungal triazole. Bioorg Med Chem Lett 2003;13:191–6.

107. Schmitt-Hoffmann A, Roos B, Peterfai E, et al. Pharmacokinetics of isavuconazole in liver impairment. Preliminary data. (abstract A-007). In: abstracts of the 48th Annual Interscience Conference on Antimicrobial Agents and Chemotherapy. Washington, DC: October 25–28, 2008.

108. Warn PA, Sharp A, Mosquera J, et al. Comparative in vivo activity of BAL4815, the active component of the prodrug BAL8557, in a neutropenic murine model of disseminated Aspergillus flavus. J Antimicrob Chemother 2006;58:1198–207.

109. Majithiya J, Sharp A, Parmar A, et al. Efficacy of isavuconazole, voriconazole, and fluconazole in temporarily neutropenic murine models of disseminated Candida tropicalis and Candida krusei. J Antimicrob Chemother 2009;63:161–6.

110. Viljoen JJ, Mitha I, Heep M, et al. Efficacy, safety, and tolerability of three different dosing regimens of BAL8557 vs. fluconazole in a double-blind, randomized, multicenter trial for the treatment of esophageal candidiasis in immunocompromised hosts (abstract LB2-32). In: abstracts of the 45th Annual Interscience Conference on Antimicrobial Agents and Chemotherapy. Washington, DC: December 16–19, 2005.

111. Cornely OA, Bohme A, Reichert D, et al. Pharmacokinetics, safety, and tolerability results from a dose-escalation study of isavuconazole in neutropenic patients (abstract M-2137). In: abstracts of the 48th Annual Interscience Conference on Antimicrobial Agents and Chemotherapy. Washington, DC: October 25–28, 2008.

112. Schmitt-Hoffmann A, Roos B, Sauer J, et al. Effect of BAL8557, a water-soluble azole pro-drug, on the pharmacokinetics of ciclosporin (abstract P-0136). In: abstracts of The 16th Congress of the International Society for Human and Animal Mycology. Paris: June 26–29, 2006.

113. Schmitt-Hoffmann A, Roos B, Sauer J, et al. Effectof BAL8557, a water-soluble azole pro-drug, on the pharmacokinetics of tacrolimus. (abstract P-0320). In: abstracts of The 16th Congress of the International Society for Human and Animal Mycology. Paris: June 26–29, 2006.

114. Schmitt-Hoffmann A, Roos B, Sauer J, et al. Effect of BAL8557, a water-soluble azole pro-drug, on the pharmacokinetics of S- and R-warfarin (abstract P-0321). In: abstracts of The 16th Congress of the International Society for Human and Animal Mycology. Paris: June 26–29, 2006.

115. Schmitt-Hoffmann A, Roos B, Sauer J, et al. Effectof ketoconazole on the pharmacokinetics of BAL4815 at steady state after multiple oral daily doses of BAL8557 (WSA) and ketoconazole (abstract P-0318). In: abstracts of The 16th Congress of the International Society for Human and Animal Mycology. Paris: June 26–29, 2006.

116. Schmitt-Hoffmann A, Roos B, Sauer J, et al. Effectof rifampicin on the pharmacokinetics of BAL4815 at steady state after multiple oral daily doses of BAL8557 and rifampicin. (abstract P-0319). In: abstracts of The 16th Congress of the International Society for Human and Animal Mycology. Paris: June 26–29, 2006.

117. Pasqualetto AC, Denning DW. New and emerging treatments for fungal infections. J Antimicrob Chemother 2008;61(suppl. 1):i19–30.

Antimicrobial Stewardship: Application in the Intensive Care Unit

Robert C. Owens, Jr, PharmD[a,b],*

KEYWORDS

• Intensive care unit • C difficile • Antimicrobial stewardship

Because microbes account for 90% of the cells in the human body, it is of the essence to avoid perturbation of normal flora when possible.[1] It is indisputable that, for certain infections, particularly those seen in the intensive care unit (ICU), antimicrobials provide great benefit. The flipside is: at what cost? Given the number of cells in our body that are not our own, antimicrobial therapy will inevitably result in collateral damage that will occur to those bacteria that comprise each host's colonization resistance. The two most common consequences of altering colonization resistance are the development of potentially life-threatening *Clostridium difficile* infection and the emergence of resistance.[2,3] ICU clinicians balance these each day as they weigh risk versus benefit.

The prophecy made decades ago could not be further from being fulfilled. In 1956, noted microbiologist Ernest Jawetz[4] wrote: "On the whole, the position of antimicrobial agents in medical therapy is highly satisfactory. The majority of bacterial infections can be cured simply, effectively, and cheaply. The mortality and morbidity from bacterial diseases has fallen so low that they are no longer among the important unsolved problems of medicine. These accomplishments are widely known and appreciated..." In the current antimicrobial era, 60-plus years after these initially optimistic observations were made, an increasing number of infections are no longer easily treated, morbidity and mortality are appreciable, many infectious diseases (IDs) have become unsolved problems of modern medicine, and novel antimicrobials have stopped pouring out of the once fertile antimicrobial pipeline.[5]

[a] Department of Clinical Pharmacy Services and Division of Infectious Diseases, Maine Medical Center, 22 Bramhall Street, Portland, ME 04102, USA
[b] Department of Medicine, University of Vermont, College of Medicine, Burlington, VT 05401, USA
* Department of Clinical Pharmacy Services, Maine Medical Center, 22 Bramhall Street, Portland, ME 04102.
E-mail address: owensr@mmc.org

Infect Dis Clin N Am 23 (2009) 683–702
doi:10.1016/j.idc.2009.04.015
0891-5520/09/$ – see front matter © 2009 Elsevier Inc. All rights reserved.

id.theclinics.com

Jawetz[4] also, however, prophesized about something that has plagued both inpatient and outpatient antimicrobial use since antimicrobials were made widely available: "... the author wishes to call attention to the abuse of antibiotics, its causes and results..." Published data note that many prescribers still do not fully value the importance of preserving these therapeutic resources. Twenty-five million pounds of antibiotics are produced yearly for human consumption and are administered to 30% to 50% of hospitalized patients. Nonhospitalized Americans receive 160 million courses.[6] Superimposed on this, data suggest that as much as 50% to 99% of antimicrobial use is inappropriate.[7,8] Use in the ICU is not exempt from this. One paper noted that, of nearly 2000 antibiotic-use days in an ICU setting, nearly one third of antimicrobial use was inappropriate.[9] The most common reasons? Treatment duration was too excessive and treatment of noninfectious entities, such as colonization or what some term "furosemide-responsive pneumonia". Several recent papers have called attention to the facts that we are running out of therapeutic options to treat bacterial infections, and that infections are becoming increasingly resistant.[5,10] Established principles are established for optimizing antimicrobial use.[11] The biggest issue I have witnessed is that these principles are not consistently being applied with appropriate patients in the ICU or throughout the hospital. For a variety of reasons, stewarding our precious antimicrobial resources has become a priority for many organizations—particularly following the publication of stewardship guidelines from the Infectious Diseases Society of America (IDSA), the Society of Healthcare Epidemiology of America (SHEA), the Society of Infectious Diseases Pharmacists, the Alliance for the Prudent Use of Antimicrobials, the Centers for Disease Control and Prevention, and the World Health Organization, Surgical Infection Society.[11,12]

Since the pioneering work of Finland and McGowan, a variety of interventional strategies have been shown to reduce unnecessary antimicrobial use, to optimize the dose and duration, and to minimize the collateral adverse effects of their use.[13–17] Most studies have evaluated the impact of interventions on inpatient antimicrobial use and, to a lesser degree, outpatient antimicrobial use. The intention of this article is to focus on interventions germane to the ICU setting, where patients are more likely to receive antimicrobials and are more likely to suffer the consequences of inappropriate therapy.

OPTIMIZING ANTIMICROBIAL USE
Antimicrobial Resistance

Data have demonstrated misuse of antimicrobials and have clearly shown that infections due to resistant organisms are increasing.[10] Optimizing antimicrobial use through appropriate selection, dosing, and duration can be viewed as a strategy to minimize the development of resistance among clinically important pathogens.[18] Factors promoting resistance are complex, numerous, and extend beyond the use of antimicrobial agents in humans. As such, it is not surprising that they do not allow for a prompt resolution.[19] An underappreciated role in all of this is the environment where C difficile, methicillin-resistant Staphylococcus aureus (MRSA), vancomycin-resistant Enterococci, multiple-drug resistant gram-negative bacilli such as extended-spectrum β-lactamase–producing Escherichia coli and Klebsiella spp, and Acinetobacter spp and Pseudomonas aeruginosa lurk.[20,21] Thus, although antimicrobial stewardship interventions are crucial, they cannot displace or be unbundled from the infection-prevention initiatives of increased cleaning of both the environment and our hands.

For the establishment of antimicrobial stewardship as a means to curb antimicrobial resistance, first one must understand that antimicrobial use, both appropriate and inappropriate, leads to conditions favoring the selection of antimicrobial-resistant organisms. Levy and colleagues[22] developed a biologic model that showed a clear relationship between antimicrobial use and the selection of resistance in humans. Furthermore, decades of supportive data exist, ranging from in vitro studies, ecological investigations correlating drug exposure with resistance, controlled trials in which patients with prior use of antimicrobials were more likely to be colonized or infected with resistant bacteria, and prospective studies in which drug use was associated with the development of resistant flora.[22-24]

For health care-acquired infections, antimicrobial resistance is a significant impediment to the empirical treatment of infections. Though treatment may be appropriate, the dose may be incorrect or the antimicrobial regimen may not be employed in a timely manner. Selection of the wrong antimicrobial at the incorrect dose has measurable effects on patient outcomes as reviewed and highlighted by several recent studies.[25-27] The most common reason for these medical errors is antimicrobial-resistant organisms that were not anticipated by the prescriber. Thus, oversight and accountability of antimicrobials makes sense in order to ascertain why this is occurring and how to fix it—within a particular hospital or a particular unit or groups of units.

Patient Safety

Antimicrobials, whether being used appropriately or inappropriately, have the potential for causing serious harm to patients beyond to the previously discussed harm of antimicrobial resistance. QT-interval prolongation, metabolic liability (P450 inhibition, induction), severe dermal manifestation (Stevens-Johnson syndrome, toxic epidermal necrolysis), and, finally, C difficile infection.[3,28-31] Disturbingly, the rate and severity of C difficile infection is increasing and traditional treatment options appear to be less effective.[32,33]

The potential harm caused by antimicrobials should incentivize even the most temerarious clinicians to not casually prescribe antimicrobials for a clinically stable patient with a suspicion of nonbacterial infection (eg, positive influenza swab); or to stop therapy in a timely manner.[2] The patient safety movement in the United States should consider patient safety issues in the context of medical errors (ie, infecting pathogen is resistant to the empirically prescribed treatment). Exclusion of this discussion from any patient safety initiative only sweeps this under the carpet for later generations to deal with.

PROGRAMS TO OPTIMIZE ANTIMICROBIAL USE
Hospital-Based Antimicrobial Stewardship Programs

While more research is needed, a variety of studies evaluating the impact of interventions on antimicrobial use in health care systems already exists. These studies have been conducted using a wide range of resources, methodologies, interventions (often multiple), and outcome measures (usually considering cost, antimicrobial consumption, patient safety, and, less frequently, resistance). The distillation of existing literature in this area, including studies done in the ICU, led to a guidance document developed jointly by IDSA and SHEA to provide the framework for developing, implementing, and monitoring the impact of antimicrobial stewardship programs (ASP).[11]

Guidelines for Developing an Institutional Program to Enhance Antimicrobial Stewardship

An effective ASP is financially self-supporting and is aligned with patient safety goals.[14,34-40] For these reasons, there should be no excuse for an institution to not have a formal program dedicated to improving the quality of antimicrobial use. Realizing that institutions vary in size and type of specialty services offered, the ASP should be customized accordingly.

Interventional Strategy

Two major styles have evolved over recent years. The first is the prospective audit and feedback ("back-end") program. This entails obtaining a daily (or 2 to 3 days per week for smaller hospitals) list of patients receiving antimicrobials and determining potential interventions in a supplemental strategy session. Recommendations are provided to the prescriber in written form or by direct conversation. Written forms of communication typically take place on nonpermanent forms placed in the patient's medical record that are removed at discharge. This allows flexibility in what can be written and allows the ASP team member to communicate educational messages effectively and to provide citations or references as to why the intervention is being recommended. The benefits of this type of program are its customizability to smaller or larger health care facilities[15,36,38] and maintenance of the prescriber's autonomy (increasing "buy-in"). Additionally, it circumvents the potential for delays in initiating timely antimicrobial therapy. The downside is that recommendations are optional. However, there are methods for correcting antimicrobial misuse, which is why a close relationship with the pharmacy and therapeutics committee—ultimately ascending to the medical executive committee, critical care committee, patient safety committee, etc—is essential. The program at Maine Medical Center has successfully employed this primary strategy for nearly a decade in a community hospital setting,[14,36,37] and others have been existence for far longer.[35]

With preauthorization ("front-end") strategy, most antimicrobials are restricted to an approval process. Here, a team member carries a pager or telephone and receives approval requests for restricted antimicrobials. At the time of interaction, the use of the antimicrobial is justified or an alternative recommendation is given. This strategy has traditionally been employed at larger teaching hospitals.[41–44] The benefits of this strategy include the ability to funnel all initial antimicrobial prescribing through experts versed in antimicrobial therapy, and immediate and significant cost savings. Numerous downsides to this strategy exist, including: (1) loss of prescriptive autonomy that often leads to "gaming the system"[45] and fosters potentially adversarial relationships, (2) potential for delays in initially appropriate therapy, (3) intensive resource use, usually 7-days per week with contingency plans for night coverage, (4) decisions are made when the least amount of information is known about the actual infection (culture and susceptibility results often are not available for 2 to 3 days), and (5) the quality of information relayed to the ASP team member by prescriber can be suspect.[46,47] Also, it typically ties up all resources and does not allow focus on any type of back-end stewardship intervention such as de-escalation and stopping antibiotics, perhaps some of the most important interventions of all.

Although ASPs may lean toward one of the two primary strategies, overlap often exists. For example, our program, while relying primarily on prospective audit and feedback, does incorporate a limited number of antimicrobials that require approval (not consultation).[14] To help the clinician navigate the empirical antibiotic-selection process, a trend toward the use of computerized decision support is beginning to take the place of preauthorization. Thus, what is being used more often is a blend of the former strategy (prospective audit with feedback) with the use of computerized decision support to provide expertise on both the front and back ends of antimicrobial prescribing.

Team Members

The IDSA-SHEA guidelines for developing an institutional program to enhance antimicrobial stewardship are very clear about the following: the ASP is directed or codirected by the two core team members, an ID physician and an ID-trained pharmacist, both receiving remuneration for their time.[11] The pharmacist should have formal training in IDs or be knowledgeable in the appropriate use of antimicrobials with training available to maintain competency. In the critical care arena, it is more commonplace to have intensivists, surgeons, and critical care pharmacists capable of doing day-to-day operations within their units. However, nothing replaces the accountability and additional expertise of dedicated, hospital-wide physicians and pharmacists whose job it is to oversee the utilization of antimicrobials. Other team members would optimally include a dedicated computer information support specialist, microbiologist, an infection control practitioner or hospital epidemiologist, and leaders knowledgeable in high-volume antimicrobial-use areas such as the ICU, surgery, and the emergency department. In fact, running an ASP is daunting because relying on colleagues in particular areas to ensure interventions are performed is almost an absolute necessity at any moderate- to large-size hospital. Most would argue to avoid duplication of efforts, so long as the interventions are being done. Administrative and committee support (eg, pharmacy and therapeutics committee) is critical. The particular interventional philosophy, responsibilities, remuneration, and reporting measures should be discussed in advance of implementation so that expectations and resources can be addressed. Effective communication between the ASP and administration and an appropriate committee should be maintained to facilitate dialogue as the health care environment continues to change.

PROSPECTIVE AUDIT AND FEEDBACK, AND PREAUTHORIZATION STUDIES
Prospective Audit and Feedback Strategy

Fraser and colleagues[36] designed a prospective, randomized, controlled study of interventions for targeted antimicrobials in hospitalized patients in a community teaching hospital (600 beds). The team included a part-time ID physician and a Doctor of Pharmacy (PharmD) with antimicrobial expertise. The intervention group (n = 141) received suggestions (written or verbal), but the control group (n = 111) did not. Controlling for severity of illness between groups, outcomes were similar with respect to clinical and microbiological response to therapy, adverse events, inpatient mortality, and readmission rates. Interventions included change to oral therapy (31%), regimen or dosing changes (42%), stopping therapy (10%), ordering additional laboratory tests (18%); and 85% of the suggestions were instituted. Multiple logistic regression models identified the intervention group as the sole predictor of lower antimicrobial expenditures. A conservative annual reduction in antimicrobial expenditures of $97,500 was realized. The intervention group also showed a trend toward reduced mean length of stay compared to control (20 days versus 24 days, respectively). Fifty percent of patients receiving targeted regimens had their treatment refined on the third day of therapy resulting in narrower spectrum therapy, lower antimicrobial costs, and most importantly, reducing antimicrobial use did not adversely affect patient outcomes. This study was later used as a platform to implement an ASP that is more robust in terms of the types of activities and numbers of patients served by the program. The original study excluded patients from the ICU. It is mentioned here because of the template it provides. The systematic program that resulted from this study does include the ICU. The team currently includes a part-time ID physician (2 hours per day, 5 days per week) and a full-time ID PharmD.

At the other end of the spectrum, at a large (1000 bed) teaching facility, Srinivasan and colleagues[48] studied the impact of an antimicrobial management program on antimicrobial expenditures. Prior to the introduction of a comprehensive ASP, the hospital utilized a closed formulary system and employed prior approval requirements on a number of antimicrobials. The ASP consisted of a hospital-funded ID physician, ID PharmD, and data analyst. The team concurrently reviewed antimicrobial therapy in all areas of the hospital except pediatrics and oncology. Their interventions included a survey, use of institution specific guidelines, concurrent antimicrobial review, and educational sessions. A "knowledge, attitude, and beliefs" survey was used to determine awareness of antimicrobial use and resistance, and to detect deficiencies in knowledge that could lead to targeted education among staff. Only 18% viewed the program as an obstacle to patient care and 70% wanted additional feedback on antimicrobial choices. Hospital guidelines were published and updated annually. Antimicrobial therapy interventions occurred before culture and susceptibility results were available only when actively solicited, or when prior authorization of an antimicrobial agent was called for. For all others, interventions were suggested at the time the microbiological data became available. Compliance with recommendations by the ASP was 79%. Costs for antimicrobial agents for the covered areas decreased by 6.4% the first year and 2.2% the second year. Assuming a steady inflation rate of 4.5%, savings translated to $224,753 and $413,998 for fiscal years 2002 and 2003.

Bantar and colleagues[49] demonstrated the impact of their ASP's interventional program on antimicrobial use, cost savings, and antimicrobial resistance. The ASP consisted of an ID physician, two pharmacists, a microbiologist and laboratory technologist, an internal medicine physician, and a computer systems analyst. The strategy selected in this multiphase study was one of education with human intervention rather than use of restrictions. The program periods were associated with declining cost savings as time advanced (periods II, III, and IV were associated with a reduction of $261,955, $57,245, and $12,881, respectively). Comparison of antibiotic order forms from period I (voluntary form and preintervention, n = 450) with period IV (mandatory form with active intervention, n = 349) showed an increase in microbiologically-based treatment intent (27% versus 62.8%, respectively, P<.0001). Twenty-seven percent of the period IV antibiotic order forms were intervened on by the team. Of the interventions, either the dose or duration (not specified) was reduced in 11.5%, 86.1% were associated with cost reduction, and 47% involved streamlining therapy to a narrower choice. In terms of impact on nosocomial infection, length of hospitalization, and mortality, only length of stay was impacted significantly (P = .04). The increased rate of cefepime use relative to third-generation cephalosporins was associated with declining third-generation cephalosporin-resistance rates among Proteus mirabilis and Enterobacter cloacae but not to E coli and K pneumoniae. The increased rate of aminopenicillin or sulbactam use relative to the third-generation cephalosporins in conjunction with a sustained reduction in vancomycin use was associated with a reduction in MRSA rates. In addition, P aeruginosa-resistance rates to carbapenems declined to 0%. This was strongly associated with the reduction in carbapenem consumption over time.

The inclusion of this study serves to provide an example of a staggered implementation. Though the cost reduction appeared to dwindle significantly with each newly introduced period, one cannot ignore the cumulative effect of the overall impact on cost. In addition, the final period offers a comprehensive mechanism for long-standing success and serves as a template to introduce other initiatives as deemed necessary. Part of the success related to reduction in resistance rates noted by this program is related to the high rate of carbapenem and ceftriaxone use and the "seldom"-ordered cefepime and aminopenicillin or sulbactam in conjunction with the types of problem pathogens noted at the hospital (eg, AmpC phenotypes and carbapenem-resistant *P aeruginosa*). Penicillin-based inhibitor combinations and cefepime have been noted to more often favorably impact the environment in contrast to high usage rates of carbapenem and third-generation cephalosporin.[15,50,51]

Another study demonstrated the impact of a multidisciplinary ASP using a blend of interventions including minimal formulary restrictions, comprehensive education (direct communication, antibiograms, peer feedback every 6 months), rounding with medical teams, and introduction of guidelines (appropriate initial empirical therapy, transitional therapy, duration of therapy).[40] All adult patients admitted to the medicine service were consecutively evaluated prior to the introduction of the program (n = 500 patients) and postimplementation. Using defined daily dose (DDD) data and hospital expenditure data, they showed a 36% reduction in overall antimicrobial use (P<.001), intravenous antimicrobial use (46%, P<.01), and overall expenditures (53%, P = .001)—all without compromising the quality of patient care (determined by inpatient survival, clinical improvement or cure, duration of hospitalization, and readmission rates within 30 days). These benefits were sustained for the 4-year period evaluated.

Carling and colleagues[35] evaluated their ASP over a 7-year period at a smaller community hospital. Their ASP consists of a physician (one-quarter time support) and PharmD (full-time support), both with specialty training in ID. Antimicrobial consumption was measured by using DDD/1000 patient days for targeted antimicrobial agents. This program operated 8 hours per day and 5 days per week, and, during this time, new orders are typically evaluated within 4 hours of their entry. Orders falling outside of the 8-hour day are reviewed as a priority the next time the PharmD is on duty. Informal written notes are generated when the team identifies a problematic regimen and are then placed in the patient's chart. This study is most commonly used as an example of sustained impact of an ASP over time on antimicrobial use, cost, and antimicrobials resistance or superinfections. It evaluated the impact on vancomycin-resistant *Enterococci*, MRSA, and *C difficile* disease by means of internal benchmarks and external benchmarks from similar hospitals within the National Nosocomial Infections Surveillance System. A 22% reduction in parenteral broad-spectrum antibiotics occurred (P<.0001) during a time when they observed a 15% increase in the acuity of their patient population over the 7-year period. Reductions in nosocomial infections caused by *C difficile* (P =.002) and resistant *Enterobacteriaceae* (P = .02) were reported. MRSA rates remained unaffected.

An example of a smaller hospital (120-bed community hospital) successfully implementing an ASP using a prospective audit and feedback strategy was published.[38] The ASP involved an ID-specialist physician, a clinical pharmacist, and representatives from the infection control and the microbiology laboratory. The ID physician was involved approximately 8 to 12 hours per week. Antimicrobial therapy in patients receiving targeted drugs or prolonged durations of therapy was reviewed 3 days a week. Recommendations were conveyed using a form that was temporarily placed in the patient's chart or by telephone if necessary. During the first year, 488 recommendations were made with a 69% acceptance rate. Antimicrobial expenditures were reduced by 19%, saving an estimated $177,000. Common interventions were discontinuation of redundant antimicrobial therapy, discontinuation of treatment because of inappropriate use or excessive duration, transition from intravenous to oral therapy, and substitution or addition of an antibiotic to the regimen.

Preauthorization Strategy

White and colleagues[44] implemented an ASP, restricting the use of antimicrobials based on cost or spectra of activity. A 24-hour-per-day, 7-day-per-week on call system was established using a dedicated pager that clinicians called to receive approval for restricted agents. In their quasi-experimental study, patients in the preimplementation period were similar to those in the postimplementation period in terms of severity of illness. Outcome measures that were not statistically significant between groups were survival (P = .49), infection-related length of stay for bacteremia (P>.05), and time to administration of the antimicrobial (P>.05). Benefits received in the post-ASP implementation group were improved susceptibilities to a number of bug-drug combinations primarily involving nonfermenting gram-negative rods and *Enterobacteriaceae*, significant reduction in the use of a number of broad spectrum agents, and a significant reduction in annualized antimicrobial costs ($803,910) and costs per patient day ($18 to $14.4).

A variety of well-conducted studies at the University of Pennsylvania over the last two decades have contributed to our current knowledge of ASPs in general.[52,53] Gross and colleagues[41] initially employed a dedicated-beeper schedule for weekdays during normal business hours which was covered by an antimicrobial management team member (an ID PharmD or ID physician). Second-year ID fellows covered evenings and weekends. At night, restricted drugs were released pending next morning follow-up. Taking advantage of their existing program, they evaluated interventions performed by the ID fellows versus those made by the ID PharmD or ID ASP attending. They concluded that interventions performed by the veteran ASP team members (ID PharmD or ID physician) were more cost-effective and resulted in narrower spectrum therapy compared to those made by ID fellows. Based on the results of their study, the ID fellows have been more fully incorporated into their ASP and work with the PharmD and ID physician attending more directly. With regard to intranet or Internet resources, they also have published their list of restricted antimicrobials and guidelines on a Web site that can be accessed, at least in part, by outside institutions (www.uphs.upenn.edu/bugdrug). In addition to the preauthorization method for active interventions, they also work closely with the hospital epidemiologist, are involved in establishing guidelines for antimicrobial use and dosing, are proactively involved in the antimicrobial formulary, work closely with the pharmacy and therapeutics committee, and provide education and continuously evaluate antimicrobial consumption trends.[52]

Potential Barriers

The literature is helpful to point out pitfalls that some have experienced. Delays in the approval for a necessary antimicrobial agent can be detrimental to critically ill patients in need of initial broad-spectrum antimicrobial therapy. White and colleagues[44] showed no delay in the administration of antimicrobial agents prior to and after the introduction of their program. However, approval times and time to antibiotic administration must be monitored as a process measure. The perception of "threatened autonomy" can be a significant impediment to the efficacy of the program. LaRocco[38] and colleagues[14] found that using the prospective audit and feedback strategy with few restricted antimicrobials promotes education at the point of intervention, neutralizing negative emotions. Thus, regardless of approach, education and constant communication with frontline prescribers are vital. The concept of "gaming the system" cannot be ignored and is a function of human nature. For example, one program reported an outbreak of nosocomial infection following the introduction of their ASP.[45] A 30% relative increase in documentation of infection in the medical record occurred (incidence of infection increased from 11 to 14.3 per 1000 patient care days, P<.05).[45] After further investigation into this counterintuitive finding, the outbreak was termed a "pseudo-outbreak". Clinicians were required to document infection in the medical record in order to justify antimicrobial use; thus, more clinicians were documenting infections in an attempt to use particular restricted antimicrobials. The perception that ASPs are solely financially driven can also be an impediment. However, the IDSA-SHEA guidelines and other authorities endorse these programs based not on the potential for cost savings, but as a means to improve patient safety and to reduce the selective pressure exerted by unnecessary antimicrobial use that facilitates the evolution of antimicrobial resistance. Typically, as a side effect of interventions to optimize antimicrobial use to improve efficacy and reduce resistance, cost saving is observed that financially justifies the program. Administrators need to be cognizant of this when helping to develop ASPs. Program funding can be a barrier for some institutions, but as mentioned in IDSA-SHEA guidelines and as numerous studies point out, ASPs typically pay for themselves as a side effect of their existence.

SUPPLEMENTAL PROGRAMS TO THE PRIMARY ANTIMICROBIAL STEWARDSHIP PROGRAM STRATEGY
Formulary Interventions

A survey of teaching hospitals suggests that 80% limit prescriber access to antibiotics using a variety of mechanisms.[54] Formulary restriction, although the most direct way to influence antimicrobial use and central to the primary preauthorization ASP strategy, is a waning concept. In place of this, most hospitals now are turning back to their pharmacy and therapeutics committees to provide them the optimal antimicrobial formulary for their institution. Drugs are excluded that are more harmful than other class members (based on toxicity or greater probability to evoke bacterial resistance than other class or nonclass members) and those that might be more expensive while providing no incremental benefit. This, in essence, limits access to the numbers of drugs within a class. Limiting the number of available antimicrobials within a class is a passive intervention strategy; enforcement through ASPs shifts this to an active intervention.

Although leveraging contracts is a useful tool, cost evaluation should extend beyond purchase prices.[55] The overall cost of care should be considered when evaluating an antimicrobial but this is not always done because of the compartmentalization of costs within an institution (also referred to as the "silo mentality"). For example, although 8-to10-fold more expensive than intravenous vancomycin in purchase cost, the use of oral linezolid has been shown to decrease the length of stay and improve discharge dynamics for patients with MRSA infections.[56–59] This is particularly financially appealing for institutions operating at maximal census (because bed costs far outweigh drug costs) and with high rates of MRSA. It is also valuable from the infection-control perspective because of reduced transmission dynamics when length of stay is shortened and, most important, from the patient's perspective of being home rather than hospitalized.

Practical, evidence-based examples exist of preferentially replacing drugs with increased resistance evoking potential (eg, ceftazidime) with a member of the same class, that has demonstrated a reduced ability to select for resistance (eg, cefepime).[29,49,57,59] For hospitals still characterized by high third-generation cephalosporin use, a number of studies have demonstrated that their replacement with cefepime or piperacillin-tazobactam are effective strategies (particularly in concert with infection control intervention) to minimize the selective pressure that facilitates the appearance of problematic β-lactamases (eg, AmpC enzymes, extended spectrum β-lactamases) and vancomycin-resistant enterococci.[8,15,16,47] Another example that highlights the point that not all drugs are created equal with regard to their potential to select for antimicrobial resistance is the contrast between vancomycin and daptomycin. Fewer high-level vancomycin-resistant S aureus strains have been reported than daptomycin-nonsusceptible S aureus strains. The difference is that vancomycin has been used in severely ill patients with bacteremia, endocarditis, and meningitis, for examples, for over 3 decades. As many (6) daptomycin-resistant strains were selected during therapy in a single endocarditis trial. Observations that linezolid resistance can occur more readily in enterococci than in staphylococci have been noted.[17] However, staphylococcal resistance to linezolid remains low after 6 years of use. Nuances related to the propensity for the antimicrobial to become resistant to the pathogens of interest within a particular institution's patient population should be considered from a formulary perspective. Monitoring the drug's susceptibility performance in a perpetual manner is an important component of an ASP working directly with the hospital epidemiologist and the microbiology laboratory.[60]

Finally, where an antimicrobial may fit into order sets and guidelines and how its use will be monitored completes a comprehensive evaluation of how the antimicrobial will be most effectively utilized within the institution. With regard to following up on an antimicrobial's utilization in the institution, the support of the pharmacy and therapeutics committee is vital because it provides a mechanism to report back inappropriate use of the drug and has the power (in many places) to intervene, making it an effective countermeasure to correct inappropriate use.

Sometimes, two generic products, if made easier to use, will provide a benefit in terms of reintroducing lesser-used drugs and ultimately leading to greater antimicrobial heterogeneity. For example, some hospitals seem to use only piperacillin-tazobactam, for the simple reason that clinicians do not have to think when prescribing. We made it just as easy to think about not prescribing it by providing the combination of two generic antimicrobials (cefepime plus metronidazole, combined in the same minibag), administered as a single product, after doing stability and compatibility studies. While it provided a cheaper alternative to piperacillin-tazobactam, it also covered the most common pathogens equally, while being administered half as many times per day.[61]

Pharmacodynamic Dose Optimization

Dose optimization interventions are likely to be one of the most common interventions from an ASP. Although formerly viewed as a means to efficiently trim excess drug exposure secondary to renal dysfunction, the modern application of pharmacodynamic principles is important in order to maximize drug exposure for organisms with elevated MICs, patients with excess body mass indices, and for closed-space or otherwise difficult to penetrate sites of infection (eg, meningitis, endocarditis, pneumonia, bone and joint infections). A recent paper provides a more in-depth review of the subject and serves as a primer for all ASPs incorporating optimal dosing strategies.[62] Although we approached our program with the thought that may patients would receive downward dose adjustments for renal impairment, we found that a significant proportion of patients required increased drug exposure.[14,37] Other examples of pharmacodynamic dose-optimization that can be incorporated include regimens intended to treat higher MIC pathogens more effectively such as continuous or prolonged infusion of short half-life β-lactams (eg, piperacillin-tazobactam, cefepime, meropenem), and extended-interval aminoglycoside dosing. Lodise and colleagues,[63] found decreased mortality in patients with high APACHE II scores when prolonged infusions of piperacillin-tazobactam were used versus standard infusion piperacillin-tazobactam. Most recently, a double-blind, randomized, controlled trial was carried out evaluating the administration of doripenem infused over 4 hours, in a prolonged fashion, compared with standard infusion imipenem for patients with ventilator-associated pneumonia, capitalizing on the concept that it is more difficult to maintain adequate time above the MIC (T > MIC) such as doripenem against higher MIC pathogens (such as *P aeruginosa*).[64] Although outcomes numerically favor the doripenem-treated patients, the difference was not statistically significant. Because of trends in difference favoring prolonged infusion, larger studies are indicated to corroborate this. Rather than waiting for these trials, common sense has led many institutions to adopt this method of administration based on the time-dependent manner in which they kill bacteria, the simple fact carbapenems have a short half life, and that MICs of hospital-acquired pathogens are elevated compared to those patients without prior hospitalization and prior antibiotic use. In some instances, computerized physician-order entry systems can be tied into smart pumps, so that when the drug is ordered, the infusion is carried out as intended with minim operational dysfunction (**Fig. 1**).

A disturbing realization that we are not even accounting for the most basic of dosing services was brought about by a paper indicating that a substantial proportion of obese patients who received vancomycin intravenously did not receive adequate exposures to this drug.[65] For a drug like vancomycin, it is relatively easy to determine a patient's drug exposure following its administration because of therapeutic drug monitoring. However, for most antimicrobials, the optimal dose remains more of an art than a science. As an example, Chen and colleagues[66] evaluated the drug exposures following ertapenem in normal-body-weight individuals and those with increasing degrees of body mass. Furthermore, they plotted the serum concentrations

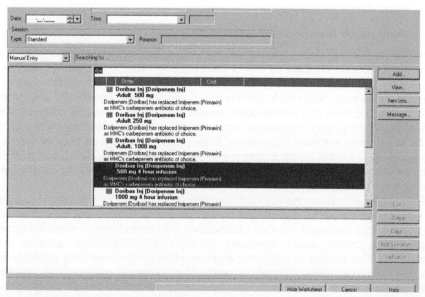

Fig. 1. Computerized physician-order entry system screenshot facilitating ordering of prolonged infusions of a short half-life β-lactam.

achieved after standard doses were administered versus T > MIC of several common organisms. What they found should not be too shocking—that it is difficult if not impossible to give a time-dependent killing drug with a 4-hour half-life once a day. Seldom was adequate T > MIC attained at standard doses, even for normal-body-weight individuals, much less for higher-body-weight ones. Discussions have occurred around other drugs, such as voriconazole, for other reasons, primarily dealing with their metabolism with or without concurrent drug interactions.[67] However, because we do not routinely monitor serum concentrations, most are unaware what is occurring when dosing as a function of body weight, MIC, pharmacogenetics, or drug interactions are considered. As was pointed out by the seminal reference in this area, patients suffer because of this.[62]

Educational Efforts

Development and dissemination of pertinent information is the first step in any process leading to change. Early attempts at influencing prescribing behaviors relied heavily on educational efforts—it was simplistically believed that the reason physicians frequently inappropriately prescribed antibiotics was that they were "therapeutically undereducated."[68] The assumption was that misuse of antibiotics was more often the result of insufficient information rather than inappropriate behavior.

Over the years that we have taught antibiotic principles and specifics of therapy at our hospital, we have been impressed by the intense interest both physicians-in-training and established practitioners have in learning more about antibiotics. Equally impressive is the "laissez-faire" and even fatalistic attitude towards retaining and applying lessons learned in these educational sessions. Without direct application to current patients, prescribers often refer to antibiotics as "alphabet soup" and "impossible to understand." These impressions are supported in the literature. Although a supplemental cornerstone to any ASP, educational efforts when applied alone are the least effective, and certainly the shortest lasting, way to affect prescriber behaviors. Active intervention that is supplemented by education is a synergistic method for changing behavior.

Computer-Assisted Decision Support Programs

Direct computer-based physician-order entry is rapidly becoming the standard of care, and has been adopted as one of the Leapfrog initiatives to avoid medication errors and improve the quality of care.[37] Computer-assisted decision-support programs have been designed to provide real-time integrated patient and institutional data including culture and susceptibility results, laboratory measures of organ function, allergy history, drug interactions, and cumulative or customized location-specific antibiogram data, and cost information. They provide therapeutic choices for clinicians and allow for the incorporation of clinical judgment by overriding suggestions. Autonomy is preserved while insuring that important variables in the choice of antimicrobial therapy are considered.

Most published data on the effect of computer-assisted decision-support programs on antibiotic use are from researchers at the Latter Day Saints Hospital in Salt Lake City, Utah. This approach has been associated with reductions in antibiotic doses, inappropriate orders, costs, treatment duration, and associated adverse drug events.[69–71] This degree of computer sophistication is not universally available but has been made available through a variety of commercial systems.[72,73] We have used our own computerized physician-order entry system to design a logic-based algorithm to optimize the treatment of pneumonia (community-, health care-, and hospital-acquired). The only randomized, controlled trial of clinical-decision support versus education alone on the appropriateness of antimicrobial prescribing demonstrated improved appropriateness of use and reduced overall use of antimicrobials for respiratory tract infections.[74] Although a variety of commercial programs can be purchased currently, each typically offering something for infection-control programs and, most recently, for ASPs, it is still possible to develop "homegrown" solutions while the budgeters determine whether these systems will be purchased or not. For example, Thiel and colleagues[75] evaluated the impact of hospital-wide standardized order sets on the management of patients with severe bacteremic sepsis. Antimicrobial therapy was improved, in addition to other markers for improved outcome. Similarly, we have developed a semi-standardized way of treating patients with pneumonia who present to the emergency department (**Fig. 2**). In an effort to guide early initial antimicrobial therapy, we ask that the clinicians utilize a "living" order set, where antimicrobial therapy is guided by a series of five questions that are answered by the prescriber. In reward, the prescriber can order up to three antimicrobials and adjust all of their doses, order the chest radiograph, and lab work, all on one screen, minimizing the time required to do all of these tasks in our computerized physician-order entry system. This is based on medical logic module coding that enables "if-then" logic to be employed. Our evaluation of this, using interrupted-time series methods in patients over the span of 4 years demonstrated a reduction in quinolone use, increase in appropriateness of therapy, and improvement in Centers for Medicare & Medicaid Services core measures in patients over the age of 65 years with respect to timing of antimicrobial therapy and appropriateness of therapy in accordance with national guidelines.

Adaptation of Locally Customized, Published Guidelines

National guidelines put forth by the IDSA and SHEA are available and are useful to construct clinical pathways locally for a variety of infections. In some cases where

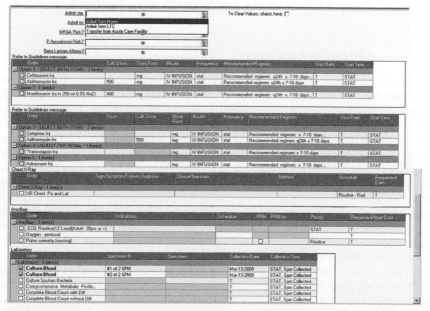

Fig. 2. Computerized decision support system for hospitalized community-acquired pneumonia using medical logic module coding ("if-then" logic).

significant time has passed between the publication of national guidelines and where the disease process has changed significantly, an institution should have a mechanism to develop evidence-based guidelines. A good example of this is the management of *C difficile*-infection (CDI). Being one of the first identified institutions in North America with a hypervirulent strain (BI/NAP1) of CDI, we saw the clinical and prescribing impact almost immediately. Shortly thereafter, we intervened by developing consensus among feuding specialties as to the proper approach to managing CDAD and created guidelines, a clinical pathway, and a follow-up order set—all of which could be accessed on our intranet site or in our computerized physician-order entry system.[31] From the identification of the BI/NAP1 strain of *C difficile* to its proper management, the ASP in conjunction with our department of epidemiology and infection prevention, environmental services, and administration, we spearheaded an institutional approach to managing this high morbidity-associated infection. We also evaluated and reported the impact of the CDAD guidelines that supplemented active interventions made by our ASP on the use of nonevidence-based treatment strategies and demonstrated a significant improvement in the treatment variability of this infection.[76]

Guidelines published by the American Thoracic Society and the IDSA for the management of hospital-acquired, and health care- and ventilator-associated pneumonia suggest a broad spectrum approach for the empirical treatment of these infections because of the high probability of mortality associated with inadequate therapy. In addition, they recommend shortened durations of therapy. From these recommendations, we developed consensus, published locally customized (per our susceptibility patterns) guidelines, and continue to meet monthly to discuss the tracking of process measures. One difficulty with just creating and making guidelines available to clinicians is that compliance is voluntary. We have found that without active follow-up, clinicians fall back on old habits. Thus, one benefit of having an ASP is having the resources to provide active intervention in the ICU whether for recommending streamlining or de-escalation when culture and susceptibility results are known, or stopping antimicrobial therapy at day 7 or 8 instead of the traditional 14, or longer, days.

PROCESS AND OUTCOME MEASUREMENTS

The IDSA-SHEA guidelines for developing an institutional program to enhance antimicrobial stewardship recommend that outcomes be measured.[11] This is the reason for having a data system and an information specialist to assist the ASP members in quantifying their impact. Without this support, the ASP team members can spend more time justifying their positions and measuring outcomes than on their primary purpose: the day-to-day management of the program and evaluation of antimicrobial therapy. Antimicrobial consumption can be measured for targeted (or all) antimicrobials. Using antimicrobial expenditure data has significant limitations, but is helpful to evaluate where the dollars are being spent. A more meaningful measure of antimicrobial consumption is the use of DDD data. Standardized definitions are available at: http://www.whocc.no/atcddd/. Converting grams of antibiotic used to DDD per 1000 patient days allows for a useful internal and external benchmark of antimicrobial consumption. Other measures include antimicrobial days of therapy. Regardless of mechanism chosen, establishing a baseline of antimicrobial use before program implementation allows one to track the progress of interventions on use over time. These measures can also be used to quantify the impact of parenteral to oral conversions. In addition, reporting to the pharmacy and therapeutics committee or another committee structure periodically as locally agreed on allows other clinicians and administrators to be aware of both the successes and challenges the ASP has faced over the reporting period.

SUMMARY

A public health crisis has emerged from the trend in antimicrobial-resistant infections and the precipitous drop in the number of approved antimicrobials over the last 2 decades—specifically, the dearth of novel agents covering multiple-drug resistant gram-negative bacilli. Because of the intensity of antimicrobial use in institutional settings, particularly the ICU, they are target-rich environments for proactive interventions to more effectively steward antimicrobial use. A variety of studies have demonstrated that systematic means to optimize antimicrobial use results in improved patient safety, increased probability of minimizing antimicrobial resistance, fewer instances of unnecessary antimicrobial use, and, as a side effect of all of this, they reduce cost. Although we are in need of more data that examines the impact of ASPs on the care of patients, there is already enough data to act. At this point, failing to act with interventions such as de-escalation based on culture and susceptibility results for patients with pneumonia is ridiculous. In the same vein, for us to continue to excessively treat ICU patients with pneumonia (eg, longer than 7 to 8 days in a responding patient), puts a patient at risk for infection due to resistant organisms. The IDSA-SHEA guidelines for developing an institutional program to enhance antimicrobial stewardship serve as a starting place for institutions considering adopting an ASP. Finally, as Calvin Kunin, MD,[77] stated "there are simply too many physicians prescribing antibiotics casually... The issues need to be presented forcefully to the medical community and the public. Third-party payers must get the message that these programs [antimicrobial stewardship] can save lives as well as money."

REFERENCES

1. Schiff GD, Wisniewski M, Bult J, et al. Improving inpatient antibiotic prescribing: insights from participation in a national collaborative. Jt Comm J Qual Improv 2001;27(8):387–402.
2. McDonald LC, Killgore GE, Thompson A, et al. An epidemic, toxin gene-variant strain of Clostridium difficile. N Engl J Med 2005;353(23):2433–41.
3. Owens RC Jr. QT prolongation with antimicrobial agents: understanding the significance. Drugs 2004;64(10):1091–124.
4. Jawetz E. Antimicrobial chemotherapy. Annu Rev Microbiol 1956;10:85–114.
5. Boucher HW, Talbot GH, Bradley JS, et al. Bad bugs, no drugs: no ESKAPE! An update from the Infectious Diseases Society of America. Clin Infect Dis 2009; 48(1):1–12.
6. Wenzel RP, Edmond MB. Managing antibiotic resistance. N Engl J Med 2000; 343(26):1961–3.
7. Lautenbach E, LaRosa LA, Kasbekar N, et al. Fluoroquinolone utilization in the emergency departments of academic medical centers: prevalence of, and risk factors for, inappropriate use. Arch Intern Med 2003;163(5):601–5.
8. Lautenbach E, LaRosa LA, Marr AM, et al. Changes in the prevalence of vancomycin-resistant Enterococci in response to antimicrobial formulary interventions: impact of progressive restrictions on use of vancomycin and third-generation cephalosporins. Clin Infect Dis 2003;36(4):440–6.

9. Hecker MT, Aron DC, Patel NP, et al. Unnecessary use of antimicrobials in hospitalized patients: current patterns of misuse with an emphasis on the antianaerobic spectrum of activity. Arch Intern Med 2003;163(8):972–8.

10. Hidron AI, Edwards JR, Patel J, et al. NHSN annual update: antimicrobial-resistant pathogens associated with healthcare-associated infections: annual summary of data reported to the National Healthcare Safety Network at the Centers for Disease Control and Prevention, 2006–2007. Infect Control Hosp Epidemiol 2008;29(11):996–1011.

11. Dellit TH, Owens RC, McGowan JE Jr, et al. Infectious Diseases Society of America and the Society For Healthcare Epidemiology of America guidelines for developing an institutional program to enhance antimicrobial stewardship. Clin Infect Dis 2007;44(2):159–77.

12. Drew RH, White R, MacDougall C, et al. Insights from the Society of Infectious Diseases Pharmacists on antimicrobial stewardship guidelines from the Infectious Diseases Society of America and the Society for Healthcare Epidemiology of America. Pharmacotherapy 2009;29(5):593–607.

13. Davey P, Brown E, Fenelon L, et al. Interventions to improve antibiotic prescribing practices for hospital inpatients. Cochrane Database Syst Rev 2005;(4): CD003543.

14. Owens RC Jr, Fraser GL, Stogsdill P. Antimicrobial stewardship programs as a means to optimize antimicrobial use. Insights from the Society of Infectious Diseases pharmacists. Pharmacotherapy 2004;24(7):896–908.

15. Owens RC Jr, Rice L. Hospital-based strategies for combating resistance. Clin Infect Dis 2006;42(Suppl 4):S173–81.

16. Owens RC Jr., Ambrose PG, Jones RN. The antimicrobial formulary: reevaluating parenteral cephalosporins in the context of emerging resistance. In: Owens RC Jr., Ambrose PG, Nightingale CH, editors. Antibiotic optimization: concepts and strategies in clinical practice. 1st edition. (Infectious Diseases and Therapy). New York: Marcel Dekker; 2005. p. 383–430.

17. Pai MP, Rodvold KA, Schreckenberger PC, et al. Risk factors associated with the development of infection with linezolid- and vancomycin-resistant Enterococcus faecium. Clin Infect Dis 2002;35(10):1269–72.

18. Glowacki RC, Schwartz DN, Itokazu GS, et al. Antibiotic combinations with redundant antimicrobial spectra: clinical epidemiology and pilot intervention of computer-assisted surveillance. Clin Infect Dis 2003;37(1):59–64.

19. McGowan JE Jr. Do intensive hospital antibiotic control programs prevent the spread of antibiotic resistance? Infect Control Hosp Epidemiol 1994;15(7): 478–83.

20. Carling PC, Parry MF, Von Beheren SM. Identifying opportunities to enhance environmental cleaning in 23 acute care hospitals. Infect Control Hosp Epidemiol 2008;29(1):1–7.

21. Owens RC Jr. Antimicrobial stewardship: concepts and strategies in the 21st century. Diagn Microbiol Infect Dis 2008;61(1):110–28.

22. Levy SB, FitzGerald GB, Macone AB. Changes in intestinal flora of farm personnel after introduction of a tetracycline-supplemented feed on a farm. N Engl J Med 1976;295(11):583–8.

23. Bell DM. Promoting appropriate antimicrobial drug use: perspective from the Centers for Disease Control and Prevention. Clin Infect Dis 2001;33(Suppl 3): S245–50.

24. Dinubile MJ, Friedland I, Chan CY, et al. Bowel colonization with resistant gram-negative bacilli after antimicrobial therapy of intra-abdominal infections: observations

from two randomized comparative clinical trials of ertapenem therapy. Eur J Clin Microbiol Infect Dis 2005;24(7):443–9.

25. Kollef MH. Inadequate antimicrobial treatment: an important determinant of outcome for hospitalized patients. Clin Infect Dis 2000;31(Suppl 4):S131–8.

26. Kollef MH. Broad-spectrum antimicrobials and the treatment of serious bacterial infections: getting it right up front. Clin Infect Dis 2008;47(Suppl 1):S3–13.

27. Osmon S, Ward S, Fraser VJ, et al. Hospital mortality for patients with bacteremia due to *Staphylococcus aureus* or *Pseudomonas aeruginosa*. Chest 2004;125(2): 607–16.

28. Owens RC Jr, Ambrose PG. Antimicrobial safety: focus on fluoroquinolones. Clin Infect Dis 2005;41(Suppl 2):S144–57.

29. Owens RC Jr, Ambrose PG, Quintiliani R. Ceftazidime to cefepime formulary switch: pharmacodynamic and pharmacoeconomic rationale. Conn Med 1997; 61(4):225–7.

30. Owens RC Jr, Nolin TD. Antimicrobial-associated QT interval prolongation: points of interest. Clin Infect Dis 2006;43(12):1603–11.

31. Owens RC. *Clostridium difficile*-associated disease: an emerging threat to patient safety: insights from the Society of Infectious Diseases pharmacists. Pharmacotherapy 2006;26(3):299–311.

32. Pepin J, Routhier S, Gagnon S, et al. Management and outcomes of a first recurrence of *Clostridium difficile*-associated disease in Quebec, Canada. Clin Infect Dis 2006;42(6):758–64.

33. Pepin J, Valiquette L, Alary ME, et al. *Clostridium difficile*-associated diarrhea in a region of Quebec from 1991 to 2003: a changing pattern of disease severity. CMAJ 2004;171(5):466–72.

34. Ansari F, Gray K, Nathwani D, et al. Outcomes of an intervention to improve hospital antibiotic prescribing: interrupted time series with segmented regression analysis. J Antimicrob Chemother 2003;52(5):842–8.

35. Carling P, Fung T, Killion A, et al. Favorable impact of a multidisciplinary antibiotic management program conducted during 7 years. Infect Control Hosp Epidemiol 2003;24(9):699–706.

36. Fraser GL, Stogsdill P, Dickens JD Jr, et al. Antibiotic optimization. An evaluation of patient safety and economic outcomes. Arch Intern Med 1997;157(15): 1689–94.

37. Fraser GL, Stogsdill P, Owens RC Jr. Antimicrobial stewardship initiatives: a programmatic approach to optimizing antimicrobial use. In: Owens RC Jr, Ambrose PG, Nightingale CH, editors. Antibiotic optimization: concepts and strategies in clinical practice. (Infectious Disease and Therapy). 1st edition. New York: Marcel Dekker; 2005. p. 261–326.

38. LaRocco A Jr. Concurrent antibiotic review programs—a role for infectious diseases specialists at small community hospitals. Clin Infect Dis 2003;37(5): 742–3.

39. Lutters M, Harbarth S, Janssens JP, et al. Effect of a comprehensive, multidisciplinary, educational program on the use of antibiotics in a geriatric university hospital. J Am Geriatr Soc 2004;52(1):112–6.

40. Ruttimann S, Keck B, Hartmeier C, et al. Long-term antibiotic cost savings from a comprehensive intervention program in a medical department of a university-affiliated teaching hospital. Clin Infect Dis 2004;38(3):348–56.

41. Gross R, Morgan AS, Kinky DE, et al. Impact of a hospital-based antimicrobial management program on clinical and economic outcomes. Clin Infect Dis 2001;33(3):289–95.

42. John JF Jr, Fishman NO. Programmatic role of the infectious diseases physician in controlling antimicrobial costs in the hospital. Clin Infect Dis 1997;24(3):471–85.

43. Paterson DL. The role of antimicrobial management programs in optimizing antibiotic prescribing within hospitals. Clin Infect Dis 2006;42(Suppl 2):S90–5.

44. White AC Jr, Atmar RL, Wilson J, et al. Effects of requiring prior authorization for selected antimicrobials: expenditures, susceptibilities, and clinical outcomes. Clin Infect Dis 1997;25(2):230–9.

45. Calfee DP, Brooks J, Zirk NM, et al. A pseudo-outbreak of nosocomial infections associated with the introduction of an antibiotic management programme. J Hosp Infect 2003;55(1):26–32.

46. Linkin DR, Paris S, Fishman NO, et al. Inaccurate communications in telephone calls to an antimicrobial stewardship program. Infect Control Hosp Epidemiol 2006;27(7):688–94.

47. Lipworth AD, Hyle EP, Fishman NO, et al. Limiting the emergence of extended-spectrum beta-lactamase-producing enterobacteriaceae: influence of patient population characteristics on the response to antimicrobial formulary interventions. Infect Control Hosp Epidemiol 2006;27(3):279–86.

48. Srinivasan A, Song X, Richards A, et al. A survey of knowledge, attitudes, and beliefs of house staff physicians from various specialties concerning antimicrobial use and resistance. Arch Intern Med 2004;164(13):1451–6.

49. Bantar C, Sartori B, Vesco E, et al. A hospitalwide intervention program to optimize the quality of antibiotic use: impact on prescribing practice, antibiotic consumption, cost savings, and bacterial resistance. Clin Infect Dis 2003;37(2):180–6.

50. Georges B, Conil JM, Dubouix A, et al. Risk of emergence of *Pseudomonas aeruginosa* resistance to beta-lactam antibiotics in intensive care units. Crit Care Med 2006;34(6):1636–41.

51. Harris AD, Smith D, Johnson JA, et al. Risk factors for imipenem-resistant *Pseudomonas aeruginosa* among hospitalized patients. Clin Infect Dis 2002;34(3):340–5.

52. Fishman N. Antimicrobial stewardship. Am J Med 2006;119(6 Suppl 1):S53–61.

53. Fowler VG Jr, Boucher HW, Corey GR, et al. Daptomycin versus standard therapy for bacteremia and endocarditis caused by *Staphylococcus aureus*. N Engl J Med 2006;355(7):653–65.

54. Lesar TS, Briceland LL. Survey of antibiotic control policies in university-affiliated teaching institutions. Ann Pharmacother 1996;30(1):31–4.

55. Scott RD, Solomon SL, Cordell R, et al. Measuring the attributable costs of resistant infections in hospital settings. In: Owens RC Jr, Ambrose PG, Nightingale CH, editors. Antibiotic optimization: concepts and strategies in clinical practice. (Infectious Disease and Therapy). 1st edition. New York: Marcel Dekker; 2005. p. 141–79.

56. Itani KM, Weigelt J, Li JZ, et al. Linezolid reduces length of stay and duration of intravenous treatment compared with vancomycin for complicated skin and soft tissue infections due to suspected or proven methicillin-resistant *Staphylococcus aureus* (MRSA). Int J Antimicrob Agents 2005;26(6):442–8.

57. Li Z, Willke RJ, Pinto LA, et al. Comparison of length of hospital stay for patients with known or suspected methicillin-resistant *Staphylococcus* species infections treated with linezolid or vancomycin: a randomized, multicenter trial. Pharmacotherapy 2001;21(3):263–74.

58. McKinnon PS, Sorensen SV, Liu LZ, et al. Impact of linezolid on economic outcomes and determinants of cost in a clinical trial evaluating patients with

MRSA complicated skin and soft-tissue infections. Ann Pharmacother 2006; 40(6):1017–23.

59. Parodi S, Rhew DC, Goetz MB. Early switch and early discharge opportunities in intravenous vancomycin treatment of suspected methicillin-resistant *Staphylococcal* species infections. J Manag Care Pharm 2003;9(4):317–26.

60. Valenti AJ. The role of infection control and hospital epidemiology in the optimization of antibiotic use. In: Owens RC Jr, Ambrose PG, Nightingale CH, editors. Antibiotic optimization: concepts and strategies in clinical practice. (Infectious Disease and Therapy). 1st edition. New York: Marcel Dekker; 2005. p. 209–59.

61. Nolin TD, Lambert DA, Owens RC Jr. Stability of cefepime and metronidazole prepared for simplified administration as a single product. Diagn Microbiol Infect Dis 2006;56(2):179–84.

62. Ambrose PG, Bhavnani SM, Rubino CM, et al. Pharmacokinetics-pharmacodynamics of antimicrobial therapy: it's not just for mice anymore. Clin Infect Dis 2007;44(1):79–86.

63. Lodise TP Jr, Lomaestro B, Drusano GL. Piperacillin-tazobactam for *Pseudomonas aeruginosa* infection: clinical implications of an extended-infusion dosing strategy. Clin Infect Dis 2007;44(3):357–63.

64. Chastre J, Wunderink R, Prokocimer P, et al. Efficacy and safety of intravenous infusion of doripenem versus imipenem in ventilator-associated pneumonia: a multicenter, randomized study. Crit Care Med 2008;36(4):1089–96.

65. Hall RG, Payne KD, Bain AM, et al. Multicenter evaluation of vancomycin dosing: emphasis on obesity. Am J Med 2008;121(6):515–8.

66. Chen M, Nafziger AN, Drusano GL, et al. Comparative pharmacokinetics and pharmacodynamic target attainment of ertapenem in normal-weight, obese, and extremely obese adults. Antimicrob Agents Chemother 2006;50(4):1222–7.

67. Smith J, Safdar N, Knasinski V, et al. Voriconazole therapeutic drug monitoring. Antimicrob Agents Chemother 2006;50(4):1570–2.

68. Melmon KL, Blaschke TF. The undereducated physician's therapeutic decisions. N Engl J Med 1983;308(24):1473–4.

69. Evans RS, Pestotnik SL, Classen DC, et al. Evaluation of a computer-assisted antibiotic-dose monitor. Ann Pharmacother 1999;33(10):1026–31.

70. Evans RS, Pestotnik SL, Classen DC, et al. A computer-assisted management program for antibiotics and other antiinfective agents. N Engl J Med 1998; 338(4):232–8.

71. Pestotnik SL, Classen DC, Evans RS, et al. Implementing antibiotic practice guidelines through computer-assisted decision support: clinical and financial outcomes. Ann Intern Med 1996;124(10):884–90.

72. Burke JP, Mehta RR. Role of computer-assisted programs in optimizing the use of antimicrobial agents. In: Owens RC Jr, Ambrose PG, Nightingale CH, editors. Antibiotic optimization: concepts and strategies in clinical practice. (Infectious Disease and Therapy). 1st edition. New York: Marcel Dekker; 2005. p. 327–52.

73. Pestotnik SL. Expert clinical decision support systems to enhance antimicrobial stewardship programs: insights from the society of infectious diseases pharmacists. Pharmacotherapy 2005;25(8):1116–25.

74. Samore MH, Bateman K, Alder SC, et al. Clinical decision support and appropriateness of antimicrobial prescribing: a randomized trial. JAMA 2005;294(18): 2305–14.

75. Thiel SW, Asghar MF, Micek ST, et al. Hospital-wide impact of a standardized order set for the management of bacteremic severe sepsis. Crit Care Med 2009;37(3):819–24.

76. Owens RC Jr, Loew B, Soni S, et al. Impact of interventions on non-evidence based treatment strategies during an outbreak of Clostridium difficile-associated disease due to BI/NAP1. [Abstr. 687]. In: Program and abstracts of the 44th Annual Infectious Diseases Society of America, Toronto, Ontario, CA. 60. 10–13-2006. Ref Type: abstract.
77. Kunin CM. Antibiotic armageddon. Clin Infect Dis 1997;25(2):240–1.

Infection Prevention in the Intensive Care Unit

Mary C. Barsanti, MD, Keith F. Woeltje, MD, PhD*

KEYWORDS

- Infection control • Infection prevention
- Health care–associated infections • Intensive care unit
- Catheter-associated bloodstream infection
- Ventilator-associated pneumonia
- Catheter-associated urinary tract infection

Managing infections in the intensive care unit (ICU) can be a daunting challenge to any practitioner. In the United States, more than 5 million patients are admitted to an ICU every year.[1,2] ICU-related infections increase the cost of hospitalization, morbidity, mortality, and hospital length of stay.[3–6] Infection prevention measures can help improve these outcomes by limiting the incidence and spread of hospital-acquired infections.

The past several decades have seen an increased effort in characterizing the epidemiology of health care–associated infections and in advancing the knowledge of infection-prevention practices. The goal of this article is to discuss risk factors and specific nosocomial infections, particularly ventilator-associated pneumonia (VAP), central line–associated bloodstream infections (CLABSIs), catheter-associated urinary tract infections (CAUTIs), and *Clostridium difficile* infections (CDIs). Antimicrobial stewardship will also be discussed briefly.

RISK FACTORS FOR NOSOCOMIAL INTENSIVE CARE UNIT INFECTIONS

Estimates from the National Nosocomial Infections Surveillance (NNIS, now the National Healthcare Safety Network [NHSN]) system found approximately 1.7 million nosocomial infections occurred in United States hospitals in 2002 with 24% of these infections in the ICU, a rate of 13 per 1000 patient days.[7] ICU patients have numerous insults to normal host mechanisms. Skin integrity is compromised by peripheral and central venous access devices or postoperative wounds. Immunosuppressive medications decrease the ability of humoral and cell-mediated immunity defenses to function properly. Underlying medical conditions, such as diabetes, may predispose

Division of Infectious Diseases, Department of Internal Medicine, Washington University School of Medicine, 660 S. Euclid Avenue, Campus Box 8051, St. Louis, MO 63110, USA
* Corresponding author.
E-mail address: kwoeltje@dom.wustl.edu (K.F. Woeltje).

Infect Dis Clin N Am 23 (2009) 703–725
doi:10.1016/j.idc.2009.04.012
0891-5520/09/$ – see front matter © 2009 Elsevier Inc. All rights reserved.

id.theclinics.com

patients to infectious complications. Potentially modifiable risk factors are related to nutrition, health care personnel, and the hospital environment.

Malnutrition

Numerous studies have delineated the connection between poor nutrition and deficiencies in immune function.[8–12] Hospitalized patients with hypoalbuminemia are noted to have impaired cellular immunity.[9] Immune system function is reduced because of a decrease in lymphocyte, cytokine, and complement production, and an attenuated response to antigenic stimuli.[9,12,13] This reduced immune system function impedes normal host responses to infection. A low albumin level in cardiac surgery patients correlates with increased risk of postoperative infections,[14] while malnutrition is a risk factor for surgical site infections.[15] Medical ICU patients who receive less than 25% of the daily recommended calories have a significantly increased risk of nosocomial bloodstream infections.[16] These studies all indicate the importance of appropriate nutrition in critically ill patients.

Supplemental Nutrition

To counteract the effects of malnutrition on the immune system, nutritional support in ICU patients is vital. Although necessary, the mode of nutritional support may also have an impact on nosocomial infections. Parenteral feeding requires long-term central venous access catheters, which are a potential source for bacterial colonization and CLABSI. This method of feeding also increases gut mucosal permeability compared with enteral nutrition, increasing the risk of bacterial translocation.[17] However, enteral feeding has also been shown to increase the risk of VAP.[18–20] This is especially seen in patients who remain in the supine position.[21]

In a recent meta-analysis of enteral versus parenteral feeding in critically ill adult patients, enteral feeding significantly decreased the risk of overall infections, but had no impact on mortality.[22] This increased risk of infections in parenteral feeding was also seen in a second meta-analysis, although there was a mortality benefit to this feeding method.[18] The mortality benefit may be explained in this series by its comparison of delayed enteral nutrition to parenteral nutrition. When comparing early parenteral versus early enteral nutrition, the incidence of sepsis or septic shock was significantly lower in the early enteral feeding group.[23] Similarly, when comparing early versus late enteral feeding alone, early feeding results in improved ICU mortality.[20]

Hyperglycemia

There has been significant recent interest in the role of glucose control in ICU patients and its relation to the immune system.[24] Hyperglycemia has been found to affect neutrophil function, phagocytosis, and cytokine activity.[24–27] This may lead to an increased risk of infectious complications, especially in critically ill patients. Diabetics undergoing cardiovascular surgery have more postoperative wound infections than nondiabetics.[28] Trauma patients admitted to the ICU with hyperglycemia have increased risk of infections, particularly respiratory and bloodstream.[29] In a study of 61 surgical ICU patients randomly assigned to tight or standard glycemic control, 34 patients in the strict glucose control group experienced significantly fewer nosocomial infections.[30]

Initiation of a continuous insulin drip protocol significantly decreases the incidence of postoperative wound infections in diabetic patients undergoing cardiovascular surgery.[31,32] However, recent studies revealed intensive glycemic control (between 80 and 110 mg/dL) did not show a mortality benefit[33,34] and only a nonsignificant reduction in bacteremia.[33] A subgroup analysis of patients staying less that 3 days in the ICU even indicated increased mortality with intensive glycemic control.[33,34] More studies are needed to determine the optimal method of controlling hyperglycemia in ICU patients.

Health Care Personnel

The complex care of an ICU patient relies upon the interaction of many individuals, including physicians, nurses, and support staff. An appropriate ICU organizational structure is vital to proper and effective patient care. One study of postoperative patients staying in an ICU that did not institute daily rounds by an ICU physician indicated increased rates of mortality and sepsis.[35] Interventions to improve communication amongst all ICU staff consisting of daily multidisciplinary rounds with discussions on mechanical ventilator, central line, and urinary catheter protocols can significantly decrease the rate of VAP and CLABSI with a downward trend in CAUTI.[36-38] Periodic educational interventions for ICU staff with reminders of infection-prevention policies can also result in the decline of hospital-acquired infection rates.[39-43]

In addition, adequate nursing and support staff is necessary. A higher patient-to-nurse ratio increases the risk of nosocomial infection,[44] including late-onset VAP[45] and CLABSI.[46] The difficulties of nurse staffing, including understaffing and the different levels of nurse training, have an impact on risk of infection.[47-49] Patients cared for by a registered nurse for longer periods of time rather than by a nurse with less education have a decreased risk of developing pneumonia or urinary tract infections while in the hospital.[50,51] Greater use of float pool nurses may also increase the risk of nosocomial infections.[52,53] These studies show that improved nurse staffing can have a significant impact in decreasing adverse events in hospitalized patients.

Hospital Environment

The hospital environment plays a crucial role in exposing patients to various pathogens, including bacterial, fungal, and viral. These organisms may be found on the hands of caretakers,[54-56] on the knobs of doors,[57] on keyboards,[58,59] or in the structure and environment of the room itself,[58,60,61] increasing the chances of a nosocomial infection. Measures to decrease the environmental burden of pathogens and subsequently lower the rates of hospital-acquired infections have been studied.

Hand hygiene

Appropriate hand hygiene is vital to patient care and is extremely cost-effective. A study evaluating the cost-effectiveness of a hand hygiene educational program found the total cost of providing alcohol-based foam and the campaign itself was less than 1% of the cost of a nosocomial infection.[62] Compliance rates of health care workers using proper hand hygiene before and after patient care activities vary, ranging from 24% to 89% (an average of 56.6%) in a recent survey of 40 hospitals.[63] This survey was conducted after the publication of new guidelines by the Association of Professionals in Infection Control, Healthcare Infection Control Practices Advisory Committee (HICPAC), Society for Healthcare Epidemiology of America (SHEA), and Infectious Diseases Society of America (IDSA) on appropriate hand hygiene practices.[64] Even with the wide gap in compliance, the overall rates of CLABSI did significantly decline in the 40 hospitals surveyed after the new guidelines were published.[63] Other studies found similar results when an educational program was instituted resulting in improved hand hygiene compliance and decreased rates of hospital-acquired infections.[65-67] Continuous encouragement and monitoring with reinforcement of hand hygiene policies are important to maintain improvement in compliance rates.[68]

In addition, appropriate placement of alcohol-based hand-rubbing solutions or hand-washing sinks is essential to increased compliance rates.[64]

Alcohol-based foam has been shown to reduce bacterial counts recovered on health care workers' hands over hand washing.[69] In a separate study, no significant difference was found in bacterial colony counts on hands of health care workers who used a chlorhexidine-containing antiseptic wash versus alcohol-based foam.[70] Investigators did note, however, that using the alcohol foam significantly decreased workers' skin damage along with time and cost compared with chlorhexidine wash. Skin damage may itself lead to increased pathogen colonization and decrease the desire for workers to perform hand hygiene. Appropriate emollients or lotions may help.[64] In addition, use of alcohol foam for hand hygiene is fast and easily accessible, which therefore can increase compliance with hand hygiene practices.[71]

Other factors may contribute to pathogen carriage on health care workers' hands. Fingernail length over 2 mm past the fingertip is associated with significantly more microorganisms recovered on the hands of workers compared with lengths of 0 to 1 mm.[71] Wearing a ring also increases the number of microorganisms recovered.[71,72]

The Hand Hygiene Task Force compiled the trials comparing soap to alcohol-based foam and determined that alcohol-based foams are more effective in decreasing bacterial colony counts and in decreasing the number of multidrug-resistant pathogens than traditional hand washing.[64] Many viruses and fungi are also susceptible to alcohol formulas; however, bacterial spores, protozoa, and some nonenveloped viruses are not affected.[64] Overall, the Hand Hygiene Task Force has compiled numerous recommendations on this subject and is a valued reference.

Hand colonization

Once health care workers' hands are colonized with a pathogen, the organism can be transferred to the environment of a patient's room or to another patient. In a study of vancomycin-resistent *Enterococcus* (VRE)–colonized patients, some environmental cultures negative before a health care worker entered the room turned positive after the worker performed patient care activities.[73] Another study of ICU patients evaluated bacterial colonization of methicillin-resistant *Staphylococcus aureus* (MRSA) or ceftazidime-resistant gram-negative bacilli on admission and at discharge. At discharge, 21.6% of patients had acquired colonization of one organism and 2.4% with both organisms, which were not present on admission.[74] While evaluating an *Acinetobacter baumannii* outbreak leading to sepsis and the death of three ICU patients, the study investigators discovered the same isolates by culturing health care workers' hands and patients' rooms.[55] After 10 days of cleaning, the ICU had 1 month without *A baumannii* infections.

Patient rooms

Patient rooms may harbor significant pathogens long after the source patient was moved. One study found that, if a previous ICU room occupant or environmental sample within the past 2 weeks was VRE positive, then the next occupant had an increased risk of VRE acquisition after 48 hours of hospitalization.[75] MRSA patient colonization may also have similar risks.[76]

Recent studies looking at terminal room-cleaning methods used a mark visible only by UV light in prespecified areas as a surrogate for transmissible pathogens, such as MRSA or multidrug-resistant gram-negative bacilli. At baseline, two studies found 44% and 49% of marks remained after completion of room cleaning by environmental services staff.[77,78] Doorknobs, sinks, toilet handles, and light switches were the most common missed surfaces.[77,78] An educational campaign with continued feedback and cleaning-regimen change resulted in a significant decline in positive surfaces.[77] Another small study used culture methods to detect VRE or *C difficile* in terminally cleaned rooms whose occupants were colonized or infected with these organisms. After cleaning, 71% to 78% of the rooms remained culture-positive.[79] An educational intervention led to significant reductions in positive cultures. Combining environmental cleaning with a hand hygiene educational campaign can significantly decrease both environmental and hand contamination rates.[80]

Other environmental factors

Besides a patient's room, air and water filtration systems provide other sources for pathogen contamination and increased risk of infection. Aspergillus has been found in hospital and ICU air samples.[81–84] *Legionella pneumophila* can colonize a hospital water system and cause pneumonia in hospitalized patients.[85,86] Tap water in a patient room can be contaminated with *Pseudomonas aeruginosa*, but placing water filters can decrease infections with this organism.[87] Caution should be taken in any ICU that plumbing, water, and air-filtration systems are closely monitored.

Patient screening

The NNIS System Report in 2004 found the percentage of antimicrobial-resistant pathogens in ICU patients increased.[88] The percentage of *S aureus* that was MRSA in 2003 was 59.5%, an increase of 11% over the mean resistance rates 5 years previously. VRE percentage increased 12% while some gram-negative bacilli, including *Klebsiella pneumoniae* and *P aeruginosa*, also noted increased resistance to third-generation cephalosporins and carbapenems.[88] With increasing resistance, it is even more important to find strategies to contain and eradicate these organisms.

Patients newly admitted to an ICU who are colonized with multidrug-resistant pathogens are a constant reservoir for transmission and subsequent infection. Surveillance cultures to detect MRSA and VRE have been implemented at many hospitals with significant success in decreasing the rate of colonization and infection with these organisms.[89–103] The Centers for Disease Control and Prevention's statement on isolation precautions state surveillance strategies prefer targeting the patients or locations at highest risk as opposed to hospital-wide surveillance for best use of resources. However, hospital-wide surveillance measures may be needed for certain organisms or situations.[104]

It remains controversial whether admission to the hospital or an ICU constitutes an appropriate indication for a surveillance culture, and how to handle a hospital outbreak of a multidrug-resistant pathogen. A multiyear study evaluated baseline levels of MRSA colonization for 12 months, then 12 months of ICU surveillance, and finally 21 months of hospital-wide MRSA testing. The rate per 10,000 days was 8.9, 7.4, and 3.9 respectively for baseline, ICU, and hospital-wide surveillance. The transition from baseline to hospital-wide surveillance significantly improved infections rates.[105] However, a study of surgical patients found no significant difference in the rate of nosocomial MRSA infection between universal versus no screening on admission.[106]

Consideration of risk factors for MRSA colonization may improve the use of hospital resources and infection-prevention strategies. Known risk factors for MRSA colonization or infection include male sex, age over 75 years, recent receipt of certain antibiotics or intravenous therapy, recent hospitalization, intrahospital transfer, HIV infection, a current skin or soft tissue infection, or presence of a urinary catheter.[107,108] Cost-benefit analyses of VRE and MRSA surveillance appear to favor surveillance as a cost-saving measure,[109–111] but it remains questionable whether all patients or a subset of patients, possibly ICU admissions, are the best target for this intervention.

Isolation measures

Use of gowns and gloves is a standard procedure for staff caring for patients with multidrug-resistant infections. Recent studies have evaluated the effectiveness of using isolation measures on patients colonized but not currently infected with these organisms. A study of glove use by 50 health care workers who care for VRE-positive patients found the use of gloves decreased the risk of the health care worker acquiring VRE by 71%. Even with glove use, five subjects with VRE cultured from their gloves also had positive VRE cultures on their hands.[112] Another study found the use of gloves upon room entry of VRE-positive patients resulted in only 5% of health care workers becoming colonized compared with 37% who did not wear gloves.[113]

A study comparing the use of gowns and gloves in eight ICU beds versus gloves only in eight separate ICU beds for all patients irrespective of pathogen colonization found no significant difference in acquiring VRE between the two groups. However, the investigators concluded that gown and glove use may improve overall compliance with isolation precautions.[114] Recent studies have found advantages in using both gowns and gloves to decrease the risk of transmitting both MRSA and VRE.[89,93,115,116] In addition, both HICPAC and SHEA guidelines encourage both gown and glove use upon entering rooms of patients colonized with antibiotic-resistant pathogens.[96,104] Cost-benefit analyses of gown use show a temporary increase in costs, but the long-term decrease in VRE or MRSA colonization and infections overall decreases hospital costs.[106,116,117]

Patient decolonization or prevention of colonization

Methods to treat or prevent MRSA and VRE colonization are under investigation. Use of 2% chlorhexidine cloths to bathe patients has been shown to decrease VRE colonization and rates of CLABSI.[118,119] The results are mixed with MRSA, one study failing to show improved decolonization rates with a 4% chlorhexidine bathing solution,[120] while others show chlorhexidine could improve decolonization rates.[121,122] The positive studies often combine chlorhexidine with nasal mupirocin and oral antibiotics, including rifampin or doxycycline. One effective program to reduce MRSA colonization included chlorhexidine, oral rinses, oral antibiotics, urinary tract decolonization, gastrointestinal tract decolonization, and vaginal decolonization.[123] Unfortunately, health care workers may have difficulty completing this intensive program.[124] At this time, the best combination remains speculative and ongoing studies may answer this question.

NOSOCOMIAL INFECTIONS
Ventilator-Associated Pneumonia

VAP occurs in 9% to 27% of all intubated patients or 2.1 to 10.7 episodes of VAP per 1000 ventilator days[6,125–128] with a crude mortality rate that may exceed 20% or greater if a high-risk pathogen is involved.[125] Patients with VAP are twice as likely to die compared with those without VAP.[6] Also, patients with VAP have a significantly longer duration of mechanical ventilation and hospital length of stay[3,128] accompanied by costlier medical bills ranging from $10,000 to over $40,000 more than patients who do not acquire VAP.[3,6,128] Knowing the tremendous personal and economic consequences of VAP necessitates increasing the knowledge of health care workers of this problem and working to improve prevention strategies.

Risk factors

A review of risk factors found postsurgical patients, presence of multiple organ failure, age greater than 60 years, supine patient positioning, decrease of gastric pH, cardiopulmonary resuscitation, continuous sedation, reintubation, presence of naso-gastric tube, enteral feeding, sinusitis, and patients transported out of the ICU had increased risk of developing VAP.[6] In a separate review, other nonmodifiable risk factors include the presence of acute respiratory distress syndrome, chronic obstructive pulmonary disease, coma, head trauma, and male patients.[19] Some studies looking at the ventilator circuit found that a lower cuff pressure, less frequent subglottic aspiration, and fewer circuit changes may also contribute to higher rates of VAP.[129] Use of systemic antibiotics remains controversial with mixed results.[6,129]

Methods of prevention

Many strategies have been studied to prevent VAP and SHEA/IDSA recently published a concise set of recommendations regarding this topic.[130] Most of the modifiable risk factors involve basic infection-prevention principles, medications, and the ventilator equipment. As previously discussed, hospital staff education of the problem,[40] proper surveillance for multidrug-resistant pathogens, appropriate isolation of patients, hand hygiene, and environmental and equipment cleaning can decrease the risk of VAP.[129] In addition, a high nurse-to-patient ratio was found in one study to decrease the rates of VAP.[45] These daily strategies can have a significant impact.

Mechanical ventilation is an inherent component to the development of VAP. This basic fact leads to the conclusion that fewer intubated patients will decrease the numbers of VAP. Use of noninvasive ventilation and fewer reintubations is preferred when possible.[129] Semirecumbent positioning appears to give some protection from pulmonary aspiration and is the recommended position for intubated patients when possible;[129,131,132] however, one study found 45° to be difficult to achieve.[133] The many components of the ventilator circuit can harbor bacterial pathogens if not frequently and properly cleaned. Continuous aspiration of subglottic secretions appears to significantly decrease the risk of VAP[134–136] along with maintaining the endotracheal intracuff pressure over 20 cm H_2O.[136,137] In addition, a review of 10 studies found no difference in the risk for VAP in open versus closed endotracheal suction systems.[138] Lastly, a recently published study found the use of silver-coated endotracheal tubes decreased the incidence of VAP among patients who used these experimental tubes.[139]

Other modifications besides respiratory care can improve VAP rates. A summary of eight trials for stress ulcer prophylaxis compared sucralfate to ranitidine with results showing a slightly decreased risk of VAP when using sucralfate, although use of this medication may increase the risk of gastrointestinal bleeding.[19] Daily interruption of sedation medication in ventilated patients can decrease the time of ventilation and in a small study decrease the incidence of VAP.[140,141] A nurse-implemented sedation protocol with around-the-clock adjustments can significantly decrease days of ventilation and decrease risk of VAP.[142] Use of oral chlorhexidine decreases bacterial colonization of oropharyngeal secretions;[143] however, a recent meta-analysis found oral chlorhexidine use only decreases the incidence of VAP when intubated for less than 48 hours.[144] More studies are needed to gather information for long-term ventilated patients.

Antibiotic use remains a controversial subject. The standard use of antibiotics for all intubated patients may select for multidrug-resistant pathogens. As a result, the American Thoracic Society (ATS)/IDSA guidelines to date do not routinely recommend antibiotic use without signs of infection.[129] Selective decontamination of the digestive system with oral or intravenous antibiotics (which are not actually selective for the digestive system) has been found in some studies to lessen the risk of VAP;[145] however, the same concern remains that the use of antibiotics will select for multidrug-resistant pathogens. At this time, selective decontamination of the digestive system is not routinely recommended.[129]

Bloodstream Infection

Use of central venous catheters is essential to the care of many ICU patients. Every catheter, though, increases the risk of a CLABSI with an estimated number of 87,500 to 350,000 in the United States per year or 1.0 to 5.6 CLABSIs per 1000 catheter days.[126,146] CLABSIs increase the length of stay and incur excess costs of hospitalization ranging from $3,400 to $56,000; however, the evidence is mixed on whether mortality rates are increased.[4,5,147–151] Because of the clinical and economic impact of CLABSI, there is an urgent need to study and reorganize infection-prevention practices.

Risk factors

The most important element in a CLABSI is the presence of a catheter. The longer a catheter remains in place, the greater is the risk of infection.[152] The presence of more than one catheter, use of a catheter with more than one lumen, use of total parenteral nutrition or chemotherapy, or the presence of a surgical wound except a noted clean wound are all noted risk factors for bloodstream infection.[152] Patients in the ICU cared by "float pool" nurses for over 60% of the time the CVC was in place, unarousable over 70% of the time, and those who had no antibiotics given within 48 hours of CVC placement had a higher risk of CLABSI.[53] Other studies have found evidence that age younger than 65 years, a low hematocrit and low white blood cell count on admission increases the risk of bloodstream infection.[153] A case-control study found the number of previous infections, older age, duration of immunosuppressive medications, number of comorbidities, and presence of neutropenia are additional risk factors.[154] One study found a majority of the pathogens causing CLABSI correlated to a culture of the patient's skin.[155] This places extra emphasis on skin colonization and need for proper antisepsis.

Methods of prevention

Implementation of an intensive infection-prevention program with emphasis on patient safety and communication among health care workers can decrease rates of CLABSI.[42,43,156,157] A compendium published by SHEA and IDSA describes in detail current recommendations.[158] Additionally, maintaining educated nursing staff with fewer pool nurses[46,52] may contribute to decreased infection rates. Some studies have even looked at the establishment of "IV (intravenous) teams," which standardize care of central venous catheter (CVC) and may lead to decreased rates of infection.[159,160]

A meta-analysis looking at use of iodine-based versus chlorhexidine skin-prepping solutions before arterial catheter placement shows a trend toward decreased rates of CLABSI.[161] Chlorhexidine also decreases catheter colonization rates[161] and appears to be the antiseptic solution of choice at this time.[162] Specific precautions during catheter insertion are recommended, such as the use of sterile drapes, masks, caps, sterile gowns, and sterile gloves, along with a checklist to ensure proper protocols have been performed.[158] A review article of 34 studies evaluated the risk of catheter-related bloodstream infections from heparin-coated, antibiotic- and antiseptic-impregnanted catheters. The results showed significant reduction in CLABSI with the use of chlorhexidine/silver sulfadiazine catheters and even further risk reduction with minocycline-rifampicin–coated catheters.[163] These catheters, though, are not routinely recommended unless the patient is at higher risk of CLABSI.[158] In regards to type of catheter, a peripherally inserted catheter is not preferred over other catheters at this time.

Steps taken after line insertion may also decrease infection rates. Such steps include disinfecting the catheter hub before its access.[158,164] Thrombus formation in the catheter can become colonized with bacterial pathogens and lead to infection. A meta-analysis found heparin flushes significantly reduced the incidence of thrombus formation with a trend toward reducing the risk of CLABSI.[165] The use of urokinase locks may also decrease the rate of CLABSI, as noted in a recent study.[166] These findings need to be further substantiated before advocating the general use of urokinase locks.

Antibiotic lock prophylaxis has been proposed to decrease CLABSI rates. A meta-analysis evaluated infusion of vancomycin with heparin to dwell in the intravascular device lumen and found a significant decrease in the risk of CLABSI among high-risk patients, particularly adults with malignancy or infants in a neonatal ICU.[167] As of this time, antibiotic lock prophylaxis is not a standard recommendation, but a consideration in particularly high-risk or difficult-access patients.

Catheters should be removed as soon as possible once they are no longer necessary. In addition, they should have the least amount of lumens needed for the patient's medications. Of course, it is often difficult to predict long term what is needed in a critically ill patient, but, when possible, these guidelines should be followed.[151,158]

Urinary Tract Infection

Approximately 23% of nosocomial infections in the ICU are urinary tract infections with 97% of those CAUTIs or 3.1 to 7.7 CAUTIs per 1000 urinary catheter days.[126,168] A CAUTI costs an additional $589 per incidence.[169] It is a common infection, but does not appear to be linked with excess patient mortality.[170] The outcomes are less severe than those for VAP or CLABSI, but the significant number of infections makes it important to find ways to decrease their incidence.

Risk factors

The most important risk factor in the development of a CAUTI is the presence of a urinary catheter with other factors being female gender, obesity, immunodeficiency, duration of catheter use, and length of stay in an ICU.[171-175] Inappropriate placement of urinary catheters when not needed also increases the risk of patients developing a CAUTI.[175]

Methods of prevention

Any patient in the ICU with a urinary catheter should have it removed as quickly as possible. To assist with this, ongoing evaluation for continued need and discussion on rounds are helpful reminders to ICU staff and can decrease the rates of CAUTI.[176] Even before this point, the need of a urinary catheter should be confirmed before initial placement, which should be done under aseptic conditions. Once placed, it should be maintained in a closed drainage system.[177]

There is no specific material recommended for catheters. Silver alloy catheters may decrease the risk of CAUTI for patients catheterized less than 1 week.[178] A meta-analysis found a possible decrease in incidence of asymptomatic bacteriuria when using silver alloy or nitrofurazone-coated catheters for the short term.[179] The evidence is unclear at this time and more studies are necessary. A summary of preventative strategies by the IDSA/SHEA is a good reference for further information.[177]

Clostridium Difficile Infection

CDI is an important source of hospital-acquired infections in the ICU and is associated with increased morbidity, length of hospital stay, cost of hospitalization, a trend toward increased mortality in the ICU, and overall increase in cause of death in the

United States.[180–183] The emergence of more virulent strains of *C difficile* increases the need to expand research of this pathogen.

Risk factors
One of the key risk factors of acquiring CDI is greater colonization pressure.[183,184] A recent study found only 1 out of 382 patients with CDI had no prior exposure to CDI before developing infection.[184] Other potential risk factors are older age, recent hospitalization, hematologic malignancy, taking medications that decrease gastric acid, and numerous antibiotics, particularly fluoroquinolones and broad-spectrum antibiotics.[185–190]

Methods of prevention
C difficile forms spores that can remain in the environment for a prolonged period of time. Appropriate hand hygiene with soap and water and thorough environmental cleaning decreases the spore burden and is essential.[191] One study showed the incidence of CDI decreased from 7.7 cases per 1000 discharges to 1.5 cases per 1000 discharges when hospital staff wore gloves while handling any body substance while also reducing carriage rates.[192] At this time, there is little evidence that using antibiotic prophylaxis to treat colonization decreases the rate of nosocomial CDI.[191]

Proper surveillance for CDI in symptomatic patients is necessary to isolate affected patients. It may be reasonable to instigate general surveillance of patients during a CDI outbreak or endemic setting.[193] General infection-prevention measures with isolation of affected patients help prevent spread of CDI.[191,193] Besides infection-prevention programs, restricting antibiotic use with antimicrobial stewardship and limiting the number of patients who receive perioperative antibacterial prophylaxis may also help decrease rates of the infection.[194–198] Strategies to identify and prevent CDI are compiled in the new SHEA/IDSA guidelines.[198]

ANTIMICROBIAL STEWARDSHIP IN THE ERA OF MULTIDRUG-RESISTANT ORGANISMS

Given the association between antimicrobial use and the selection of resistant pathogens, the frequency of inappropriate antimicrobial use is often used as a surrogate marker for the avoidable impact on antimicrobial resistance. The combination of effective antimicrobial stewardship with a comprehensive infection control program has been shown to limit the emergence and transmission of antimicrobial-resistant bacteria. A secondary goal of antimicrobial stewardship is to reduce health care costs without adversely impacting quality of care.[199]

Antibiotic resistance in the ICU is more prevalent than in the general hospital ward.[200,201] Resistance rates to most bacterial pathogens are increasing, as shown in the NNIS System Report from 2004.[88] This increase is therefore especially important in the ICU where critically ill patients have the highest risk of infection. The cause of antibiotic resistance is multifactorial, but one of the most critical and possibly amenable reasons is antibiotic disuse.[199,202–206]

Establishing guidelines or interventions for appropriate antibiotic use have been shown to significantly reduce the number of antibiotics used and decrease hospital costs.[207] A Cochrane review of 66 studies found improvement in optimization of antibacterial use and microbiologic outcomes when hospitals put forth interventions to improve antibiotic policies.[208] Many hospitals have added multidisciplinary measures, including antimicrobial stewardship programs, to decrease inappropriate usage of antibiotics with success in decreasing broad-spectrum antibiotic usage, decreasing medication costs, and likely improvement in antimicrobial susceptibility profiles.[209–215] With increasing antibiotic resistance, risk of CDI from antibiotic use, and constant need to find new cost-saving health care measures, comprehensive antimicrobial plans are essential to further improve patient care.

SUMMARY

It is vital to recognize and understand the impact of nosocomial infections on ICU patients. The social, economic, and personal costs to patients and hospitals are overwhelming, but researchers have found many interventions to decrease infection rates. A multidirectional approach, including continuing staff education, minimizing risk factors, and implementing guidelines established by national committees, is needed. Infection-prevention committees can assist in implementing policies. This is an active area of research and we anticipate continued advancements to improve patient care.

REFERENCES

1. Joint Commission Resources. Improving care in the ICU. 1st edition. Oakbrook Terrace (IL): Joint Commission Resources; 2004.
2. Society of Critical Care Medicine. Critical care units: a descriptive analysis. 1st edition. Des Plaines (IL): Society of Critical Care Medicine; 2005.
3. Warren DK, Shukla SJ, Olsen MA, et al. Outcome and attributable cost of ventilator-associated pneumonia among intensive care unit patients in a suburban medical center. Crit Care Med 2003;31(5):1312–7.
4. Blot SI, Depuydt P, Annemans L, et al. Clinical and economic outcomes in critically ill patients with nosocomial catheter-related bloodstream infections. Clin Infect Dis 2005;41:1591–8.
5. Warren DK, Quadir WW, Hollenbeak CS, et al. Attributable cost of catheter-associated bloodstream infections among intensive care patients in a nonteaching hospital. Crit Care Med 2006;34(8):2084–9.
6. Safdar N, Dezfulian C, Collard HR, et al. Clinical and economic consequences of ventilator associated pneumonia: a systematic review. Crit Care Med 2005; 33(10):2184–93.
7. Klevens RM, Edwards JR, Richards CL, et al. Estimating health care-associated infections and deaths in U.S. hospitals, 2002. Public Health Rep 2007;122: 160–6.
8. Dempsey DT, Mullen JL, Buzby GP. The link between nutritional status and clinical outcome: can nutritional intervention modify it? Am J Clin Nutr 1988;47: 352–6.
9. Bistrian BR, Blackburn GL, Scrimshaw NS, et al. Cellular immunited in semi-starved states in hospitalized adults. Am J Clin Nutr 1975;28:1148–55.
10. Cunningham-Rundles S. Analytical methods for evaluation of immune response in nutrient intervention. Nutr Rev 1998;56(1 Pt 2):S27–37.
11. Scrimshaw NS. Historical concepts of interactions, synergism and antagonism between nutrition and infection. J Nutr 2003;133(1):316S–21S.
12. Keusch GT. The history of nutrition: malnutrition, infection and immunity. J Nutr 2003;133(1):336S–40S.
13. Chandra RK, Kumari S. Symposium: dietary nucleotides: a recently demonstrated requirement for cellular development and immune function. J Nutr 1994;124(8 Suppl):1433S–5S.
14. Rapp-Kesek D, Ståhle E, Karlsson T. Body mass index and albumin in the preoperative evaluation of cardiac surgery patients. Clin Nutr 2004;23:1398–404.

15. Kaya E, Yetim I, Dervisoglu A, et al. Risk factors for and effect of a one-year surveillance program on a surgical site infection at a university hospital in Turkey. Surg Infect (Larchmt) 2006;7(6):519–26.
16. Rubinson L, Diette GB, Song X, et al. Low caloric intake is associated with nosocomial bloodstream infections in patients in the medial intensive care unit. Crit Care Med 2004;32(2):350–7.
17. Hadfield RJ, Sinclair DG, Houldsworth PE, et al. Effects of enteral and parenteral nutrition on gut mucosal permeability in the critically ill. Am J Respir Crit Care Med 1995;152:1545–8.
18. Simpson F, Doig GS. Parenteral vs. enteral nutrition in the critically ill patient: a meta-analysis of trials using the intention to treat principle. Intensive Care Med 2005;31(1):12–23.
19. Bonten MJ, Kollef MH, Hall JB. Risk factors for ventilator-associated pneumonia: from epidemiology to patient management. Clin Infect Dis 2004;38:1141–9.
20. Vasken A, Krayem H, DiGiovine B. Effects of early enteral feeding on the outcome of critically ill mechanically ventilated medical patients. Chest 2006; 129:960–7.
21. Drakulovic MB, Torres A, Bauer TT, et al. Supine body position as a risk factor for nosocomial pneumonia in mechanically ventilated patients: a randomized trial. Lancet 1999;354(9193):1851–8.
22. Gramlich L, Kichian K, Pinilla J, et al. Does enteral nutrition compared to parenteral nutrition result in better outcomes in critically ill adult patients? A systematic review of the literature. Nutrition 2004;20(10):843–8.
23. Radrizzani D, Bertolini G, Facchini R, et al. Early enteral immunonutrition vs. parenteral nutrition in critically ill patients without severe sepsis: a randomized clinical trial. Intensive Care Med 2006;32:1191–8.
24. Blondet JJ, Beilman GJ. Glycemic control and prevention of perioperative infection. Curr Opin Crit Care 2007;13:421–7.
25. Black CT, Hennessey PJ, Andrassy RJ. Short-term hyperglycemia depresses immunity through nonenzymatic glycosylation of circulating immunoglobulin. J Trauma 1990;30(7):830–2.
26. Delamaire M, Maugendre D, Moreno M, et al. Impaired leucocyte functions in diabetic patients. Diabet Med 1997;14(1):29–34.
27. Esposito K, Nappo F, Marfella R, et al. Inflammatory cytokine concentrations are acutely increased by hyperglycemia in humans: role of oxidative stress. Circulation 2002;106(16):2067–72.
28. Latham R, Lancaster AD, Covington JF, et al. The association of diabetes and glucose control with surgical-site infections among cardiothoracic surgery patients. Infect Control Hosp Epidemiol 2001;22(10):607–12.
29. Bochicchio GV, Sung J, Joshi M, et al. Persistent hyperglycemia is predictive of outcome in critically ill trauma patients. J Trauma 2005;58(5):921–4.
30. Grey NJ, Perdrizet GA. Reduction of nosocomial infections in the surgical intensive-care unit by strict glycemic control. Endocr Pract 2004;10(Suppl 2):46–52.
31. Hruska LA, Smith JM, Hendy MP, et al. Continuous insulin infusion reduces infectious complications in diabetics following coronary surgery. J Card Surg 2005; 20(5):403–7.
32. Furnary AP, Wu Y. Eliminating the diabetic disadvantage: the Portland Diabetic Project. Semin Thorac Cardiovasc Surg 2006;18(4):302–8.
33. Van den Berghe G, Wilmer A, Hermans G, et al. Intensive insulin therapy in the medical ICU. N Engl J Med 2006;354(5):449–61.

34. Treggiari MM, Karir V, Yanez ND, et al. Intensive insulin therapy and mortality in critically ill patients. Crit Care 2008;12(1):R29.
35. Pronovost PJ, Jenckes MW, Dorman T, et al. Organizational characteristics of intensive care units related to outcomes of abdominal aortic surgery. JAMA 1999;281(14):1310–7.
36. Jain M, Miller L, Belt D, et al. Decline in ICU adverse events, nosocomial infections and cost through a quality improvement initiative focusing on teamwork and culture change. Qual Saf Health Care 2006;15(4):235–9.
37. Berriel-Cass D, Adkins FW, Jones P, et al. Eliminating nosocomial infections at Ascension Health. Jt Comm J Qual Patient Saf 2006;32(11):612–20.
38. Harrigan S, Hurst D, Lee C, et al. Developing and implementing quality initiatives in the ICU: strategies and outcomes. Crit Care Nurs Clin North Am 2006;18(4): 469–79.
39. Misset B, Timsit JF, Dumay MF, et al. A continuous quality-improvement program reduces nosocomial infection rates in the ICU. Intensive Care Med 2004;30(3): 395–400.
40. Apisarnthanarak A, Pinitchai U, Thongphubeth K, et al. Effectiveness of an educational program to reduce ventilator-associated pneumonia in a tertiary care center in Thailand: a 4-year study. Clin Infect Dis 2007;45(6):704–11.
41. Zack JE, Garrison T, Trovillion E, et al. Effect of an education program aimed at reducing the occurrence of ventilator-associated pneumonia. Crit Care Med 2002;30(11):2407–12.
42. Pronovost P, Needham D, Berenholtz S, et al. An intervention to decrease catheter-related bloodstream infections in the ICU. N Engl J Med 2006;355(26): 2725–32.
43. Lobo RD, Levin AS, Gomes LM, et al. Impact of an educational program and policy changes on decreasing catheter-associated bloodstream infections in a medical intensive care unit in Brazil. Am J Infect Control 2005;33(2):83–7.
44. Hugonnet S, Chevrolet J, Pittet D. The effect of workload on infection risk in critically ill patients. Crit Care Med 2007;35(1):76–81.
45. Hugonnet S, Uçkay I, Pittet D. Staffing level: a determinant of late-onset ventilator-associated pneumonia. Crit Care 2007;11(4):R80.
46. Fridkin SK, Pear SM, Williamson TH, et al. The role of understaffing in central venous catheter-associated bloodstream infections. Infect Control Hosp Epidemiol 1996;17(3):150–8.
47. Hugonnet S, Harbarth S, Sax H, et al. Nursing resources: a major determinant of nosocomial infection? Curr Opin Infect Dis 2004;17:329–33.
48. Kovner C, Gergen PJ. Nurse staffing levels and adverse events following surgery in U.S. hospitals. Image J Nurs Sch 1998;30(4):315–21.
49. Kane RL, Shamliyan TA, Mueller C, et al. The association of registered nurse staffing levels and patient outcomes: systematic review and meta-analysis. Med Care 2007;45(12):1195–204.
50. Cho SH, Ketefian S, Barkauskas VH, et al. The effects of nurse staffing on adverse events, morbidity, mortality and medical costs. Nurse Res 2003;52(2): 71–9.
51. Needleman J, Buerhaus P, Mattke S, et al. Nurse-staffing levels and the quality of care in hospitals. N Engl J Med 2002;346(22):1715–22.
52. Robert J, Fridkin SK, Blumberg HM, et al. The influence of the composition of the nursing staff on primary bloodstream infection rates in a surgical intensive care unit. Infect Control Hosp Epidemiol 2000;21(1):12–7.

53. Alonso-Echanove J, Edwards JR, Richards MJ, et al. Effect of nurse staffing and anti-microbial-impregnated central venous catheters on the risk for bloodstream infections in intensive care units. Infect Control Hosp Epidemiol 2003;24(12):916–25.
54. Pittet D, Dharan S, Touveneau S, et al. Bacterial contamination of the hands of hospital staff during routine patient care. Arch Intern Med 1999;159(8):821–6.
55. Markogiannakis A, Fildisis G, Tsiplakou S, et al. Cross-transmission of multidrug-resistant Acinetobacter baumannii clonal strains causing episodes of sepsis in a trauma intensive care unit. Infect Control Hosp Epidemiol 2008;29(5):410–7.
56. Ojajärvi J. Effectiveness of hand washing and disinfection methods in removing transient bacteria after patient nursing. J Hyg (Lond) 1980;85(2):193–203.
57. Oelberg DG, Joyner SE, Jiang X, et al. Detection of pathogen transmission in neonatal nurseries using DNA markers as surrogate indicators. Pediatrics 2000;105(2):311–5.
58. Bures S, Fishbain JT, Uyehara CF, et al. Computer keyboards and faucet handles as reservoirs of nosocomial pathogens in the intensive care unit. Am J Infect Control 2000;28(6):465–71.
59. Hartmann B, Benson M, Junger A, et al. Computer keyboard and mouse as a reservoir of pathogens in an intensive care unit. J Clin Monit Comput 2004; 18(1):7–12.
60. Curtis L, Cali S, Conroy L, et al. Aspergillus surveillance project at a large tertiary-care hospital. J Hosp Infect 2005;59(3):188–96.
61. Lee LD, Berkheiser M, Jiang Y, et al. Risk of bioaerosol contamination with Aspergillus species before and after cleaning in rooms filtered with high-efficiency particulate air filters that house patients with hematologic malignancy. Infect Control Hosp Epidemiol 2007;28(9):1066–70.
62. Pittet D, Sax H, Hugonnet S, et al. Cost implications of successful hand hygiene promotion. Infect Control Hosp Epidemiol 2004;25(3):264–6.
63. Larson EL, Quiros D, Lin SX. Dissemination of the CDC's Hand Hygiene Guideline and impact on infection rates. Am J Infect Control 2007;35(10):666–75.
64. Boyce JM, Pittet D, Healthcare Infection Control Practices Advisory Committee, Society for Healthcare Epidemiology of America. Association for Professionals in Infection Control, Infectious Diseases Society of America. Hand Hygiene Task Force. Guideline for hand hygiene in health-care settings: recommendations of the Healthcare Infection Control Practices Advisory Committee and the HIC-PAC/SHEA/APIC/IDSA Hand Hygiene Task Force. Infect Control Hosp Epidemiol 2002;23(12 Suppl):S3–40.
65. Rosenthal VD, Guzman S, Safdar N. Reduction in nosocomial infection with improved hand hygiene in intensive care units of a tertiary care hospital in Argentina. Am J Infect Control 2005;33(7):392–7.
66. Pittet D, Hugonnet S, Harbarth S, et al. Effectiveness of a hospital-wide programme to improve compliance with hand hygiene. Infection Control Programme. Lancet 2000;356(9238):1307–12.
67. Aragon D, Sole ML, Brown S. Outcomes of an infection prevention project focusing on hand hygiene and isolation practices. AACN Clin Issues 2005; 16(2):121–32.
68. Eldridge NE, Woods SS, Bonello RS, et al. Using the six sigma process to implement the Centers for Disease Control and Prevention Guideline for Hand Hygiene in 4 intensive care units. J Gen Intern Med 2006;21(Suppl 2):S35–42.
69. Girou E, Loyeau S, Legrand P, et al. Efficacy of handrubbing with alcohol based solution versus standard handwashing with antiseptic soap: randomized clinical trial. BMJ 2002;325(7360):362–6.

70. Larson EL, Aiello AE, Bastyr J, et al. Assessment of two hand hygiene regimens for intensive care unit personnel. Crit Care Med 2001;29(5):944–51.
71. Rupp ME, Fitzgerald T, Puumala S, et al. Prospective, controlled, cross-over trial of alcohol-based hand gel in critical care units. Infect Control Hosp Epidemiol 2008;29(1):8–15.
72. Trick WE, Vernon MO, Hayes RA, et al. Impact of ring wearing on hand contamination and comparison of hand hygiene agents in a hospital. Clin Infect Dis 2003;36(11):1383–90.
73. Duckro AN, Blom DW, Lyle EA, et al. Transfer of vancomycin-resistant *Enterococci* via health care worker hands. Arch Intern Med 2005;165(3):302–7.
74. Ho PL, For the Hong Kong intensive care unit antimicrobial resistance study (HK-ICARE) Group. Carriage of methicillin-resistant *Staphylococcus aureus*, ceftazidime-resistant gram-negative bacilli, and vancomycin-resistant *Enterococci* before and after intensive care unit admission. Crit Care Med 2003;31(4): 1175–82.
75. Drees M, Snydman DR, Schmid CH, et al. Prior environmental contamination increases the risk of acquisition of vancomycin-resistant *Enterococci*. Clin Infect Dis 2008;46(5):678–85.
76. Huang S, Datta R, Platt R. Risk of acquiring antibiotic-resistant bacteria from previous room occupants. Arch Intern Med 2006;166:1945–51.
77. Goodman ER, Platt R, Bass R, et al. Impact of an environmental cleaning intervention on the presence of methicillin-resistant *Staphylococcus aureus* and vancomycin-resistant *Enterococci* on surfaces in intensive care unit rooms. Infect Control Hosp Epidemiol 2008;29(7):593–9.
78. Carling PC, Parry MF, Von Beheren SM, Healthcare Environmental Hygiene Study Group. Identifying opportunities to enhance environmental cleaning in 23 acute care hospitals. Infect Control Hosp Epidemiol 2008;29(1):1–7.
79. Eckstein BC, Adams DA, Eckstein EC, et al. Reduction of *Clostridium difficile* and vancomycin-resistant *Enterococcus* contamination of environmental surfaces after an intervention to improve cleaning methods. BMC Infect Dis 2007;7:61.
80. Hayden MK, Bonten MJ, Blom DW, et al. Reduction in acquisition of vancoycin-resistant *Enterococcus* after enforcement of routine environmental cleaning measures. Clin Infect Dis 2006;42(11):1552–60.
81. Haiduven D. Nosocomial aspergillosis and building construction. Med Mycol 2009;47:S210–6.
82. Gniadek A, Macura AB. Intensive care unit environment contamination with fungi. Adv Med Sci 2007;52:283–7.
83. Crimi P, Argellati F, Macrina G, et al. Microbiological surveillance of hospital ventilation systems in departments at high risk of nosocomial infections. J Prev Med Hyg 2006;47(3):105–9.
84. Oren I, Haddad N, Finkelstein R, et al. Invasive pulmonary aspergillosis in neutropenic patients during hospital construction: before and after chemoprophylaxis and institution of HEPA filters. Am J Hematol 2001;66(4):257–62.
85. Stout JE, Muder RR, Mietzner S, et al. Role of environmental surveillance in determining the risk of hospital-acquired legionellosis: a national surveillance study with clinical correlations. Infect Control Hosp Epidemiol 2007;28(7): 818–24.
86. Sabriá M, Mòdol JM, Garcia-Nuñez M, et al. Environmental cultures and hospital-acquired Legionnaires' disease: a 5-year prospective study in 20 hospitals in Catalonia, Spain. Infect Control Hosp Epidemiol 2004;25(12):1072–6.

87. Trautmann M, Halder S, Hoegel J, et al. Point-of-use water filtration reduces endemic *Pseudomonas aeruginosa* infections on a surgical intensive care unit. Am J Infect Control 2008;36(6):421–9.

88. National Nosocomial Infections Surveillance System. National Nosocomial Infections Surveillance (NNIS) System Report, data summary from January 1992 through June 2004, issued October 2004. Am J Infect Control 2004;32(8):470–85.

89. Jernigan JA, Titus MG, Gröschel DH, et al. Effectiveness of contact isolation during a hospital outbreak of methicillin-resistant *Staphylococcus aureus*. Am J Epidemiol 1996;143(5):496–504.

90. Haley RW, Cushion NB, Tenover FC, et al. Eradication of endemic methicillin-resistant *Staphylococcus aureus* infections from a neonatal intensive care unit. J Infect Dis 1995;171(3):614–24.

91. Safdar N, Marx J, Meyer NA, et al. Effectiveness of preemptive barrier precautions in controlling nosocomial colonization and infection by methicillin-resistant *Staphylococcus aureus* in a burn unit. Am J Infect Control 2006;34(8):476–83.

92. Mangini E, Segal-Maurer S, Burns J, et al. Impact of contact and droplet precautions on the incidence of hospital-acquired methicillin-resistant *Staphylococcus aureus* infection. Infect Control Hosp Epidemiol 2007;28(11):1261–6.

93. Rubinovitch B, Pittet D. Screening for methicillin-resistant *Staphylococcus aureus* in the endemic hospital: What have we learned? J Hosp Infect 2001; 47(1):9–18.

94. Lucet JC, Paoletti X, Lolom I, et al. Successful long-term program for controlling methicillin-resistant *Staphylococcus aureus* in intensive care units. Intensive Care Med 2005;31(8):1051–7.

95. Huang SS, Yokoe DS, Hinrichsen VL, et al. Impact of routine intensive care unit surveillance cultures and resultant barrier precautions on hospital-wide methicillin-resistant *Staphylococcus aureus* bacteremia. Clin Infect Dis 2006;43(8): 971–8.

96. Muto CA, Jernigan JA, Ostrowsky BE, et al. SHEA guideline for preventing nosocomial transmission of multidrug-resistant strains of *Staphylococcus aureus* and *Enterococcus*. Infect Control Hosp Epidemiol 2003;24(5):362–86.

97. Calfee DP, Giannetta ET, Durbin LJ, et al. Control of endemic vancomycin-resistant Enterococcus among inpatients at a university hospital. Clin Infect Dis 2003; 37(3):326–32.

98. Boyce JM, Mermel LA, Zervos MJ, et al. Controlling vancomycin-resistant *Enterococci*. Infect Control Hosp Epidemiol 1995;16(11):634–7.

99. Ostrowsky BE, Trick WE, Sohn AH, et al. Control of vancomycin-resistant *Enterococcus* in health care facilities in a region. N Engl J Med 2001;344(19):1427–33.

100. Perencevich EN, Fisman DN, Lipsitch M, et al. Projected benefits of active surveillance for vancomycin-resistant *Enterococci* in intensive care units. Clin Infect Dis 2004;38(8):1108–15.

101. Kurup A, Chlebicki MP, Ling ML, et al. Control of a hospital-wide vancomycin-resistant *Enterococci* outbreak. Am J Infect Control 2008;36(3):206–11.

102. Mascini EM, Troelstra A, Beitsma M, et al. Genotyping and preemptive isolation to control an outbreak of vancomycin-resistant *Enterococcus faecium*. Clin Infect Dis 2006;42(6):739–46.

103. Byers KE, Anglim AM, Anneski CJ, et al. A hospital epidemic of vancomycin-resistant *Enterococcus*: risk factors and control. Infect Control Hosp Epidemiol 2001;22(3):140–7.

104. Siegel JD, Rhinehart E, Jackson M, et al. 2007 guideline for isolation precautions: preventing transmission of infectious agents in healthcare settings.

Available at: http://www.cdc.gov/ncidod/dhqp/pdf/isolation2007.pdf. Accessed January 13, 2009.

105. Robicsek A, Beaumont JL, Paule SM, et al. Universal surveillance for methicillin-resistant *Staphylococcus aureus* in 3 affiliated hospitals. Ann Intern Med 2008; 148(6):409–18.

106. Harbarth S, Fankhauser C, Schrenzel J, et al. Universal screening for methicillin-resistant *Staphylococcus aureus* at hospital admission and nosocomial infection in surgical patients. JAMA 2008;299(10):1149–57.

107. Harbarth S, Sax H, Frankhauser-Rodriguez C, et al. Evaluating the probability of previously unknown carriage of MRSA at hospital admission. Am J Med 2006; 119(3):e15–23, 275.

108. Hidron AI, Kourbatova EV, Halvosa JS, et al. Risk factors for colonization with methicillin-resistant *Staphylococcus aureus* (MRSA) in patients admitted to an urban hospital: emergence of community-associated MRSA nasal carriage. Clin Infect Dis 2005;41(2):159–66.

109. Karchmer TB, Durbin LJ, Simonton BM, et al. Cost-effectiveness of active surveillance cultures and contact/droplet precautions for control of methicillin-resistant *Staphylococcus aureus*. J Hosp Infect 2002;51(2):126–32.

110. Muto CA, Giannetta ET, Durbin LJ, et al. Cost-effectiveness of perirectal surveillance cultures for controlling vancomycin-resistant *Enterococcus*. Infect Control Hosp Epidemiol 2002;23(8):429–35.

111. Tenorio A, Badri S, Sahgal N, et al. Effectiveness of gloves in the prevention of hand carriage of vancomycin-resistant *Enterococcus* species by health care workers after patient care. Clin Infect Dis 2001;32:826–9.

112. Hayden M, Blom D, Lyle E, et al. Risk of hand or glove contamination after contact with patients colonized with vancomycin-resistant *Enterococcus* or the colonized patients' environment. Infect Control Hosp Epidemiol 2008;29(2): 149–54.

113. Slaughter S, Hayden M, Nathan C, et al. A comparison of the effect of universal use of gloves and gowns with that of glove use alone on acquisition of vancomycin-resistant *Enterococci* in a medical intensive care unit. Ann Intern Med 1996;125(6):448–56.

114. Puzniak LA, Leet T, Mayfield J, et al. To gown or not to gown: the effect on acquisition of vancomycin-resistant *Enterococci*. Clin Infect Dis 2002;35(1):18–25.

115. Srinivasan A, Song X, Ross T, et al. A prospective study to determine whether cover gowns in addition to gloves decrease nosocomial transmission of vancomycin-resistant *Enterococci* in an intensive care unit. Infect Control Hosp Epidemiol 2002;23(8):424–8.

116. Puzniak LA, Gillespie KN, Leet T, et al. A cost-benefit analysis of gown use in controlling vancomycin-resistant *Enterococcus* transmission: Is it worth the price? Infect Control Hosp Epidemiol 2004;25(5):418–24.

117. Montecalvo MA, Jarvis WR, Uman J, et al. Costs and savings associated with infection control measures that reduced transmission of vancomycin-resistant *Enterococci* in an endemic setting. Infect Control Hosp Epidemiol 2001;22(7):437–42.

118. Vernon MO, Hayden MK, Trick WE, et al. Chlorhexidine gluconate to cleanse patients in a medical intensive care unit: the effectiveness of source control to reduce the bioburden of vancomycin-resistant *Enterococci*. Arch Intern Med 2006;166(3):306–12.

119. Bleasdale SC, Trick WE, Gonzalez IM, et al. Effectiveness of chlorhexidine bathing to reduce catheter-associated bloodstream infections in medical intensive care unit patients. Arch Intern Med 2007;167(19):2073–9.

120. Wendt C, Schinke S, Württemberger M, et al. Value of whole-body washing with chlorhexidine for the eradication of methicillin-resistant *Staphylococcus aureus*: a randomized, placebo-controlled, double-blind clinical trial. Infect Control Hosp Epidemiol 2007;28(9):1036–43.

121. Simor AE, Phillips E, McGeer A, et al. Randomized controlled trial of chlorhexidine gluconate for washing, intranasal mupirocin, and rifampin and doxycycline versus no treatment for the eradication of methicillin-resistant *Staphylococus aureus* colonization. Clin Infect Dis 2007;44(2):178–85.

122. Ridenour G, Lampen R, Federspiel J, et al. Selective use of intranasal mupirocin and chlorhexidine bathing and the incidence of methicillin-resistant *Staphylococcus aureus* colonization and infection among intensive care unit patients. Infect Control Hosp Epidemiol 2007;28(10):1155–61.

123. Buehlmann M, Frei R, Fenner L, et al. Highly effective regimen for decolonization of methicillin-resistant *Staphylococcus aureus* carriers. Infect Control Hosp Epidemiol 2008;29(6):510–6.

124. Hansen D, Patzke PI, Werfel U, et al. Success of MRSA eradication in hospital routine: depends on compliance. Infection 2007;35(4):260–4.

125. Chastre J, Fagon JY. Ventilator-associated pneumonia. Am J Respir Crit Care Med 2002;165(7):867–903.

126. Edwards JR, Peterson KD, Andrus ML, et al. National Healthcare Safety Network (NHSN) Report, data summary for 2006 through 2007, issued November 2008. Am J Infect Control 2008;36:609–26.

127. Hyllienmark P, Gårdlund B, Persson JO, et al. Nosocomial pneumonia in the ICU: a prospective cohort study. Scand J Infect Dis 2007;39(8):676–82.

128. Rello J, Ollendorf DA, Oster G, et al. Epidemiology and outcomes of ventilator-associated pneumonia in a large US database. Chest 2002;122(6):2115–21.

129. American Thoracic Society; Infectious Diseases Society of America. Guidelines for the management of adults with hospital-acquired, ventilator-associated, and healthcare-associated pneumonia. Am J Respir Crit Care Med 2005;171(4): 388–416.

130. Coffin SE, Klompas M, Classen D, et al. Strategies to prevent ventilator-associated pneumonia in acute care hospitals. Infect Control Hosp Epidemiol 2008; 29(Suppl 1):S31–40.

131. Orozco-Levi M, Torres A, Ferrer M, et al. Semirecumbent position protects from pulmonary aspiration but not completely from gastroesophageal reflux in mechanically ventilated patients. Am J Respir Crit Care Med 1995;152(4 Pt 1): 1387–90.

132. Ferrer R, Artigas A. Clinical review: non-antibiotic strategies for preventing ventilator-associated pneumonia. Crit Care 2002;6(1):45–51.

133. van Nieuwenhoven CA, Vandenbroucke-Grauls C, van Tiel FH, et al. Feasibility and effects of the semirecumbent position to prevent ventilator-associated pneumonia: a randomized study. Crit Care Med 2006;34(2):396–402.

134. Bouza E, Jesús Pérez M, Muñoz P, et al. Continuous Aspiration of Subglottic Secretions (CASS) in the prevention of ventilator-associated pneumonia in the postoperative period of major heart surgery. Chest 2008;134:938–46.

135. Vallés J, Artigas A, Rello J, et al. Continuous aspiration of subglottic secretions in preventing ventilator-associated pneumonia. Ann Intern Med 1995;122(3): 179–86.

136. Diaz E, Rodríguez AH, Rello J. Ventilator-associated pneumonia: issues related to the artificial airway. Respir Care 2005;50(7):900–6.

137. Rello J, Soñora R, Jubert P, et al. Pneumonia in intubated patients: role of respiratory airway care. Am J Respir Crit Care Med 1996;154(1):111–5.
138. Niël-Weise BS, Snoeren RL, van den Broek PJ. Policies for endotracheal suctioning of patients receiving mechanical ventilation: a systematic review of randomized controlled trials. Infect Control Hosp Epidemiol 2007;28(5): 531–6.
139. Kollef MH, Afessa B, Anzueto A, et al. Silver-coated endotracheal tubes and incidence of ventilator-associated pneumonia: the NASCENT randomized trial. JAMA 2008;300(7):805–13.
140. Schweickert WD, Gehlbach BK, Pohlman AS, et al. Daily interruption of sedative infusions and complications of critical illness in mechanically ventilated patients. Crit Care Med 2004;32(6):1272–6.
141. Kress JP, Pohlman AS, O'Connor MF, et al. Daily interruption of sedative infusions in critically ill patients undergoing mechanical ventilation. N Engl J Med 2000;342(20):1471–7.
142. Quenot JP, Ladoire S, Devoucoux F, et al. Effect of a nurse-implemented sedation protocol on the incidence of ventilator-associated pneumonia. Crit Care Med 2007;35(9):2031–6.
143. Fourrier F, Dubois D, Pronnier P, et al. Effect of gingival and dental plaque antiseptic decontamination on nosocomial infections acquired in the intensive care unit: a double-blind placebo-controlled multicenter study. Crit Care Med 2005; 33(8):1728–35.
144. Kola A, Gastmeier P. Efficacy of oral chlorhexidine in preventing lower respiratory tract infections. Meta-analysis of randomized controlled trials. J Hosp Infect 2007;66(3):207–16.
145. Liberati A, D'Amico R, Pifferi, et al. Antibiotic prophylaxis to reduce respiratory tract infections and mortality in adults receiving intensive care. Cochrane Database Syst Rev 2004;(1):CD000022.
146. Wenzel RP, Edmond MB. The impact of hospital-acquired bloodstream infections. Emerg Infect Dis 2001;7(2):174–7.
147. Digiovine B, Chenoweth C, Watts C, et al. The attributable mortality and costs of primary nosocomial bloodstream infections in the intensive care unit. Am J Respir Crit Care Med 1999;160(3):976–81.
148. Laupland KB, Lee H, Gregson DB, et al. Cost of intensive care unit-acquired bloodstream infections. J Hosp Infect 2006;63(2):124–32.
149. Rello J, Ochagavia A, Sabanes E, et al. Evaluation of outcome of intravenous catheter-related infections in critically ill patients. Am J Respir Crit Care Med 2000;162(3 Pt 1):1027–30.
150. Garrouste-Orgeas M, Timsit JF, Tafflet M, et al. Excess risk of death from intensive care unit-acquired nosocomial bloodstream infections: a reappraisal. Clin Infect Dis 2006;42(8):1118–26.
151. O'Grady NP, Alexander M, Dellinger EP, et al. Guidelines for the prevention of intravascular catheter-related infections. Infect Control Hosp Epidemiol 2002; 23(12):759–69.
152. Holton D, Paton S, Conly J, et al. Central venous catheter-associated bloodstream infections occurring in Canadian intensive care units: a six-month cohort study. Can J Infect Dis Med Microbiol 2006;17(3):169–76.
153. Laupland KB, Zygun DA, Davies HD, et al. Population-based assessment of intensive care unit-acquired bloodstream infections in adults: incidence, risk factors, and associated mortality rate. Crit Care Med 2002;30(11):2462–7.

154. Jamulitrat S, Meknavin U, Thongpiyapoom S. Factors affecting mortality outcome and risk of developing nosocomial bloodstream infection. Infect Control Hosp Epidemiol 1994;15(3):163–70.
155. Safdar N, Maki DG. The pathogenesis of catheter-related bloodstream infection with noncuffed short-term central venous catheters. Intensive Care Med 2004; 30(1):62–7.
156. Berenholtz SM, Pronovost PJ, Lipsett PA, et al. Eliminating catheter-related bloodstream infections in the intensive care unit. Crit Care Med 2004;32(10): 2014–20.
157. Racco M, Horn K. Central catheter infections: use of a multidisciplinary team to find simple solutions. Crit Care Nurse 2007;27(1):80, 78–9.
158. Marschall J, Mermel LA, Classen D, et al. Strategies to prevent central line-associated bloodstream infections in acute care hospitals. Infect Control Hosp Epidemiol 2008;29(Suppl 1):S22–30.
159. Brunelle D. Impact of a dedicated infusion therapy team on the reduction of catheter-related nosocomial infections. J Infus Nurs 2003;26(6):362–6.
160. Meier PA, Fredrickson M, Catney M, et al. Impact of a dedicated intravenous therapy team on nosocomial bloodstream infections rates. Am J Infect Control 1998;26(4):388–92.
161. Crnich CJ, Maki DG. The promise of novel technology for the prevention of intravascular device-related bloodstream infection. I. Pathogenesis and short-term devices. Clin Infect Dis 2002;34(9):1232–42.
162. O'Grady NP, Alexander M, Dellinger EP, et al. Guidelines for the prevention of intravascular catheter-related infections. Clin Infect Dis 2002;35:1281–307.
163. Ramritu P, Halton K, Collignon P, et al. A systematic review comparing the relative effectiveness of antimicrobial-coated catheters in intensive care units. Am J Infect Control 2008;36(2):104–17.
164. Salzman MB, Isenberg HD, Rubin LG. Use of disinfectants to reduce microbial contamination of hubs of vascular catheters. J Clin Microbiol 1993;31(3):475–9.
165. Randolph AG, Cook DJ, Gonzales CA, et al. Benefit of heparin in central venous and pulmonary artery catheters: a meta-analysis of randomized controlled trials. Chest 1998;113(1):165–71.
166. Kethireddy S, Safdar N. Urokinase lock or flush solution for prevention of bloodstream infections associated with central venous catheters for chemotherapy: a meta-analysis of prospective randomized trials. J Vasc Access 2008;9(1):51–7.
167. Safdar N, Maki DG. Use of vancomycin-containing lock or flush solutions for prevention of bloodstream infection associated with central venous access devices: a meta-analysis of prospective, randomized trials. Clin Infect Dis 2006;43(4):474–84.
168. Richards MJ, Edwards JR, Culver DH, et al. Nosocomial infections in combined medical-surgical intensive care units in the United States. Infect Control Hosp Epidemiol 2000;21(8):510–5.
169. Tambyah PA, Knasinski V, Maki DG. The direct costs of nosocomial catheter-associated urinary tract infection in the era of managed care. Infect Control Hosp Epidemiol 2002;23(1):27–31.
170. Clec'h C, Schwebel C, Français A, et al. Does catheter-associated urinary tract infection increase mortality in critically ill patients? Infect Control Hosp Epidemiol 2007;28(12):1367–73.
171. Laupland KB, Bagshaw SM, Gregson DB, et al. Intensive care unit-acquired urinary tract infections in a regional critical care system. Crit Care 2005;9(2): R60–5.

172. Savas L, Guvel S, Onlen Y, et al. Nosocomial urinary tract infections: micro-organisms, antibiotic sensitivities and risk factors. West Indian Med J 2006; 55(3):188–93.
173. van der Kooi TI, de Boer AS, Manniën J, et al. Incidence and risk factors of device-associated infections and associated mortality at the intensive care in the Dutch surveillance system. Intensive Care Med 2007;33(2):271–8.
174. Bochicchio GV, Joshi M, Shih D, et al. Reclassification of urinary tract infections in critically ill trauma patients: a time-dependent analysis. Surg Infect (Larchmt) 2003;4(4):379–85.
175. Apisarnthanarak A, Rutjanawech S, Wichansawakun S, et al. Initial inappropriate urinary catheters use in a tertiary-care center: incidence, risk factors, and outcomes. Am J Infect Control 2007;35(9):594–9.
176. Apisarnthanarak A, Thongphubeth K, Sirinvaravong S, et al. Effectiveness of multifaceted hospitalwide quality improvement programs featuring an intervention to remove unnecessary urinary catheters at a tertiary care center in Thailand. Infect Control Hosp Epidemiol 2007;28(7):791–8.
177. Lo E, Nicolle L, Classen D, et al. Strategies to prevent catheter-associated urinary tract infections in acute care hospitals. Infect Control Hosp Epidemiol 2008;29(Suppl 1):S41–50.
178. Brosnahan J, Jull A, Tracy C. Types of urethral catheters for management of short-term voiding problems in hospitalized adults. Cochrane Database Syst Rev 2004;(1):CD004013.
179. Johnson JR, Kuskowski MA, Wilt TJ. Systematic review: antimicrobial urinary catheters to prevent catheter-associated urinary tract infection in hospitalized patients. Ann Intern Med 2006;144(2):116–26.
180. Kenneally C, Rosini JM, Skrupky LP, et al. Analysis of 30-day mortality for *Clostridium difficile*-associated disease in the ICU setting. Chest 2007;132:418–24.
181. Dubberke ER, Reske KA, Olsen MA, et al. Short- and long-term attributable costs of *Clostridium difficile*-associated disease in nonsurgical inpatients. Clin Infect Dis 2008;46(4):497–504.
182. Redelings MD, Sorvillo F, Mascola L. Increase in *Clostridium difficile*–related mortality rates, United States, 1999–2004. Emerg Infect Dis 2007;13(9):1417–9.
183. Lawrence SJ, Puzniak LA, Shadel BN, et al. *Clostridium difficile* in the intensive care unit: epidemiology, costs, and colonization pressure. Infect Control Hosp Epidemiol 2007;28(2):123–30.
184. Dubberke ER, Reske KA, Olsen MA, et al. Evaluation of *Clostridium difficile*-associated disease pressure as a risk factor for *C. difficile*-associated disease. Arch Intern Med 2007;167:1092–7.
185. Dubberke ER, Reske KA, Yan Y, et al. *Clostridium difficile*-associated disease in a setting of endemicity: identification of novel risk factors. Clin Infect Dis 2007; 45:1543–9.
186. Pépin J, Saheb N, Coulombe MA, et al. Emergence of fluoroquinolones as the predominant risk factor for *Clostridium difficile*-associated diarrhea: a cohort study during an epidemic in Quebec. Clin Infect Dis 2005;41(9):1254–60.
187. Dial S, Delaney JA, Barkun AN, et al. Use of gastric acid-suppressive agents and the risk of community-acquired *Clostridium difficile*-associated disease. JAMA 2005;294(23):2989–95.
188. Kyne L, Merry C, O'Connell B, et al. Community-acquired *Clostridium difficile* infection. J Infect 1998;36(3):287–8.
189. Bignardi GE. Risk factors for *Clostridium difficile* infection. J Hosp Infect 1998; 40(1):1–15.

190. Kelly CP, Pothoulakis C, LaMont JT. *Clostridium difficile* colitis. N Engl J Med 1994;330(4):257–62.
191. Gerding DN, Muto CA, Owens RC. Measures to control and prevent *Clostridium difficile* infection. Clin Infect Dis 2008;46(Suppl 1):S43–9.
192. Johnson S, Gerding DN, Olson MM, et al. Prospective, controlled study of vinyl glove use to interrupt *Clostridium difficile* nosocomial transmission. Am J Med 1990;88(2):137–40.
193. Vonberg RP, Kuijper EJ, Wilcox MH, et al. Infection control measures to limit the spread of *Clostridium difficile*. Clin Microbiol Infect 2008;14(Suppl 5):2–20.
194. McNulty C, Logan M, Donald IP, et al. Successful control of *Clostridium difficile* infection in an elderly care unit through use of a restrictive antibiotic policy. J Antimicrob Chemother 1997;40(5):707–11.
195. Climo MW, Israel DS, Wong ES, et al. Hospital-wide restriction of clindamycin: effect on the incidence of *Clostridium difficile*-associated diarrhea and cost. Ann Intern Med 1998;128(12 Pt 1):989–95.
196. Starks I, Ayub G, Walley G, et al. Single-dose cefuroxime with gentamicin reduces *Clostridium difficile*-associated disease in hip-fracture patients. J Hosp Infect 2008;70(1):21–6.
197. Carignan A, Allard C, Pépin J, et al. Risk of *Clostridium difficile* infection after perioperative antibacterial prophylaxis before and during an outbreak of infection due to a hypervirulent strain. Clin Infect Dis 2008;46:1838–43.
198. Dubberke E, Gerding DN, Classen D, et al. Strategies to prevent clostridium difficile infections in acute care hospitals. Infect Control Hosp Epidemiol 2008; 29(Suppl 1):S81–92.
199. Dellit TH, Owens RC, McGowan JE, et al. Infectious Diseases Society of America and the Society for Healthcare Epidemiology of America guidelines for developing an institutional program to enhance antimicrobial stewardship. Clin Infect Dis 2007;15(44):159–77.
200. Bryce EA, Smith JA. Focused microbiological surveillance and gram-negative beta-lactamase–mediated resistance in an intensive care unit. Infect Control Hosp Epidemiol 1995;16(6):331–4.
201. Rhomberg PR, Fritsche TR, Sader HS, et al. Antimicrobial susceptibility pattern comparisons among intensive care unit and general ward gram-negative isolates from the Meropenem Yearly Susceptibility Test Information Collection Program (USA). Diagn Microbiol Infect Dis 2006;56(1):57–62.
202. Barbosa TM, Levy SB. The impact of antibiotic use on resistance development and persistence. Drug Resist Updat 2000;3(5):303–11.
203. McGowan JE Jr. Antimicrobial resistance in hospital organisms and its relation to antibiotic use. Rev Infect Dis 1983;5(6):1033–48.
204. Gaynes R. The impact of antimicrobial use on the emergence of antimicrobial-resistant bacteria in hospitals. Infect Dis Clin North Am 1997;11(4):757–65.
205. Monroe S, Polk R. Antimicrobial use and bacterial resistance. Curr Opin Microbiol 2000;3(5):496–501.
206. Archibald L, Phillips L, Monnet D, et al. Antimicrobial resistance in isolates from inpatients and outpatients in the United States: increasing importance of the intensive care unit. Clin Infect Dis 1997;24(2):211–5.
207. Lutters M, Harbarth S, Janssens JP, et al. Effect of a comprehensive, multidisciplinary, educational program on the use of antibiotics in a geriatric university hospital. J Am Geriatr Soc 2004;52(1):112–6.

208. Davey P, Brown E, Fenelon L, et al. Interventions to improve antibiotic prescribing practices for hospital inpatients. Cochrane Database Syst Rev 2005;(4): CD003543.

209. Buising KL, Thursky KA, Robertson MB, et al. Electronic antibiotic stewardship–reduced consumption of broad-spectrum antibiotics using a computerized antimicrobial approval system in a hospital setting. J Antimicrob Chemother 2008; 62:608–16.

210. Carling P, Fung T, Killion A, et al. Favorable impact of a multidisciplinary antibiotic management program conducted during 7 years. Infect Control Hosp Epidemiol 2003;24(9):699–706.

211. Ansari F, Gray K, Nathwani D, et al. Outcomes of an intervention to improve hospital antibiotic prescribing: interrupted time series with segmented regression analysis. J Antimicrob Chemother 2003;52(5):842–8.

212. Rüttimann S, Keck B, Hartmeier C, et al. Long-term antibiotic cost savings from a comprehensive intervention program in a medical department of a university-affiliated teaching hospital. Clin Infect Dis 2004;38(3):348–56.

213. Ozkurt Z, Erol S, Kadanali A, et al. Changes in antibiotic use, cost and consumption after an antibiotic restriction policy applied by infectious disease specialists. Jpn J Infect Dis 2005;58(6):338–43.

214. Mach R, Vlcek J, Prusova M, et al. Impact of a multidisciplinary approach on antibiotic consumption, cost and microbial resistance in a Czech hospital. Pharm World Sci 2007;29(5):565–72.

215. Feucht CL, Rice LB. An interventional program to improve antibiotic use. Ann Pharmacother 2003;37(5):646–51.

Clostridium difficile Infection in the Intensive Care Unit

David J. Riddle, MD[a], Erik R. Dubberke, MD, MSPH[b],*

KEYWORDS

• Nosocomial infection • Pseudomembranous colitis
• Intensive care • Critical care • Clostridium difficile

Diarrhea is a common problem in critically ill patients regardless of the disease process that necessitated admission to the intensive care unit (ICU). Overall, up to 40% of patients develop diarrhea after admission to the ICU.[1] Certain patient populations, such as those suffering extensive burns, may have an incidence of diarrhea greater than 90%.[2] Furthermore, patients who develop diarrhea are at risk of other complications, such as dehydration, hemodynamic instability, malnutrition, electrolyte imbalances, and skin breakdown.[3] Enteral feeding is the most common cause of diarrhea in the intensive care setting; however, other noninfectious causes include hypoalbuminemia, intestinal ischemia, and medications.[4,5] Clostridium difficile infection (CDI) is the most common infectious cause of diarrhea in the ICU.[4]

First discovered in 1935,[6] C difficile was not identified as a cause of pseudomembranous colitis in humans until 1978.[7] Since that time, C difficile has been recognized as the most common cause of nosocomial infectious diarrhea.[8] Recent changes in CDI epidemiology have had a significant impact in the ICU setting. The incidence of CDI is increasing in the ICU, as well as in the hospitalized population as a whole.[9] The severity of CDI also is increasing, prompting more admissions to the ICU for management of CDI-related complications.[10] Recent data indicate outcomes may be improved by recognizing patients with more severe CDI and by prompt initiation of the most appropriate therapy.

This work was supported by grant T32 HD007507 from the NICHD and 1 UL1 RR024992-01 (PI: Polonsky); 1 KL2 RR024994-01 (PI: Fraser) from the NCRR.
[a] Division of Infectious Diseases, Departments of Medicine and Pediatrics, Washington University School of Medicine, 660 S. Euclid Avenue, Campus Box 8051, St. Louis, MO 63110-1093, USA
[b] Division of Infectious Diseases, Department of Medicine, Washington University School of Medicine, 660 S. Euclid, Box 8051, St. Louis, MO 63110-1093, USA
* Corresponding author.
E-mail address: edubberk@im.wustl.edu (E.R. Dubberke).

Infect Dis Clin N Am 23 (2009) 727–743
doi:10.1016/j.idc.2009.04.011
0891-5520/09/$ – see front matter © 2009 Elsevier Inc. All rights reserved.
id.theclinics.com

PATHOGENESIS AND EPIDEMIOLOGY

C difficile causes diarrhea through the secretion of exotoxins within the gastrointestinal tract. The production of toxin is necessary for *C difficile* to cause disease and invasion of *C difficile* across the colonic mucosa is exceedingly rare. Toxin A causes neutrophilic infiltration and damage to the colonic mucosa.[11,12] Toxin B has similar destructive effects on the colonic mucosa, but appears to be roughly 10 times more cytotoxic than toxin A.[13] Necrosis and sloughing of cellular debris into the colonic lumen result from the interaction of the toxins with colonocyte surface receptors that induce the degradation of actin filaments.[14] Toxin-induced cytokine release also triggers the exudation of inflammatory cells and proteins from the resulting mucosal ulcerations.[15] The resulting inflammatory exudate forms the pseudomembrane that is nearly pathogneumonic for CDI.[13]

Roughly 3% of healthy adults are asymptomatically colonized with *C difficile*.[16] Colonization rates increase to as much as 50% in patients residing in long-term care facilities.[17] As many as 60% of patients who acquire the organism in the health care setting remain asymptomatic.[18] Generally, an individual's risk of becoming colonized with *C difficile* is directly proportional to length of the hospital stay, with mean time to acquisition of the organism of 2 weeks.[19] Additional studies have found that length of stay is a surrogate for exposure to patients with CDI, and is not an independent risk factor for CDI.[20]

Patients who lack previous or established colonization with *C difficile* are at highest risk for developing symptomatic disease after becoming infected with the organism. A review of several longitudinal studies showed that only about 1% of individuals already colonized with *C difficile* at the time of hospital admission developed diarrhea, but 5% of previously uncolonized individuals had symptomatic disease after new acquisition of the organism.[21] This disparity is thought to be due to a protective effect from antitoxin antibodies in patients with prior exposure. Patients capable of mounting a brisk antibody response to the *C difficile* toxins after exposure are also less likely to develop symptomatic disease.[22]

The overall incidence of CDI varies between centers, but generally about 1%–2% of all hospitalized patients develop symptomatic infection.[23] In the intensive care setting, CDI is more common with an overall incidence of roughly 4%.[24] Up to 20% of ICU patients who develop symptomatic disease progress to a fulminant colitis with a mortality rate of nearly 60%.[25,26]

Although numerous strains coexist within a single hospital, outbreaks are typically linked to a single strain. The spores of *C difficile* are difficult to eradicate because of resistance to many environmental cleaning detergents[27] and can be isolated from environmental swabs taken from a patient's room months after discharge.[28] Although persistence in the environment is well documented, *C difficile* is typically thought to spread through person-to-person transmission. Health care workers are often responsible for spreading the organism on their hands or medical equipment.[18]

The incidence and severity of CDI among hospitalized patients continue to increase worldwide. According to data from the National Inpatient Sample, the number of patients diagnosed with CDI in United States hospitals doubled between 2000 and 2005 to 11.2 cases per 10,000 population.[9] The age-adjusted CDI-related mortality showed a similar trend, increasing from 1.2% in 2000 to 2.2% in 2004.[9] Overall 30-day mortality in patients with CDI in the ICU was almost 40% during 2004 and 2005. Case control analysis estimated that 6% mortality was directly attributable to CDI in critically ill patients.[29]

A hypervirulent strain of *C difficile*, the North American pulse-field gel electrophoresis type 1 (NAP1) strain, has also been implicated as a cause of the increasing severity of CDI. Epidemics from this strain have occurred across the United States, Canada, and Europe.[23,30–32] Patients infected with this strain undergo a higher proportion of urgent colectomies[33] and attributable mortality is estimated to be roughly 17%.[34] A deletion in the toxin regulatory gene, *tcdC*, is thought to allow the NAP1 strain to overproduce toxin A and toxin B by as much as 15- to 20-fold.[32] The NAP1 strain also produces binary toxin, although this virulence factor's role in pathogenesis is currently unknown.[31] Outbreaks of the NAP1 strain are strongly associated with the use of fluoroquinolones, although other antibiotics are also implicated.[33,35]

RISK FACTORS

There are numerous independent risk factors reported for developing symptomatic disease after acquisition of *C difficile*. The risk factors most consistently identified in the literature include antibiotic exposure, age over 60 years, longer duration of hospital stay, severe underlying disease, and gastric acid suppression.[36] Many of these factors are often found in critically ill patients residing in the ICU, making it unsurprising that ICU stay is also a commonly cited risk factor.[37] The most pertinent, potentially modifiable risk factors for intensive care patients are discussed below.

Exposure to antimicrobials is the most important risk factor for the development of CDI.[37] Preceding antibiotic administration is demonstrated in roughly 95% of inpatient cases.[38] The disruption of the normal flora caused by antibiotics allows *C difficile* to colonize and overgrow within the gastrointestinal tract. Nearly every antibiotic has been implicated in leading to CDI. However, broad-spectrum antibiotics with anti-anaerobic activity appear to cause the greatest risk.[37] Before the epidemics from the NAP1 strain, clindamycin, ampicillin, and cephalosporins were the most frequently implicated.[37,39] With the increasing use of fluoroquinolones in hospitalized patients, these antibiotics have also emerged as an important cause of CDI.[35] Outbreaks of NAP1-related CDI are more specifically linked to the 8-methoxy fluoroquinolones, moxifloxacin, and gatifloxacin. Administration of multiple antibiotics or use of longer treatment courses also increases the risk of developing CDI.[35,37]

Several retrospective studies have shown that hospitalized patients are over twice as likely to develop CDI if prescribed proton pump inhibitors.[36,40] This is especially relevant for patients in ICUs where gastric acid suppression is a routine intervention because of the extremely high incidence of stress-related mucosal damage.[41] The usual acidic environment of the stomach is fatal to the vegetative form of *C difficile* and may make it less likely for the spore form to germinate after passing into the bowel.[42] Once the pH rises above 5, even vegetative *C difficile* is able to survive gastric exposure.[42] Proton pump inhibitors also appear to cause an alteration in the gastrointestinal flora that may also create a niche for *C difficile* colonization.[43]

Enteral feeding is another common practice in ICUs that has been implicated as a possible contributing factor in the development of CDI. Up to 60% of patients receiving enteral feeds develop diarrhea, so it is often difficult to distinguish infected from noninfected patients.[44] Several factors associated with tube feeding are thought to increase the risk of infection, including contamination of the formula or equipment during handling,[45] or an alteration of the colonic environment associated with the special formulas.[46] In a prospective cohort study involving 152 patients, enteral feeding increased the risk of *C difficile* acquisition from 8% to 20% and the risk of developing CDI from 1% to 9%.[47] The finding that enteral feeding doubles the risk of CDI has also been demonstrated in other prospective studies.[24,48] The risk appears to be greatest when the patients were fed with a postpyloric tube.[47]

Mechanical ventilation has also been demonstrated as a risk for both the development of CDI and increased disease severity in the few studies that evaluate this risk factor. Mechanical ventilation was associated with the acquisition of *C difficile* while in the ICU; however, statistical significance was not maintained after adjusting for confounders.[24] Ventilator support was found to increase the risk of developing CDI by twofold based on multivariable logistic regression on data from 36,086 patients.[36] Postoperative ICU patients who developed CDI had a median duration of ventilator support greater than 24 hours, compared with only 12 hours in the uninfected cohort.[49]

CLINICAL MANIFESTATIONS

CDI has a wide range of manifestations, causing a self-limited mild diarrheal illness to a fulminant life-threatening colitis.[50] The onset of CDI symptoms may range from 1 day to up to 10 weeks after antibiotics are administered; however, most cases begin between within 3 and 7 days of exposure.[51-54] The watery diarrhea of CDI is usually accompanied by low-grade fever and cramping abdominal pain. Although standard definitions of disease severity are lacking, systemic symptoms generally increase with the degree of colitis. Severe cases of colitis can progress to ileus or toxic megacolon that may cause a paradoxic decrease in the amount of diarrhea[51-54] or may result in an acute abdomen.[55]

DIAGNOSIS

CDI is diagnosed by confirming the presence of a toxigenic strain of *C difficile* or one of its toxins in the stool of a patient with symptoms consistent with the disease. Unlike most other bacterial infections, isolating the organism in culture is expensive, time consuming, and insufficient to prove disease because of the existence of nontoxigenic *C difficile* in the stool. The presence of nontoxigenic strains of *C difficile* can result in a false-positive rate that exceeds 10% if culture alone is used to diagnose CDI.[56] Proving the cultured organism is pathogenic requires further analysis to determine the presence of toxin A, toxin B, or the virulence factor genes.

Multiple toxin-detecting tests are commercially available for the diagnosis of CDI. The laboratory gold standard for detection of *C difficile* toxins in the stool is the cytotoxicity cell assay. When filtered diarrheal stool that contains *C difficile* toxins is added to cultured fibroblasts, a characteristic cytopathic effect is seen. The cytotoxicity cell assay is largely considered too impractical for routine use because of cost, time delays, and need for cull culture equipment, and has been replaced by ELISAs in most centers.[57] The ELISAs are relatively inexpensive and can confirm the diagnosis within several hours. Most currently available ELISAs are capable of detecting both toxin A and toxin B and have sensitivities that approach 90% in comparison to the cytotoxicity assay.[58] Another enzyme immunoassay that detects *C difficile* glutamate dehydrogenase is highly sensitive, but this assay must also be confirmed by a toxin-detecting assay since this enzyme is produced by nontoxigenic strains.[59]

Up to 20% of critically ill patients may suffer from ileus and lack the diarrhea typically associated with CDI.[60] A lack of diarrhea coupled with an inability of the critically ill patient to communicate with care providers may make diagnosis of CDI extremely difficult. Intensivists need to maintain a high index of suspicion and must often rely on physical examination and laboratory findings to make the diagnosis. Examination findings, such as fever, abdominal pain, and abdominal distention, are likely to be present in severe colitis. Hematology panels may also uncover a significant leukocytosis (often > 20,000 cells/mm^2) and bandemia.[61] Elevation in serum lactate dehydrogenase is a relatively nonspecific finding for gastrointestinal disease, but may also be a potential clue to the presence of CDI.[62,63] These findings often precede multiorgan dysfunction and should prompt urgent consideration of CDI as a possible cause.[61,64,65]

In the uncommon event that the diagnosis of CDI cannot be established through stool testing or compatible clinical syndrome, endoscopy may be a useful adjunct if the diagnosis cannot be delayed. The goal of endoscopy is to visualize the nearly pathognomic pseudomembrane. However, colonic edema, erythema, and mucosal ulcerations may also be consistent with the diagnosis.[66,67] Rectal sparing occurs in up to 25% of patients, but most lesions are visible within 60 cm from the anus so either flexible sigmoidoscopy or colonoscopy are acceptable methods.[68] Although intestinal perforation appears uncommon in patients with CDI who undergo flexible sigmoidoscopy, this remains an associated risk in severe disease, so endoscopic confirmation of the diagnosis should be performed with caution.[67]

CT is rarely used in the diagnosis of CDI; however, it may reveal patterns consistent with colitis and can also be used as supportive evidence for the diagnosis. Findings of colonic wall thickening greater than 4 mm, wall nodularity, pericolonic stranding, and ascites are common in CDI.[69,70] In a retrospective study using a combination of these criteria to diagnose CDI based on CT scan, the sensitivity was 52% and specificity was 93% compared with stool toxin assays.[69] Bowel wall thickening is the most sensitive finding, but lacks specificity if not supported by other characteristic imaging changes.[69] Less common findings also include distention of the colon, colonic fold effacement, and nodular fold thickening.[70] Characteristic imaging findings are typically associated with other clinical and laboratory abnormalities, but they do not necessarily correlate with severity of the disease.[71,72]

TREATMENT

Treatment of CDI should be based on the severity of the disease. Unfortunately, standardized definitions for disease severity are lacking and current definitions are somewhat subjective and artificial given that the illness varies along a continuous spectrum of symptoms. In general, symptoms of CDI can be grouped into three categories: mild to moderate, severe, and severe disease with complications.[73,74] Mild to moderate CDI consists only of diarrhea and abdominal cramping unaccompanied by systemic symptoms. Patients with abundant diarrhea, abdominal pain, leukocytosis, and fever or other systemic symptoms should be considered to have severe CDI. Individuals suffering from severe disease with complications may have any degree of gastrointestinal symptoms that are also accompanied by paralytic ileus, toxic megacolon, or other life-threatening conditions. The disease may become progressively more serious even after treatment has been initiated, so assessment of disease category must remain a dynamic process.

For all severities of CDI, cessation of the inciting antibiotic is the first step in treatment whenever possible. This should theoretically allow for recovery of the normal colonic flora to help combat the overgrowth of *C difficile*. Before the NAP1 epidemic, stopping the administration of antibiotics resulted in the resolution of diarrhea in nearly one quarter of patients with CDI.[75,76] Unfortunately, this intervention is rarely possible in the intensive care setting because more than 60% of patients who develop CDI have documented serious concomitant infections.[38] When it is unsafe to stop the inciting antibiotic therapy, it is prudent to change to a more narrow-spectrum regimen when possible.

Metronidazole and vancomycin are the most common antibiotics used to treat *C difficile* in patients with symptomatic infection.[77] Both antibiotics should be administered orally in patients able to tolerate that route. Metronidazole may also be given intravenously because both biliary excretion and exudation across inflamed colonic mucosa allow adequate treatment concentrations to be reached in the colon.[78] The use of intravenous metronidazole is also supported by several published case series and extensive clinical experience.[79,80] Intravenous vancomycin is not effective for CDI because there is minimal excretion of the drug into the bowel so fecal concentration is low.

Metronidazole has historically been the drug of preference in CDI because of significant cost advantage in comparison to oral vancomycin and equal efficacy demonstrated in prior studies.[81,82] There has also been reluctance to use oral vancomycin because of concern that it will result in more intestinal colonization with vancomycin-resistant enterococci, although this concern has been not been substantiated in the literature.[83,84] *C difficile* continues to be susceptible to both medications in vitro[85]; however, recent studies indicate that the choice of one drug over the other should now be based on disease severity.[74,86]

Metronidazole remains appropriate first-line therapy for mild to moderate disease. In recent studies, oral vancomycin appears to have improved clinical outcomes in patients with severe disease. The decreasing efficacy of metronidazole was illustrated in a prospective observational study of 207 patients with CDI that reported 22% of patients remained symptomatic after 10 days of metronidazole therapy and an additional 27% suffered relapse.[87] In a randomized trial that enrolled 150 patients, metronidazole therapy resulted in a cure rate of only 76%, compared with a 97% cure rate with vancomycin for the treatment of severe CDI.[74] The difference between the two antibiotics was not significant of mild to moderate disease in this study. Because of these findings, vancomycin is preferred initial therapy for patients with severe disease or with risk factors for progressing to severe disease.

In cases of severe CDI with complications, reduced or absent bowel motility may prevent adequate amounts of orally administered vancomycin from reaching the site of infection. Several case reports have supported the intracolonic administration of vancomycin when oral therapy cannot be tolerated.[88-90] Some experts also use higher doses of oral vancomycin with the goal of improving the chance that adequate fecal concentrations will be reached, although this practice has not been studied. Intravenous metronidazole may be added to either oral or intracolonic vancomycin in severely ill patients with ileus, although this approach has also not been adequately evaluated.[79,80]

When the colitis is so extreme that the efficacy of antibiotic therapy is in doubt, it is important to consider surgical consultation. Fulminant *C difficile* colitis that necessitates colectomy is rare, occurring in less than 3% of all patients with CDI.[91] In the ICU patient population, it is not surprising that the incidence of severe colitis is much higher, with 20% of patients requiring colectomy or diversion procedures.[25] Improved mortality rates are seen when surgical intervention is performed within 48 hours of lack of response to medical therapy.[92] With the increased number of rapidly progressing cases secondary to the hypervirulent NAP1 strain of *C difficile*, surgical consultation is becoming even more urgent. Elderly patients with leukocytosis and elevated lactate appear to benefit the most from early colectomy during NAP1 epidemics.[93] Admission to the hospital for a diagnosis other than CDI, mental status changes, prolongation of attempted medical treatment, and vasopressor support are all predictors of postoperative mortality.[93]

Multiple other antibiotics have been considered in the treatment of CDI, but none have demonstrated any significant clinical benefits over the current conventional therapy. Rifaximin, nitazoxanide, and fusidic acid are equally efficacious to vancomycin or metronidazole.[82,94–96] The only benefit noted with teicoplanin was a significant reduction in stool toxin levels in comparison to vancomycin and metronidazole, but there is no corresponding significant clinical benefit[82,95,97] and it is not available in the United States. Combination therapy with metronidazole and rifampin has been evaluated in a single randomized trial of 39 patients, but the only significant finding was an increase in mortality in the combination group.[98] The lack of any significant clinical benefits coupled with reduced physician experience with these medications has resulted in these other antibiotics being rarely used or advocated for CDI.

A novel macrocycle antibiotic, OPT-80, is currently in phase 3 trials evaluating its effectiveness in the treatment of CDI. OPT-80 is minimally absorbed from the gastrointestinal tract and well tolerated in most subjects.[99] Although highly effective against *C difficile*, OPT-80 leaves the majority of the gram-negative anaerobic flora of the gastrointestinal tract intact.[100] A total of 48 subjects with mild to moderate CDI participated in the trial and were randomized to receive 100 mg, 200 mg, or 400 mg per day of the medication.[100] Although only 77% of patients treated with the lower dose had resolution of diarrhea within 10 days, this climbed to 94% in the high-dose treatment group. Only two patients suffered disease relapse across all treatment groups. Unfortunately, it is currently unknown if the drug will perform well in patients with severe or complicated disease, but OPT-80 does show some early promise as a potential future alternative to the current conventional therapy.

Another commonly employed strategy in combating CDI is the administration of probiotics. The live microorganisms in the probiotic formula are intended to restore the nonpathogenic flora to the colon, inhibit *C difficile* toxin production, and stimulate the immune system.[101] The combination of *Saccharomyces* or Lactobacillus probiotics with conventional antibiotic therapy has shown no statistically significant benefit for the treatment of CDI in several randomized controlled trials.[102–105] *Saccharomyces boulardii* did appear to reduce the relapse rate of CDI when combined with conventional therapy in one randomized, placebo-controlled trial after subgroup analysis[103]; however, this result was unable to be replicated. Although adverse effects of probiotics are rare, occasional case reports of bloodstream infections in critically ill patients with central venous catheters are reported, and being critically ill, immunocompromised, or having a central venous catheter are considered contraindications for probiotics.[106] These organisms may also become aerosolized and place other patients in the ICU at risk for opportunistic infection.[107]

Neutralizing the *C difficile* toxins has been another attempted treatment strategy. Cholestyramine and colestipol bind *C difficile* toxins in vitro; however, clinical trails have shown no efficacy during acute CDI.[108] The only placebo-controlled trial evaluating these medications showed no reduction in the stool concentration of either *C difficile* or its toxins.[53] There is also a potential harm in using these medications during therapy with vancomycin because the drugs can complex with one another and may result in subtherapeutic antibiotic concentrations in the stool.[109]

Intravenous immunoglobulin (IVIG) has also been evaluated for the treatment of CDI with the goal of neutralizing the effect of the toxins. A poor humoral response to *C difficile* toxins is known to be associated with an increased risk of developing symptomatic disease and a higher incidence of relapses.[22] Anti-*C difficile* toxin antibodies are commonly present in healthy subjects and typically found in pooled immuneglobulin.[110] Although theoretically beneficial, IVIG use is currently only supported by case studies and series.[110–113] These studies are contradicted by a retrospective analysis of 18 pair-matched patients with severe CDI that did not show a clear benefit in adding IVIG to standard antibiotic therapy.[114] Unfortunately, this study suffered from methodological difficulties, such as not controlling for the length of time between onset of symptoms and administration of IVIG. Because of the insufficient evidence base, IVIG cannot be generally recommended for the treatment of CDI, although this appears to be an area worth further study, especially in patients with severe disease or multiple relapses.

Although the evidence is anecdotal, it is generally advised that any medications with an antiperistaltic effect be avoided in patients with CDI. Drugs that decrease intestinal motility are thought to increase the risk of severe complications, such as toxic megacolon.[115] Unfortunately, the critically ill patient population often requires sedatives and narcotics for pain management or mechanical ventilation. Nevertheless, it is prudent to wean medications with antiperistaltic effects if possible in patients at high risk for developing severe CDI.

TREATMENT FAILURE

Patients typically have some symptomatic improvement, including fever resolution, within 48 hours after the initiation of appropriate antibiotic therapy for CDI.[116] A significant reduction in the amount of diarrhea is expected within 6 days of starting therapy in most patients.[116] Failure to respond appropriately after treatment with metronidazole is associated with low serum albumin, continued exposure to the inciting antibiotic, and residence in the ICU.[117,118] One possible physiologic explanation for metronidazole failure comes from the observation that stool concentrations diminish as the colitis improves because of reduced exudation across the noninflamed colonic mucosa.[78] In vitro susceptibilities performed on C difficile strains obtained from the stool of patients who have failed to respond continue to be metronidazole sensitive.[119] Although the emergence of resistance to metronidazole is rare, many clinicians advocate changing therapy to oral vancomycin in this scenario. If patients continue to fail antibiotic therapy with vancomycin, surgical intervention or other less-established treatments, such as IVIG, should be considered.

RELAPSE

Intensivists are likely to encounter CDI relapses in patients who have prolonged stays within the ICU. About one third of patients develop at least one relapse to CDI regardless of initial treatment choice.[120] Relapses have been reported to occur up to several months after the initial episode, but most occur within the first 2 weeks of completing therapy. The first relapse is followed by even more episodes of recurrent disease in 50% of patients.[121] The risk factors of recurrent disease are similar to those associated with the first episode of CDI. It remains unresolved if disease relapse is secondary to reactivation of latent C difficile spores, reacquisition of the organism from the environment, or a combination of both scenarios.[122]

Treatment of recurrent disease is a difficult problem because it has not been extensively studied and current strategies have questionable effectiveness. Because antibiotic resistance does not appear to be a cause of relapse, the first recurrence is generally managed similarly to the initial disease with either metronidazole or vancomycin, depending on disease severity.[122] Treatment with longer courses of oral vancomycin in either a tapering or pulse-dosing schedule is generally thought to be an appropriate strategy for patients who suffer multiple CDI relapses, but this approach is only supported by observational studies and is not always effective.[123,124] Several recent studies used rifaximin after a standard treatment course of vancomycin was completed. All but one patient remained disease-free in a case series of eight patients with at a history of multiple CDI relapses treated with vancomycin followed by 2 weeks of rifaximin.[125] The patient who suffered the relapse had a *C difficile* strain that developed resistance to rifaximin. Another case series treated six patients with recurrent CDI with rifaximin alone and five patients had no recurrence after a mean follow-up of 310 days.[126] As noted above, combining probiotics, toxin-binding resins, or IVIG with vancomycin therapy has shown potential in reducing the incidence of multiple relapses in some small studies and these may be considered on a case-by-case basis. The investigational macrocycle, OTP-80, may also prove beneficial in treating CDI relapses in the future.

PREVENTION

The most essential aspect of CDI prevention is protecting patients from initial acquisition of the organism in the health care setting. As with many other nosocomial pathogens, strict hand hygiene and appropriate contact precautions are the cornerstones of reducing the spread of *C difficile* among patients. *C difficile* spores are not eradicated by the commonly used alcohol-based hand sanitizers; however, the use of these products has not been associated with any significant increases in the incidence of CDI within centers.[127] Contact precautions that include the use of a gown and gloves when entering a patient's room also results in a significant decrease in new CDI cases.[128,129] The combination of rigorous hand hygiene with contact precautions can decrease the incidence of CDI by as much as 80%.[128–130]

Environmental contamination with *C difficile* spores is also a potential source of disease acquisition in the hospital setting. Rapid identification and treatment of patients are essential in reducing the amount of spores released into the environment because the amount of contamination correlates with the duration of symptoms.[131] Disinfection of the patient's surroundings is difficult because the spore form of *C difficile* is resistant to standard cleaning products and may persist in patient rooms for months.[132,133] In the absence of an Environmental Protection Agency–approved liquid disinfectant with known sporicidal activity, household bleach diluted 1:10 with water may be used and has been shown rapidly fatal to *C difficile* spores.[134] There is currently no evidence that routine decontamination of patient rooms results in a decrease in CDI, but this step is reasonable to consider in outbreak situations.

Attention should also be directed at reducing each modifiable individual risk factor if possible. The most significant intervention in this area appears to be ensuring the prudent use of antibiotics through formulary restrictions and antimicrobial stewardship programs. During a NAP1 strain outbreak in Quebec, an antimicrobial stewardship program was introduced that resulted in a 54% reduction in antibiotic use and a 60% reduction in the incidence of CDI.[135] When broad-spectrum antibiotics are specifically restricted in antimicrobial stewardship programs, CDI rates also fall despite the overall antibiotic use remaining unchanged.[136] More specific interventions that restrict antibiotics highly associated with CDI, such as fluoroquinolones and clindamycin, have also proven successful.[137–140] In addition to the control of antibiotic use, prudent use of other medications, such as proton pump inhibitors, may also be beneficial.

SUMMARY

C difficile is commonly encountered in the ICU setting and critically ill patients are at significant risk for morbidity and mortality from this pathogen. The incidence and severity of CDI have been increasing with new epidemics secondary to the hypervirulent NAP1 strain. Critically ill patients share many of the risk factors for developing severe CDI, so vigilance must be maintained in this patient population to prevent and rapidly treat the disease. Clinical manifestations may be variable in the ICU setting because of the high incidence of complicated disease, so intensivists should have a high index of suspicion in patients with otherwise unexplained examination or laboratory findings associated with CDI. Treatment of choice for patients with mild to moderate disease remains metronidazole; however, patients with severe and complicated disease should be treated with vancomycin. Intracolonic administration of vancomycin, surgical intervention, and less well-established therapies, such as IVIG, may be beneficial in some patients with severe disease. Prevention efforts that focus on hand hygiene, contact precautions, and antimicrobial stewardship programs remain essential in halting the spread of this disease within medical centers.

REFERENCES

1. Kelly TW, Patrick MR, Hillman KM. Study of diarrhea in critically ill patients. Crit Care Med 1983;11:7–9.
2. Thakkar K, Kien CL, Rosenblatt JI, et al. Diarrhea in severely burned children. JPEN J Parenter Enteral Nutr 2005;29:8–11.
3. Ringel AF, Jameson GL, Foster ES. Diarrhea in the intensive care patient. Crit Care Clin 1995;11:465–77.
4. Liolios A, Oropello JM, Benjamin E. Gastrointestinal complications in the intensive care unit. Clin Chest Med 1999;20:329–45, viii.
5. Wiesen P, Van Gossum A, Preiser JC. Diarrhoea in the critically ill. Curr Opin Crit Care 2006;12:149–54.
6. Hall IC, O'Toole E. Intestinal flora in new-born infants with a description of a new pathogenic anaerobe, Bacillus difficilis. Am J Dis Child 1935;49:390–402.
7. Bartlett JG, Chang TW, Gurwith M, et al. Antibiotic-associated pseudomembranous colitis due to toxin-producing clostridia. N Engl J Med 1978;298:531–4.
8. Barbut F, Corthier G, Charpak Y, et al. Prevalence and pathogenicity of Clostridium difficile in hospitalized patients. A French multicenter study. Arch Intern Med 1996;156:1449–54.
9. Zilberberg MD. Clostridium difficile-related hospitalizations among US adults, 2006. Emerg Infect Dis 2009;15:122–4.
10. Labbe AC, Poirier L, Maccannell D, et al. Clostridium difficile infections in a Canadian tertiary care hospital before and during a regional epidemic associated with the BI/NAP1/027 strain. Antimicrob Agents Chemother 2008;52:3180–7.
11. Pothoulakis C, Sullivan R, Melnick DA, et al. Clostridium difficile toxin A stimulates intracellular calcium release and chemotactic response in human granulocytes. J Clin Invest 1988;81:1741–5.
12. Triadafilopoulos G, Pothoulakis C, O'Brien MJ, et al. Differential effects of Clostridium difficile toxins A and B on rabbit ileum. Gastroenterology 1987;93:273–9.
13. Riegler M, Sedivy R, Pothoulakis C, et al. Clostridium difficile toxin B is more potent than toxin A in damaging human colonic epithelium in vitro. J Clin Invest 1995;95:2004–11.
14. Voth DE, Ballard JD. Clostridium difficile toxins: mechanism of action and role in disease. Clin Microbiol Rev 2005;18:247–63.
15. Meyer GK, Neetz A, Brandes G, et al. Clostridium difficile toxins A and B directly stimulate human mast cells. Infect Immun 2007;75:3868–76.

16. Barbut F, Petit JC. Epidemiology of Clostridium difficile-associated infections. Clin Microbiol Infect 2001;7:405–10.
17. Riggs MM, Sethi AK, Zabarsky TF, et al. Asymptomatic carriers are a potential source for transmission of epidemic and nonepidemic Clostridium difficile strains among long-term care facility residents. Clin Infect Dis 2007;45:992–8.
18. McFarland LV, Mulligan ME, Kwok RY, et al. Nosocomial acquisition of Clostridium difficile infection. N Engl J Med 1989;320:204–10.
19. Clabots CR, Johnson S, Olson MM, et al. Acquisition of Clostridium difficile by hospitalized patients: evidence for colonized new admissions as a source of infection. J Infect Dis 1992;166:561–7.
20. Dubberke ER, Reske KA, Olsen MA, et al. Evaluation of Clostridium difficile-associated disease pressure as a risk factor for C difficile-associated disease. Arch Intern Med 2007;167:1092–7.
21. Shim JK, Johnson S, Samore MH, et al. Primary symptomless colonisation by Clostridium difficile and decreased risk of subsequent diarrhoea. Lancet 1998; 351:633–6.
22. Kyne L, Warny M, Qamar A, et al. Asymptomatic carriage of Clostridium difficile and serum levels of IgG antibody against toxin A. N Engl J Med 2000;342:390–7.
23. Loo VG, Poirier L, Miller MA, et al. A predominantly clonal multi-institutional outbreak of Clostridium difficile-associated diarrhea with high morbidity and mortality. N Engl J Med 2005;353:2442–9.
24. Lawrence SJ, Puzniak LA, Shadel BN, et al. Clostridium difficile in the intensive care unit: epidemiology, costs, and colonization pressure. Infect Control Hosp Epidemiol 2007;28:123–30.
25. Grundfest-Broniatowski S, Quader M, Alexander F, et al. Clostridium difficile colitis in the critically ill. Dis Colon Rectum 1996;39:619–23.
26. Kyne L, Merry C, O'Connell B, et al. Factors associated with prolonged symptoms and severe disease due to Clostridium difficile. Age Ageing 1999;28: 107–13.
27. Gerding DN, Muto CA, Owens RC Jr. Measures to control and prevent Clostridium difficile infection. Clin Infect Dis 2008;46(Suppl 1):S43–9.
28. Kim KH, Fekety R, Batts DH, et al. Isolation of Clostridium difficile from the environment and contacts of patients with antibiotic-associated colitis. J Infect Dis 1981;143:42–50.
29. Kenneally C, Rosini JM, Skrupky LP, et al. Analysis of 30-day mortality for clostridium difficile-associated disease in the ICU setting. Chest 2007;132:418–24.
30. Centers for Disease Control and Prevention. Severe Clostridium difficile-associated disease in populations previously at low risk—four states, 2005. MMWR Morb Mortal Wkly Rep 2005;54:1201–5.
31. McDonald LC, Killgore GE, Thompson A, et al. An epidemic, toxin gene-variant strain of Clostridium difficile. N Engl J Med 2005;353:2433–41.
32. Warny M, Pepin J, Fang A, et al. Toxin production by an emerging strain of Clostridium difficile associated with outbreaks of severe disease in North America and Europe. Lancet 2005;366:1079–84.
33. Muto CA, Pokrywka M, Shutt K, et al. A large outbreak of Clostridium difficile-associated disease with an unexpected proportion of deaths and colectomies at a teaching hospital following increased fluoroquinolone use. Infect Control Hosp Epidemiol 2005;26:273–80.
34. Pepin J, Valiquette L, Cossette B. Mortality attributable to nosocomial Clostridium difficile-associated disease during an epidemic caused by a hypervirulent strain in Quebec. CMAJ 2005;173:1037–42.

35. Pepin J, Saheb N, Coulombe MA, et al. Emergence of fluoroquinolones as the predominant risk factor for Clostridium difficile-associated diarrhea: a cohort study during an epidemic in Quebec. Clin Infect Dis 2005;41:1254–60.

36. Dubberke ER, Reske KA, Yan Y, et al. Clostridium difficile–associated disease in a setting of endemicity: identification of novel risk factors. Clin Infect Dis 2007; 45:1543–9.

37. Bignardi GE. Risk factors for Clostridium difficile infection. J Hosp Infect 1998; 40:1–15.

38. Marra AR, Edmond MB, Wenzel RP, et al. Hospital-acquired Clostridium difficile-associated disease in the intensive care unit setting: epidemiology, clinical course and outcome. BMC Infect Dis 2007;7:42.

39. Gurwith MJ, Rabin HR, Love K. Diarrhea associated with clindamycin and ampicillin therapy: preliminary results of a cooperative study. J Infect Dis 1977; 135(Suppl):S104–10.

40. Cunningham R, Dale B, Undy B, et al. Proton pump inhibitors as a risk factor for Clostridium difficile diarrhoea. J Hosp Infect 2003;54:243–5.

41. Brett S. Science review: The use of proton pump inhibitors for gastric acid suppression in critical illness. Crit Care 2005;9:45–50.

42. Jump RL, Pultz MJ, Donskey CJ. Vegetative Clostridium difficile survives in room air on moist surfaces and in gastric contents with reduced acidity: a potential mechanism to explain the association between proton pump inhibitors and C. difficile-associated diarrhea? Antimicrob Agents Chemother 2007; 51:2883–7.

43. Thorens J, Froehlich F, Schwizer W, et al. Bacterial overgrowth during treatment with omeprazole compared with cimetidine: a prospective randomised double blind study. Gut 1996;39:54–9.

44. Bliss DZ, Guenter PA, Settle RG. Defining and reporting diarrhea in tube-fed patients—what a mess. Am J Clin Nutr 1992;55:753–9.

45. Thurn J, Crossley K, Gerdts A, et al. Enteral hyperalimentation as a source of nosocomial infection. J Hosp Infect 1990;15:203–17.

46. Rolfe RD. Role of volatile fatty acids in colonization resistance to Clostridium difficile. Infect Immun 1984;45:185–91.

47. Bliss DZ, Johnson S, Savik K, et al. Acquisition of Clostridium difficile and Clostridium difficile-associated diarrhea in hospitalized patients receiving tube feeding. Ann Intern Med 1998;129:1012–9.

48. Asha NJ, Tompkins D, Wilcox MH. Comparative analysis of prevalence, risk factors, and molecular epidemiology of antibiotic-associated diarrhea due to Clostridium difficile, Clostridium perfringens, and Staphylococcus aureus. J Clin Microbiol 2006;44:2785–91.

49. Crabtree T, Aitchison D, Meyers BF, et al. Clostridium difficile in cardiac surgery: risk factors and impact on postoperative outcome. Ann Thorac Surg 2007;83: 1396–402.

50. Kelly CP, Pothoulakis C, LaMont JT. Clostridium difficile colitis. N Engl J Med 1994;330:257–62.

51. Beaulieu M, Williamson D, Pichette G, et al. Risk of Clostridium difficile-associated disease among patients receiving proton-pump inhibitors in a Quebec medical intensive care unit. Infect Control Hosp Epidemiol 2007;28:1305–7.

52. Hurley BW, Nguyen CC. The spectrum of pseudomembranous enterocolitis and antibiotic-associated diarrhea. Arch Intern Med 2002;162:2177–84.

53. Mogg GA, Burdon DW, Keighley M. Oral metronidazole in Clostridium difficile colitis. Br Med J 1979;2:335.

54. Tedesco FJ. Pseudomembranous colitis: pathogenesis and therapy. Med Clin North Am 1982;66:655–64.
55. Triadafilopoulos G, Hallstone AE. Acute abdomen as the first presentation of pseudomembranous colitis. Gastroenterology 1991;101:685–91.
56. Peterson LR, Kelly PJ. The role of the clinical microbiology laboratory in the management of Clostridium difficile-associated diarrhea. Infect Dis Clin North Am 1993;7:277–93.
57. Gelone SP, Fishman N, Gerding DN, et al: Clostridium difficile epidemiology: Results of an international web-based survey project. In SHEA '06, Chicago [abstract].
58. Musher DM, Manhas A, Jain P, et al. Detection of Clostridium difficile toxin: comparison of enzyme immunoassay results with results obtained by cytotoxicity assay. J Clin Microbiol 2007;45:2737–9.
59. Wilkins TD, Lyerly DM. Clostridium difficile testing: after 20 years, still challenging. J Clin Microbiol 2003;41:531–4.
60. Sheth SG, LaMont JT. Gastrointestinal problems in the chronically critically ill patient. Clin Chest Med 2001;22:135–47.
61. Wanahita A, Goldsmith EA, Marino BJ, et al. Clostridium difficile infection in patients with unexplained leukocytosis. Am J Med 2003;115:543–6.
62. Grossmann EM, Longo WE, Kaminski DL, et al. Clostridium difficile toxin: cytoskeletal changes and lactate dehydrogenase release in hepatocytes. J Surg Res 2000;88:165–72.
63. Lamontagne F, Labbe AC, Haeck O, et al. Impact of emergency colectomy on survival of patients with fulminant Clostridium difficile colitis during an epidemic caused by a hypervirulent strain. Ann Surg 2007;245:267–72.
64. Peled N, Pitlik S, Samra Z, et al. Predicting Clostridium difficile toxin in hospitalized patients with antibiotic-associated diarrhea. Infect Control Hosp Epidemiol 2007;28:377–81.
65. Wanahita A, Goldsmith EA, Musher DM. Conditions associated with leukocytosis in a tertiary care hospital, with particular attention to the role of infection caused by Clostridium difficile. Clin Infect Dis 2002;34:1585–92.
66. Adams SD, Mercer DW. Fulminant Clostridium difficile colitis. Curr Opin Crit Care 2007;13:450–5.
67. Mylonakis E, Ryan ET, Calderwood SB. Clostridium difficile–associated diarrhea: a review. Arch Intern Med 2001;161:525–33.
68. Tedesco FJ, Corless JK, Brownstein RE. Rectal sparing in antibiotic-associated pseudomembranous colitis: a prospective study. Gastroenterology 1982;83:1259–60.
69. Kirkpatrick ID, Greenberg HM. Evaluating the CT diagnosis of Clostridium difficile colitis: should CT guide therapy. AJR Am J Roentgenol 2001;176:635–9.
70. Kunimoto D, Thomson AB. Recurrent Clostridium difficile-associated colitis responding to cholestyramine. Digestion 1986;33:225–8.
71. Ash L, Baker ME, O'Malley CM Jr, et al. Colonic abnormalities on CT in adult hospitalized patients with Clostridium difficile colitis: prevalence and significance of findings. AJR Am J Roentgenol 2006;186:1393–400.
72. Boland GW, Lee MJ, Cats AM, et al. Clostridium difficile colitis: correlation of CT findings with severity of clinical disease. Clin Radiol 1995;50:153–6.
73. Cohen SH, Gerding DN, Johnson S, et al. Clostridium difficile infection: clinical practice guidelines by SHEA and IDSA. Oral Presentation in IDSA 45th Annual Meeting, San Diego, California.

74. Zar FA, Bakkanagari SR, Moorthi KM, et al. A comparison of vancomycin and metronidazole for the treatment of Clostridium difficile-associated diarrhea, stratified by disease severity. Clin Infect Dis 2007;45:302–7.

75. Bartlett JG. Treatment of antibiotic-associated pseudomembranous colitis. Rev Infect Dis 1984;6(Suppl 1):S235–41.

76. Olson MM, Shanholtzer CJ, Lee JT Jr, et al. Ten years of prospective Clostridium difficile-associated disease surveillance and treatment at the Minneapolis VA Medical Center, 1982–1991. Infect Control Hosp Epidemiol 1994;15: 371–81.

77. Miller MA. Clinical management of Clostridium difficile-associated disease. Clin Infect Dis 2007;45(Suppl 2):S122–8.

78. Bolton RP, Culshaw MA. Faecal metronidazole concentrations during oral and intravenous therapy for antibiotic associated colitis due to Clostridium difficile. Gut 1986;27:1169–72.

79. Friedenberg F, Fernandez A, Kaul V, et al. Intravenous metronidazole for the treatment of Clostridium difficile colitis. Dis Colon Rectum 2001;44:1176–80.

80. Johnson S, Peterson LR, Gerding DN. Intravenous metronidazole and Clostridium difficile-associated diarrhea or colitis. J Infect Dis 1989;160:1087–8.

81. Teasley DG, Gerding DN, Olson MM, et al. Prospective randomised trial of metronidazole versus vancomycin for Clostridium-difficile-associated diarrhoea and colitis. Lancet 1983;2:1043–6.

82. Wenisch C, Parschalk B, Hasenhundl M, et al. Comparison of vancomycin, teicoplanin, metronidazole, and fusidic acid for the treatment of Clostridium difficile-associated diarrhea. Clin Infect Dis 1996;22:813–8.

83. Al-Nassir WN, Sethi AK, Li Y, et al. Both oral metronidazole and oral vancomycin promote persistent overgrowth of vancomycin-resistant enterococci during treatment of Clostridium difficile-associated disease. Antimicrob Agents Chemother 2008;52:2403–6.

84. Salgado CD, Giannetta ET, Farr BM. Failure to develop vancomycin-resistant Enterococcus with oral vancomycin treatment of Clostridium difficile. Infect Control Hosp Epidemiol 2004;25:413–7.

85. Wong SS, Woo PC, Luk WK, et al. Susceptibility testing of Clostridium difficile against metronidazole and vancomycin by disk diffusion and Etest. Diagn Microbiol Infect Dis 1999;34:1–6.

86. Louie T, Gerson M, Grimard D, et al. Results of a phase III trial comparing tolevamar, vancomycin and metronidazole in patients with Clostridium difficile-associated diarrhea (CDAD). In 47th Annual ICAAC, Chicago [abstract].

87. Musher DM, Aslam S, Logan N, et al. Relatively poor outcome after treatment of Clostridium difficile colitis with metronidazole. Clin Infect Dis 2005;40:1586–90.

88. Apisarnthanarak A, Razavi B, Mundy LM. Adjunctive intracolonic vancomycin for severe Clostridium difficile colitis: case series and review of the literature. Clin Infect Dis 2002;35:690–6.

89. Malnick SD, Zimhony O. Treatment of Clostridium difficile-associated diarrhea. Ann Pharmacother 2002;36:1767–75.

90. Nathanson DR, Sheahan M, Chao L, et al. Intracolonic use of vancomycin for treatment of clostridium difficile colitis in a patient with a diverted colon: report of a case. Dis Colon Rectum 2001;44:1871–2.

91. Rubin MS, Bodenstein LE, Kent KC. Severe Clostridium difficile colitis. Dis Colon Rectum 1995;38:350–4.

92. Ali SO, Welch JP, Dring RJ. Early surgical intervention for fulminant pseudomembranous colitis. Am Surg 2008;74:20–6.

93. Byrn JC, Maun DC, Gingold DS, et al. Predictors of mortality after colectomy for fulminant Clostridium difficile colitis. Arch Surg 2008;143:150–4 [discussion: 155].

94. Musher DM, Logan N, Hamill RJ, et al. Nitazoxanide for the treatment of Clostridium difficile colitis. Clin Infect Dis 2006;43:421–7.

95. Nelson R. Antibiotic treatment for Clostridium difficile-associated diarrhea in adults. Cochrane Database Syst Rev 2007;3:CD004610.

96. Wullt M, Odenholt I. A double-blind randomized controlled trial of fusidic acid and metronidazole for treatment of an initial episode of Clostridium difficile-associated diarrhoea. J Antimicrob Chemother 2004;54:211–6.

97. de Lalla F, Nicolin R, Rinaldi E, et al. Prospective study of oral teicoplanin versus oral vancomycin for therapy of pseudomembranous colitis and Clostridium difficile-associated diarrhea. Antimicrob Agents Chemother 1992;36:2192–6.

98. Lagrotteria D, Holmes S, Smieja M, et al. Prospective, randomized inpatient study of oral metronidazole versus oral metronidazole and rifampin for treatment of primary episode of Clostridium difficile-associated diarrhea. Clin Infect Dis 2006;43:547–52.

99. Louie T, Miller M, Donskey C, et al. Clinical outcomes, safety, and pharmacokinetics of OPT-80 in a phase 2 trial with patients with Clostridium difficile infection. Antimicrob Agents Chemother 2009;53:223–8.

100. Louie TJ, Emery J, Krulicki W, et al. OPT-80 eliminates Clostridium difficile and is sparing of bacteroides species during treatment of C. difficile infection. Antimicrob Agents Chemother 2009;53:261–3.

101. Ng SC, Hart AL, Kamm MA, et al. Mechanisms of action of probiotics: recent advances. Inflamm Bowel Dis 2009;2:300–10.

102. Lawrence SJ, Korzenik JR, Mundy LM. Probiotics for recurrent Clostridium difficile disease. J Med Microbiol 2005;54:905–6.

103. McFarland LV, Surawicz CM, Greenberg RN, et al. A randomized placebo-controlled trial of Saccharomyces boulardii in combination with standard antibiotics for Clostridium difficile disease. JAMA 1994;271:1913–8.

104. Surawicz CM, McFarland LV, Greenberg RN, et al. The search for a better treatment for recurrent Clostridium difficile disease: use of high-dose vancomycin combined with Saccharomyces boulardii. Clin Infect Dis 2000;31:1012–7.

105. Wullt M, Hagslatt ML, Odenholt I. Lactobacillus plantarum 299v for the treatment of recurrent Clostridium difficile-associated diarrhoea: a double-blind, placebo-controlled trial. Scand J Infect Dis 2003;35:365–7.

106. Lherm T, Monet C, Nougiere B, et al. Seven cases of fungemia with Saccharomyces boulardii in critically ill patients. Intensive Care Med 2002;28:797–801.

107. Cassone M, Serra P, Mondello F, et al. Outbreak of Saccharomyces cerevisiae subtype boulardii fungemia in patients neighboring those treated with a probiotic preparation of the organism. J Clin Microbiol 2003;41:5340–3.

108. Ariano RE, Zhanel GG, Harding GK. The role of anion-exchange resins in the treatment of antibiotic-associated pseudomembranous colitis. CMAJ 1990;142:1049–51.

109. Taylor NS, Bartlett JG. Binding of Clostridium difficile cytotoxin and vancomycin by anion-exchange resins. J Infect Dis 1980;141:92–7.

110. Salcedo J, Keates S, Pothoulakis C, et al. Intravenous immunoglobulin therapy for severe Clostridium difficile colitis. Gut 1997;41:366–70.

111. Hassoun A, Ibrahim F. Use of intravenous immunoglobulin for the treatment of severe Clostridium difficile colitis. Am J Geriatr Pharmacother 2007;5:48–51.

112. McPherson S, Rees CJ, Ellis R, et al. Intravenous immunoglobulin for the treatment of severe, refractory, and recurrent Clostridium difficile diarrhea. Dis Colon Rectum 2006;49:640–5.
113. Warny M, Denie C, Delmee M, et al. Gamma globulin administration in relapsing Clostridium difficile-induced pseudomembranous colitis with a defective antibody response to toxin A. Acta Clin Belg 1995;50:36–9.
114. Juang P, Skledar SJ, Zgheib NK, et al. Clinical outcomes of intravenous immune globulin in severe clostridium difficile-associated diarrhea. Am J Infect Control 2007;35:131–7.
115. Bartlett JG. Clinical practice. Antibiotic-associated diarrhea. N Engl J Med 2002; 346:334–9.
116. Fekety R, Shah AB. Diagnosis and treatment of Clostridium difficile colitis. JAMA 1993;269:71–5.
117. Fernandez A, Anand G, Friedenberg F. Factors associated with failure of metronidazole in Clostridium difficile-associated disease. J Clin Gastroenterol 2004; 38:414–8.
118. Nair S, Yadav D, Corpuz M, et al. Clostridium difficile colitis: factors influencing treatment failure and relapse—a prospective evaluation. Am J Gastroenterol 1998;93:1873–6.
119. Sanchez JL, Gerding DN, Olson MM, et al. Metronidazole susceptibility in Clostridium difficile isolates recovered from cases of C. difficile–associated disease treatment failures and successes. Anaerobe 1999;5:201–4.
120. Fekety R, McFarland LV, Surawicz CM, et al. Recurrent Clostridium difficile diarrhea: characteristics of and risk factors for patients enrolled in a prospective, randomized, double-blinded trial. Clin Infect Dis 1997;24:324–33.
121. McFarland LV. Alternative treatments for Clostridium difficile disease: What really works? J Med Microbiol 2005;54:101–11.
122. Barbut F, Richard A, Hamadi K, et al. Epidemiology of recurrences or reinfections of Clostridium difficile-associated diarrhea. J Clin Microbiol 2000;38: 2386–8.
123. McFarland LV, Elmer GW, Surawicz CM. Breaking the cycle: treatment strategies for 163 cases of recurrent Clostridium difficile disease. Am J Gastroenterol 2002;97:1769–75.
124. Tedesco FJ, Gordon D, Fortson WC. Approach to patients with multiple relapses of antibiotic-associated pseudomembranous colitis. Am J Gastroenterol 1985; 80:867–8.
125. Johnson S, Schriever C, Galang M, et al. Interruption of recurrent Clostridium difficile-associated diarrhea episodes by serial therapy with vancomycin and rifaximin. Clin Infect Dis 2007;44:846–8.
126. Garey KW, Salazar M, Shah D, et al. Rifamycin antibiotics for treatment of Clostridium difficile-associated diarrhea. Ann Pharmacother 2008;42:827–35.
127. Boyce JM, Ligi C, Kohan C, et al. Lack of association between the increased incidence of Clostridium difficile-associated disease and the increasing use of alcohol-based hand rubs. Infect Control Hosp Epidemiol 2006;27:479–83.
128. Johnson S, Gerding DN, Olson MM, et al. Prospective, controlled study of vinyl glove use to interrupt Clostridium difficile nosocomial transmission. Am J Med 1990;88:137–40.
129. Zafar AB, Gaydos LA, Furlong WB, et al. Effectiveness of infection control program in controlling nosocomial Clostridium difficile. Am J Infect Control 1998;26:588–93.

130. Muto CA, Blank MK, Marsh JW, et al. Control of an outbreak of infection with the hypervirulent Clostridium difficile BI strain in a university hospital using a comprehensive "bundle" approach. Clin Infect Dis 2007;45:1266–73.
131. Gerding DN, Johnson S, Peterson LR, et al. Clostridium difficile-associated diarrhea and colitis. Infect Control Hosp Epidemiol 1995;16:459–77.
132. Kaatz GW, Gitlin SD, Schaberg DR, et al. Acquisition of Clostridium difficile from the hospital environment. Am J Epidemiol 1988;127:1289–94.
133. Wilcox MH, Fawley WN, Wigglesworth N, et al. Comparison of the effect of detergent versus hypochlorite cleaning on environmental contamination and incidence of Clostridium difficile infection. J Hosp Infect 2003;54:109–14.
134. Perez J, Springthorpe VS, Sattar SA. Activity of selected oxidizing microbicides against the spores of Clostridium difficile: relevance to environmental control. Am J Infect Control 2005;33:320–5.
135. Valiquette L, Cossette B, Garant MP, et al. Impact of a reduction in the use of high-risk antibiotics on the course of an epidemic of Clostridium difficile-associated disease caused by the hypervirulent NAP1/027 strain. Clin Infect Dis 2007; 45(Suppl 2):S112–21.
136. Fowler S, Webber A, Cooper BS, et al. Successful use of feedback to improve antibiotic prescribing and reduce Clostridium difficile infection: a controlled interrupted time series. J Antimicrob Chemother 2007;59:990–5.
137. Climo MW, Israel DS, Wong ES, et al. Hospital-wide restriction of clindamycin: effect on the incidence of Clostridium difficile-associated diarrhea and cost. Ann Intern Med 1998;128:989–95.
138. Davey P, Brown E, Fenelon L, et al. Interventions to improve antibiotic prescribing practices for hospital inpatients. Cochrane Database Syst Rev 2005;4:CD003543.
139. Khan R, Cheesbrough J. Impact of changes in antibiotic policy on Clostridium difficile-associated diarrhoea (CDAD) over a five-year period in a district general hospital. J Hosp Infect 2003;54:104–8.
140. O'Connor KA, Kingston M, O'Donovan M, et al. Antibiotic prescribing policy and Clostridium difficile diarrhoea. QJM 2004;97:423–9.

Index

Note: Page numbers of article titles are in **boldface** type.

A

Abscess(es)
    brain, 615–618. See also *Brain abscess.*
    intra-abdominal sepsis–related, management of, percutaneous drainage vs. surgery
      in, 596–597
    intracardiac, acute infective endocarditis and, 656–657
Acute infective endocarditis, **643–664.** See also *Infective endocarditis, acute.*
Anidulafungin, for candidal bloodstream infections in ICU, 637
Antibiotic(s). See also *Antimicrobial stewardship.*
    broad-spectrum, in severe community-acquired infections, 598
    for acute infective endocarditis, 648
    for brain abscess, 617
    for intra-abdominal sepsis, initiation of, 595–596
    for meningitis, 613–614
    for septic shock and severe sepsis, 487–489
    for severe CAP, 508–512
    for SSTIs, 573–574
      methicillin-resistant *Staphylococcus aureus*–related, 573–577
    for VAP
      initial, 523
      prescription at bedside, 523–528. See also *Ventilator-associated pneumonia (VAP),*
        management of, antibiotics in.
    in health care–associated intra-abdominal infections, regimens for, 599–601
    in ICU, **683–702**
      described, 683–684
      new agents, **665–681.** See also specific agents.
        ceftaroline, 665–666
        ceftobiprole, 666–667
        dalbavancin, 668
        iclaprim, 671
        isavuconazole, 672
        oritavancin, 669–670
        telavancin, 670–671
      optimizing use of, 684–685
        programs for, 685–687
      patient safety with, 685
      resistance to, 684–685
Antibiotic resistance, in ICU, 684–685
Antigenemia, CMV, fever in ICU patients due to, 479
Antimicrobial agents. See *Antibiotic(s).*

Infect Dis Clin N Am 23 (2009) 745–756
doi:10.1016/S0891-5520(09)00067-1
0891-5520/09/$ – see front matter © 2009 Elsevier Inc. All rights reserved.

id.theclinics.com

Moving?

Make sure your subscription moves with you!

To notify us of your new address, find your **Clinics Account Number** (located on your mailing label above your name), and contact customer service at:

Email: journalscustomerservice-usa@elsevier.com

800-654-2452 (subscribers in the U.S. & Canada)
314-447-8871 (subscribers outside of the U.S. & Canada)

Fax number: 314-447-8029

**Elsevier Health Sciences Division
Subscription Customer Service
3251 Riverport Lane
Maryland Heights, MO 63043**

*To ensure uninterrupted delivery of your subscription, please notify us at least 4 weeks in advance of move.

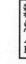

Printed and bound by CPI Group (UK) Ltd, Croydon, CR0 4YY

03/10/2024

01040462-0008